Multidisciplinary Approach to Ectodermal Dysplasia

Gianluca Tadini • John Timothy Wright
Smaïl Hadj-Rabia • Holm Schneider
Editors

Multidisciplinary Approach to Ectodermal Dysplasia

Springer

Editors
Gianluca Tadini
Center for Inherited Cutaneous Diseases
University of Milan
Milan, Italy

Smaïl Hadj-Rabia
Department of Dermatology
Necker–Enfants Malades Hospital
PARIS, France

John Timothy Wright
Department of Pediatric Dentistry and
Dental Public Health
Adams School of Dentistry
University of North Carolina
Chapel Hill, NC, USA

Holm Schneider
Department of Pediatrics
University of Erlangen-Nürnberg
Erlangen, Bayern, Germany

ISBN 978-3-031-75789-1 ISBN 978-3-031-75790-7 (eBook)
https://doi.org/10.1007/978-3-031-75790-7

This Springer imprint is published by the registered company Springer Nature Switzerland AG
The registered company address is: Gewerbestrasse 11, 6330 Cham, Switzerland

The book is dedicated to our patients and their families.

Foreword

Everything comes from a desire, a need or a great wish for knowledge.

Giulia's story is certainly similar to many other stories, where the main protagonist is an unknown pathology. Her father, born in the 1920s, was born with a strange disease, which in everyone's eyes seems like an old child. In fact, the most obvious characteristic is very, very dry skin, without fluff or hair. When he cries he has no tears, he doesn't have adequate thermoregulation and therefore he doesn't sweat. Later, even the lack of teeth makes everyday life problematic. At the time the ignorance was truly impressive, the few doctors did not know about rare diseases and therefore they blamed who knows what sin committed to conceive such a child.

Years pass and this child somehow devises methods of survival. During the hot season, he goes around with wet clothes to feel a little coolness and relief, in winter to cope with the cold he greases his skin with olive oil or animal fat, eats very cooked foods, soups, and lots of fruit.

He gets married, has four children, only one of whom has the same pathology in a more nuanced way. He regrets this and, in every way, tries to find out what this illness is if it really is an illness. No matter where he went, he always looked for a specialist to contact without any fear of asking for medical advice. Even though times had changed, no one still knew how to give a name to this disease.

Giulia experiences childhood and part of her adolescence with this heavy burden that her father experienced.

Very young she moved to Milan, where in her father's place she continued the search for a specialist who could give a name.

Although the city offered a lot, Giulia had to wait until the birth of her first child to finally come across the right specialist and finally give a name and perhaps even a cure to this pathology.

Her father will never know that this long search has finally come to an end but, precisely for the love for him and for what he has suffered in his long life, Giulia starts looking for other families and in 1999 she establishes the association with the name of A.N.D.E. (National Ectodermal Dysplasia Association). No child had to suffer anymore, be mocked, ghettoized, every family had to know not only the name of the pathology, but also how to deal with it and live their daily lives with serenity.

The information had to pass at every level, from school to doctors to friends, etc... no one should be ashamed of being dysplastic anymore, but learn to show the best part of themselves, in fact they are very intelligent and sensitive children and this is the winning card.

The work of the association was very meticulous from the start. In addition to finding other families throughout the country, the most constructive commitment was finding specialists who knew the pathology. The first doctors who embraced the association's cause began to speak at various conferences and meetings and knowledge spread all over. Today, although it is easy to recognize rare disease(s), we are still faced with unawareness and ignorance both in the medical and social fields, and there is still no adequate training.

However, despite everything, the specialists who belong to the association have set up a network and three reference centers where the patient can be followed.

The association's commitment to families, in addition to providing moral and bureaucratic support, is to help them cover implant-prosthetic expenses that the health system does not recognize as its own expense.

Since the association was born there has been exponential growth, in fact if at the time of its establishment there were only five families, now there are 310 associated families with a total of around 600 people including adults and children, grandparents and cousins, affected by anhidrotic/hypohidrotic ectodermal dysplasia but also other forms of dysplasia although in smaller numbers.

Over time the association has found a gap between the north, center, and south in having dysplasia recognized by the various medical commissions. There is no knowledge of the rare disease and there is no uniform method for the whole nation that can evaluate the dysplastic patient.

The situation at an international level is even worse; each nation adopts its own method of evaluation and treatment.

We can boast a cutting-edge team, especially in the dermatology and implantology fields. We were the first to apply mini implants to 10-year-old dysplastic patients, with a sensational result, years later, to say the least. This made everyday life normal from both a functional and aesthetic point of view, giving the boy more psychological security.

In all these years, science has also advanced; today, we can carry out genetic investigations knowing also the cases where the pathology is hidden. At an international level, a team of experts has studied an experimental method which, with simple intrauterine inoculations, improves the characteristics evident in the dysplastic child.

In almost 25 years of activity, giant strides have been made and the goal has not yet been reached.

I thank all those who have been and continue to work for this cause, doctors who have spared no effort in offering their knowledge and by going further, informing themselves, studying and applying for the best.

My wish is addressed to the many willing young doctors with a great desire to know, not to give up at the first difficulty but to carry on with small steps the studies undertaken, so that one day we will have a distant memory of rare diseases.

Italian Association of Ectodermal Dysplasias (ANDE) Giulia Fedele
Carugate, Italy

Preface

After numerous meetings over the last 20 years dedicated to the classification of ectodermal dysplasias (ED), we have taken up the challenge of summarizing the current knowledge in a book that conveys the many facets of this group of genetic disorders. The book compiles clinically relevant information on ED, organized according to the most recent revision of the classification: EDA1-, p63-, and Wnt-related ED as well as nectin- and connexin-related ED are explained in an easily understandable way from a clinical and molecular diagnostic point of view. Attention is also paid to very rare (and often unknown) ED entities, the characteristics of which are presented to facilitate their recognition.

Our book follows a "common thread" from epidemiology to diagnosis and practical management to recently introduced targeted therapies, highlighting the complexity of these genetic disorders. The first two chapters describe the prevalence of ED in different populations and recent attempts to classify the various disease entities, which is a prerequisite for accurate diagnosis and therapy. Subsequent chapters deal with the specific manifestations of ED in the eyes, nose, ears, and internal organs. Everyday aspects of the treatment of ED are detailed as well as the latest molecular therapeutic approaches. The final chapter highlights the crucial role of patient associations, with testimonies from patients and their families, providing a holistic view of living with ED.

We thank Springer for the continuous and highly appreciated support of this book and hope that it will become a very useful resource for students, trainees, pediatricians, geneticists, dermatologists, dentists, gynecologists, and many other specialists involved in diagnosing and treating ED.

Milan, Italy — Gianluca Tadini
Paris, France — Smail Hadj-Rabia
Erlangen, Germany — Holm Schneider
Chapel Hill, NC, USA — John Timothy Wright

Contents

1 **Epidemiology of Ectodermal Dysplasias** 1
Lidia Pezzani and Donatella Milani
References 3

2 **What Is and Isn't an Ectodermal Dysplasia?** 5
Nicolai Peschel and Holm Schneider
2.1 Introduction 5
2.2 Classification 7
2.3 Group 2: Wnt/β-Catenin Signaling Pathway 10
2.4 Group 6: To Be Classified Elsewhere? 15
2.5 Outlook 17
References 17

3 **X-Linked Hypohidrotic Ectodermal Dysplasia: The Pathogenic Role of the *EDA* Gene** 25
Debora Vergani, Giulia Gori, and Giovanna Traficante
3.1 Introduction 25
3.2 Ectodysplasin A (EDA): Molecular Aspects 26
3.2.1 Gene Structure 26
3.2.2 The Role of EDA in Multiple Signaling Pathways 28
3.2.3 Molecular Alterations in *EDA* 29
3.3 Clinical Characteristics 30
3.4 Diagnosis 31
3.5 Genetic Counseling 31
3.6 Prenatal Perspectives 32
3.7 Therapy Studies 33
References 33

4 **X-Linked Hypohidrotic Ectodermal Dysplasia: Clinical Features** 37
Átila Visinoni and Nina Pagnan
4.1 Historical Considerations 37
4.2 Etiology and Genetic Counseling 38

4.3 Clinical Features 39
4.3.1 Craniofacial Aspects 40
4.3.2 Hair 40
4.3.3 Teeth and Salivary Glands 41
4.3.4 Sweating. 42
4.3.5 Skin 42
4.3.6 Nails. 43
4.3.7 Nose and Throat. 44
4.3.8 Eyes 44
4.3.9 Heterozygous Females. 44
4.4 Treatment 45
4.4.1 Prenatal Diagnosis and In-Utero Treatment. 46
References. 47

5 **Incontinentia Pigmenti** 51
Alessandra Pescatore, Matilde Valeria Ursini, and Francesca Fusco
5.1 Clinical Features 51
5.2 Genetic Features. 53
5.3 The Role of NEMO Protein Loss in the Pathogenesis of IP 56
References. 57

6 **Genetic Basis and Molecular Diagnosis of p63-Associated Ectodermal Dysplasia** 61
Daniela Di Girolamo and Caterina Missero
6.1 Introduction 61
6.2 Architecture of p63 Gene and Its Protein Products 61
6.3 p63 Biological Function in Stratified Epithelium Development . . . 64
6.4 Causative Mutations in the *TP63* Gene in Syndromic and Non-syndromic Diseases. 65
6.4.1 Ankyloblepharon-Ectodermal Defects Cleft Lip/Palate Syndrome (AEC) Syndrome 65
6.4.2 Ectrodactyly, Ectodermal Dysplasia and Cleft Lip/Palate Syndrome (EEC) Syndrome 69
6.5 Clinical Manifestations 70
6.5.1 Limb-Mammary (LMS) and Acro-Dermato-Ungual-Lacrimal-Tooth (ADULT) Syndromes 71
6.5.2 Non-syndromic Diseases Associated with *TP63* Mutations 72
6.6 Molecular Diagnosis of p63-Associated Syndromes. 72
6.7 Potential Therapeutic Approaches to Treat Severe Manifestations of p63-Associated Syndromes. 74
References. 75

7 Focal Dermal Hypoplasia (FDH) and WNT10A-Related Ectodermal Dysplasia (ED) 81
Alessandra Gelmetti and Gianluca Tadini
7.1 Clinical Features 82
7.1.1 Skin, Mucosae, and Appendage Manifestations 82
7.1.2 Skeletal Malformations 85
7.1.3 Ocular Involvement 86
7.1.4 Neurologic Anomalies 87
7.1.5 Miscellaneous 88
7.2 Diagnosis 88
7.3 Novel Variants 88
7.3.1 WNT10A-Related ED 89
References 92

8 Nectinopathies: Ectodermal Dysplasia Syndromes Caused by Mutations in *PVRL1/4* Genes Encoding Cell Adhesion Molecules Nectins-1/4 95
Paola Fortugno and Francesco Brancati
8.1 History and Terminology: Toward a Molecularly Driven Dyadic Approach 95
8.2 Nectin-1 ED 96
8.3 Nectin 4-ED 98
8.4 Possible existence of genetic heterogeneity 99
8.5 Differential Diagnosis Among Families with Ectodermal Dysplasia and Syndactyly 99
8.6 Molecular Pathology of Nectinopathies 101
8.7 Role of Nectins as Viral Receptors 102
8.8 Role of Nectins in Cancer 102
References 102

9 Other Syndromes with Prominent Ectodermal Dysplasia Signs 107
Gianluca Tadini, Beatrice Carcano, and Michela Brena
9.1 KREMEN-1-Related ED 107
9.2 LEF1-Related ED 107
9.3 AXIN2-Related ED 109
9.4 LRP6 110
9.5 KDF1-Related ED 110
9.6 HELIX Syndrome 111
9.7 TSPEAR-Related ED 111
9.8 HIST1H1E-Related ED 114
9.9 MAP3K20-Related ED 115
9.10 CHAND Syndrome 115
9.11 CHUK-Related ED 115
9.12 Basan Syndrome 116
9.13 ARF1-Related ED 116

9.14 SEN (Scalp-Ear-Nipple) Syndrome 116
9.15 NEMO Syndrome 116
9.16 Sensenbrenner Syndrome 117
9.17 Tricho-Dento-Osseous Syndrome 117
9.18 Tricho-Rhino-Phalangeal Syndrome 118
9.19 "Pure Hair-Nail" ED 118
9.20 ED with Skin Fragility 118
9.21 Naegeli-Franceschetti Syndrome 119
9.22 Witkop Syndrome 119
9.23 Connexins-Related Syndromes 120
9.23.1 Clouston Syndrome 120
9.23.2 Oculo-Dento-Digital Dysplasia (ODDD) 121
9.23.3 KID Syndrome 121
References 122

10 Ectodermal Dysplasias: Orofacial Manifestations and Management 125
B. Meyer and John Timothy Wright
10.1 Introduction 125
10.2 Soft Tissues 126
10.2.1 Cleft Lip/Palate 127
10.2.2 Oral Mucosa and Gingiva 128
10.2.3 Salivary Glands 129
10.2.4 Managing the Soft Tissues 129
10.3 Hard Tissues 130
10.3.1 Face and Occlusion 130
10.3.2 Dentition 132
10.3.3 Other Hard Tissue Findings 135
10.3.4 Managing the Hard Tissues 135
10.4 Summary 139
References 140

11 Oral and Dental Phenotype of Ectodermal Dysplasias 147
Johanna Norderyd and Hilde Nordgarden
11.1 Introduction 147
11.2 Summary 160
References 160

12 Ocular Manifestation in Hypohidrotic Ectodermal Dysplasia 163
Michele Callea, Vito Romano, Stefano Bignotti, Stefano Pensiero, and Colin Eric Willoughby
12.1 Introduction 163
12.2 Hypohidrotic Ectodermal Dysplasia 164
12.3 Clinical Features 165
12.4 Ocular Features 165
12.5 Conclusion 170
References 170

13 Otorhinolaryngologic Manifestations in Hypohidrotic Ectodermal Dysplasia 173
Michele Callea, Piercesare Grimaldi, and Roberto Teggi
13.1 Ear Manifestations 173
13.2 Nose Manifestations. 174
13.3 Throat Manifestations 175
References. 176

14 Broad Phenotypic Spectrum of Ectodermal Dysplasias in Childhood and Adolescence 177
Laura Guazzarotti
References. 180

15 ED Practical Management 183
Gianluca Tadini and Michela Brena
15.1 Socio-political Issues 183
15.2 Registries 183
15.3 Medical Centers 184
15.4 Prenatal Diagnosis 184
15.5 Diagnosis and Skin Management. 184
15.6 Management of Internal Organs Disorders 187
References. 188

16 Molecular Therapies 189
Holm Schneider and Pascal Schneider
16.1 Introduction 189
16.2 EDA1 Replacement Therapy 190
16.3 Treatment of Cutaneous and Ocular Lesions Resulting from p63 Deficiency 193
References. 195

17 Patient Advocacy Organizations: One Story of Success 197
Mary Fete
17.1 NFED History 197
17.2 Knowledge Is Power 198
17.3 Education 199
17.4 Vision/Passion 199
17.5 Representing Patients. 200
17.6 National Programs/Policies 200
17.7 NFED Impact. 200
17.8 International Collaboration 201
17.9 Support Services 201
17.10 Treatment. 202
17.11 Research. 203
17.12 Conclusion 204
References. 204

Contributors

Stefano Bignotti Eye Unit, ASST Spedali Civili di Brescia, Piazzale Spedali Civili, Brescia, Italy

Eye Unit, Department of Medical and Surgical Specialties, Radiological Sciences, and Public Health, University of Brescia, Brescia, Italy

Francesco Brancati IRCCS San Raffaele Roma, Rome, Italy

Human Genetics, Department of Life, Health and Environmental Sciences, University of L'Aquila, L'Aquila, Italy

Michela Brena Pediatric Dermatology Unit, Department of Clinical Sciences and Community Health, Fondazione IRCCS Ca' Granda Ospedale Maggiore Policlinico, Milan, Italy

Center for Inherited Cutaneous Diseases, University of Milan, Milan, Italy

Michele Callea Pediatric Dentistry and Special Dental Care Unit, Meyer Children's Hospital IRCCS, Florence, Italy

Beatrice Carcano Center for Inherited Cutaneous Diseases, University of Milan, Milan, Italy

Mary Fete National Foundation for Ectodermal Dysplasias, Fairview Heights, IL, USA

Paola Fortugno Università Telematica San Raffaele, Rome, Italy

IRCCS San Raffaele Roma, Rome, Italy

Francesca Fusco Institute of Genetics and Biophysics 'Adriano Buzzati-Traverso' (CNR), Naples, Italy

Alessandra Gelmetti Department of Experimental, Diagnostic and Specialty Medicine, Alma Mater Studiorum University of Bologna, Bologna, Italy

Daniela Di Girolamo CEINGE Biotecnologie Avanzate Franco Salvatore, Naples, Italy

Biology Department, University of Naples Federico II, Naples, Italy

Giulia Gori Medical Genetics Unit, Meyer Children's Hospital IRCCS, Florence, Italy

Piercesare Grimaldi University of Turin, Turin, Italy

Laura Guazzarotti Pediatric Endocrinology Unit, University of Padova, Padova, Italy

B. Meyer Department of Pediatric Dentistry, School of Dentistry, The Ohio State University, Columbus, OH, USA

Donatella Milani Fondazione IRCCS Ca' Granda Ospedale Maggiore Policlinico, Milan, Italy

Caterina Missero Biology Department, University of Naples Federico II, Naples, Italy

Center for Genetic Engineering, CEINGE Biotecnologie Avanzate Franco Salvatore, Naples, Italy

Johanna Norderyd Centre for Oral Health, Jönköping University, Jönköping, Sweden

Hilde Nordgarden National Competence Center for Oral Health in Rare Diagnoses, The TAKO Centre, Lovisenberg Diaconal Hospital, Oslo, Norway

Nina Pagnan Department of Genetics, Federal University of Paraná, Curitiba, Brazil

Stefano Pensiero Ophthalmology Unit, IRCCS Burlo Garofolo, Trieste, Italy

Alessandra Pescatore Institute of Genetics and Biophysics 'Adriano Buzzati-Traverso' (CNR), Naples, Italy

Nicolai Peschel Department of Pediatrics, University of Erlangen-Nürnberg, Erlangen, Germany

Lidia Pezzani Fondazione IRCCS Ca' Granda Ospedale Maggiore Policlinico, Milan, Italy

UO Pediatria, ASST Papa Giovanni XXIII, Bergamo, Italy

Vito Romano Eye Unit, ASST Spedali Civili di Brescia, Piazzale Spedali Civili, Brescia, Italy

Eye Unit, Department of Medical and Surgical Specialties, Radiological Sciences, and Public Health, University of Brescia, Brescia, Italy

Holm Schneider Department of Pediatrics & Center for Ectodermal Dysplasias, University of Erlangen-Nürnberg, Erlangen, Germany

Department of Pediatrics, Center for Ectodermal Dysplasias, University Hospital, Erlangen, Germany

Pascal Schneider Department of Immunobiology, University of Lausanne, Lausanne, Switzerland

Gianluca Tadini Center for Inherited Cutaneous Diseases, University of Milan, Milan, Italy

Pediatric Dermatology Unit, Department of Clinical Sciences and Community Health, Fondazione IRCCS Ca' Granda Ospedale Maggiore Policlinico, Milan, Italy

Roberto Teggi San Raffaele Scientific Institute—"Vita e Salute" University, Milan, Italy

Giovanna Traficante Medical Genetics Unit, Meyer Children's Hospital IRCCS, Florence, Italy

Matilde Valeria Ursini Institute of Genetics and Biophysics 'Adriano Buzzati-Traverso' (CNR), Naples, Italy

Debora Vergani Medical Genetics Unit, Meyer Children's Hospital IRCCS, Florence, Italy

Átila Visinoni School of Health Sciences, Positivo University, Curitiba, Brazil

Colin Eric Willoughby Genomic Medicine, Biomedical Sciences Research Institute, Ulster University, Coleraine, UK

John Timothy Wright Division of Pediatric and Public Health, Adams School of Dentistry, University of North Carolina, Chapel Hill, NC, USA

Chapter 1
Epidemiology of Ectodermal Dysplasias

Lidia Pezzani and Donatella Milani

Keywords Ectodermal dysplasia · ED · Epidemiology · Incidence · Mortality

Ectodermal dysplasias (EDs) are a large, heterogeneous group of genetic disorders characterized by impaired formation of tissues of ectodermal derivation.

EDs belong to the genodermatoses and can be inherited in an autosomal recessive, autosomal dominant, or X-linked manner, with X-linked hypohidrotic ectodermal dysplasias (XLHED) being the most frequent form (about 70% of all EDs). It was firstly reported by Thurman [1] and then observed by Charles Darwin, who reported on a family from India in which several male members showed sparse hair, abnormal teeth, and dryness of the skin during hot weather and postulated a sex-linked inheritance [2]. EDs can occur in any race but are much more frequent in Caucasians, and especially in fair Caucasians. Caucasians might be in fact more prone to ectodermal mutations since they seem to have already modified ectodermal structures (thinner, fairer skin and fewer sweat glands) as a consequence of adaptation to their environment.

In 2010, the Ectodermal Dysplasias International Registry (EDIR), a web-based questionnaire, was launched in order to provide data for expanding knowledge of the natural history of Ectodermal Dysplasias. In a few months, 835 individuals had entered data into the EDIR, equally divided between males and females. Unfortunately, only data on XLHED have been published since data were consistent enough, as it was the primary diagnosis reported by about 27% of participants. Overall, 96% of XLHED families reported at least one other affected family member, and 21% had a positive family history of infant or childhood deaths [3]. In 2013, Nguyen-Nielsen et al. [4] performed a population-based study that aimed to

L. Pezzani (✉)
Fondazione IRCCS Ca' Granda Ospedale Maggiore Policlinico, Milan, Italy

UO Pediatria, ASST Papa Giovanni XXIII, Bergamo, Italy

D. Milani
Fondazione IRCCS Ca' Granda Ospedale Maggiore Policlinico, Milan, Italy

G. Tadini et al. (eds.), *Multidisciplinary Approach to Ectodermal Dysplasia*,
https://doi.org/10.1007/978-3-031-75790-7_1

estimate the prevalence of XLHED in the Danish population and assumed a value of 1.6–22 per 100,000 persons. Diagnosis has been made most frequently during adolescence, between the ages of 11 and 18 years, probably because all the clinical signs become (more) evident.

Several studies have shown an increase in mortality in HED cases from hyperpyrexia due to the failure to regulate body temperatures through sweating. While Clarke et al. [5] estimated a mortality rate of approximately 30% in the first year of life, Blüschke et al. [6] reported a significantly lower mortality rate of 2.1%. These data may suggest that over the last few decades, constant monitoring of the temperature in the neonatal and pediatric care units has enabled quick recognition of the presence of hyperthermia and the assessment of appropriate and immediate management, which has led to better HED prognosis [6]. However, HED still today remains a potentially life-threatening condition despite worldwide progress in neonatal/pediatric care.

Other EDs seem to be ultra-rare, as evidenced by the lack of prevalence data. To date, more than 180 different types of ED have been outlined. In 2017, a panel of experts re-classified them based on known molecular pathways rather than phenotype and lowered the number of ED entities to 97, further revised to 49 in 2022 [7, 8]. Although the aim was to facilitate clinical and molecular diagnosis of EDs, this simplification could also be a first step towards more precise prevalence estimates. To date, Orphanet (the portal for rare diseases, https://www.orpha.net) only stated theoretical and vague estimates or just the number of reported cases. For example, for ectrodactyly, ectodermal dysplasia, and orofacial clefts (EEC) syndrome, the estimated prevalence is 1–9:100.000, with “more than 300 cases described in the literature.” Incontinentia Pigmenti has an estimated prevalence at birth of about 0.7/100,000; for ankyloblepharon-ectodermal defects-cleft lip/palate (AEC) syndrome, the prevalence is simply “unknown.” Since the phenotype of EDs can be mild, however, all these diseases may be underdiagnosed and their prevalence may be underestimated.

Curiously, although generally very rare, over 21 cohorts have been described for autoimmune polyendocrinopathy-candidiasis-ectodermal dystrophy (APECED, OMIM #240300) from 1998 to 2021. APECED is also known as autoimmune polyendocrine syndrome 1 (APS-1) and has an overall prevalence of 2.6 cases/million (range 0.5–17). The highest prevalence has been reported in the Iranian Jewish population (1:9000) and Finland (1:25,000), followed by Norway (1:90,000), Poland (1:129,000), Ireland (1:130,000), and Italy (1:380,000), while the lowest prevalence has been observed in France (1:500,000) and Japan (1:10,000,000) [9].

The increase in mortality in EDs in general appears to be significant, with both disease-related causes and infections, alcohol abuse, and accidents being the main causes [10]. Children and young adults showed the highest relative increase, mostly before the age of 45 years.

In conclusion, EDs are a very large and heterogeneous group of hereditary disorders, characterized by a wide phenotypic spectrum and clinical variability that could be a frequent cause of diagnostic delay or underdiagnosis. Precise information on the occurrence of EDs in the general population is then totally unavailable, and all existing studies are only based on small or theoretical data.

Of note, the U.S. National Foundation for Ectodermal Dysplasias (NFED) (https://nfed.org/) plans to launch in the near future a new patient registry and biobank, which will be a database of important genetic, epidemiologic, and natural history information for EDs patients. In the meanwhile, in 2022, NFED founded a Work Group composed of professionals from North America and Europe with the aim to establish more accurate and valid prevalence estimates of the more common EDs.

References

1. Thurnam J. Two cases in which the skin, hair and teeth were very imperfectly developed. Med Chir Trans. 1848;31:71–82. https://doi.org/10.1177/095952874803100108. PMID: 20895907; PMCID: PMC2104055
2. Darwin C. The variations of animals and plants under domestication, vol. 2. 2nd ed. London: John Murray; 1885. p. 319–20.
3. Fete M, Hermann J, Behrens J, Huttner KM. X-linked hypohidrotic ectodermal dysplasia (XLHED): clinical and diagnostic insights from an international patient registry. Am J Med Genet A. 2014;164A(10):2437–42. https://doi.org/10.1002/ajmg.a.36436. Epub 2014 Mar 24
4. Nguyen-Nielsen M, Skovbo S, Svaneby D, Pedersen L, Fryzek J. The prevalence of X-linked hypohidrotic ectodermal dysplasia (XLHED) in Denmark, 1995-2010. Eur J Med Genet. 2013;56(5):236–42. https://doi.org/10.1016/j.ejmg.2013.01.012. Epub 2013 Feb 14
5. Clarke A, Phillips DI, Brown R, Harper PS. Clinical aspects of X-linked hypohidrotic ectodermal dysplasia. Arch Dis Child. 1987;62(10):989–96. https://doi.org/10.1136/adc.62.10.989. PMID: 2445301; PMCID: PMC1778691
6. Blüschke G, Nüsken KD, Schneider H. Prevalence and prevention of severe complications of hypohidrotic ectodermal dysplasia in infancy. Early Hum Dev. 2010;86(7):397–9. https://doi.org/10.1016/j.earlhumdev.2010.04.008. Epub 2010 Jun 1
7. Peschel N, Wright JT, Koster MI, Clarke AJ, Tadini G, Fete M, Hadj-Rabia S, Sybert VP, Norderyd J, Maier-Wohlfart S, Fete TJ, Pagnan N, Visinoni AF, Schneider H. Molecular pathway-based classification of ectodermal dysplasias: first five-yearly update. Genes (Basel). 2022;13(12):2327. https://doi.org/10.3390/genes13122327. PMID: 36553593; PMCID: PMC9778228
8. Wright JT, Fete M, Schneider H, Zinser M, Koster MI, Clarke AJ, Hadj-Rabia S, Tadini G, Pagnan N, Visinoni AF, Bergendal B, Abbott B, Fete T, Stanford C, Butcher C, D'Souza RN, Sybert VP, Morasso MI. Ectodermal dysplasias: classification and organization by phenotype, genotype and molecular pathway. Am J Med Genet A. 2019;179(3):442–7. https://doi.org/10.1002/ajmg.a.61045. Epub 2019 Jan 31. PMID: 30703280; PMCID: PMC6421567
9. Garelli S, Dalla Costa M, Sabbadin C, Barollo S, Rubin B, Scarpa R, Masiero S, Fierabracci A, Bizzarri C, Crinò A, Cappa M, Valenzise M, Meloni A, De Bellis AM, Giordano C, Presotto F, Perniola R, Capalbo D, Salerno MC, Stigliano A, Radetti G, Camozzi V, Greggio NA, Bogazzi F, Chiodini I, Pagotto U, Black SK, Chen S, Rees Smith B, Furmaniak J, Weber G, Pigliaru F, De Sanctis L, Scaroni C, Betterle C. Autoimmune polyendocrine syndrome type 1: an Italian survey on 158 patients. J Endocrinol Invest. 2021;44(11):2493–510. https://doi.org/10.1007/s40618-021-01585-6. Epub 2021 May 18. PMID: 34003463; PMCID: PMC8502131
10. Borchers J, Pukkala E, Mäkitie O, Laakso S. Patients with APECED have increased early mortality due to endocrine causes, malignancies and infections. J Clin Endocrinol Metab. 2020;105(6):e2207–13. https://doi.org/10.1210/clinem/dgaa140. PMID: 32185376; PMCID: PMC7150614

Chapter 2
What Is and Isn't an Ectodermal Dysplasia?

Nicolai Peschel and Holm Schneider

Keywords Classification · Syndromes · Criteria

2.1 Introduction

Since clinical symptoms of ectodermal dysplasia, such as missing teeth, hair, or nails, are easily recognizable with the naked eye, descriptions of affected patients were published in the medical literature as early as in the nineteenth century. In 1848, the physician John Thurnam first reported a case of hypohidrotic ectodermal dysplasia: "He was distinguished, throughout life, by the almost complete absence of hair; by the teeth being not more than four in number; by the delicate structure of the skin; and by the absence of sensible perspiration and tears" [1]. Similarly, Charles Darwin wrote about an observation made by W. Wedderburn:" ... a Hindoo family in Scinde, in which ten men, in the course of four generations, were furnished, in both jaws taken together, with only four small and weak incisor teeth and with eight posterior molars. The men thus affected have very little hair on the body, and become bald early in life. They also suffer much during hot weather from excessive dryness of the skin. It is remarkable that no instance has occurred of a daughter being thus affected" [2]. In this short section, he already mentioned some of the most important clinical features of ectodermal dysplasias that were originally used for the classification. However, the term ectodermal dysplasia was only coined by Weech in the early twentieth century, when he reported 2 cases of "Hereditary Ectodermal Dysplasia (Congenital Ectodermal Defect)" [3]. Four more decades passed before the classification and categorization of the respective disease entities

N. Peschel (✉) · H. Schneider
Department of Pediatrics, University of Erlangen-Nürnberg, Erlangen, Germany
e-mail: nicolai.peschel@fau.de; holm.schneider@uk-erlangen.de

G. Tadini et al. (eds.), *Multidisciplinary Approach to Ectodermal Dysplasia*,
https://doi.org/10.1007/978-3-031-75790-7_2

began. The Brazilian dentist, professor, and geneticist Newton Freire-Maia became involved in the study of these diseases rather by chance. While working on a different project, he noticed that there was no definition of ectodermal dysplasia. Furthermore, he found many anomalies and conditions in the medical literature that all appeared to be ectodermal dysplasias but were not classified as such—simply because neither a definition nor a classification existed. In 1971, he published a very brief paper, only three pages long, that proposed a definition and classification, featuring about 30 disease entities [4]. An ectodermal dysplasia was originally described by him as a congenital disorder characterized by the involvement of two or more structures derived from the ectodermal germ layer [5]. These include primarily the skin and its appendages, such as hair, nails, or certain glands, as well as the teeth.

In these early attempts to classify ectodermal dysplasias, the different conditions were divided into subgroups according to the anatomical structures affected, e.g., conditions in which hair, nails, teeth, and sweat glands showed abnormalities or conditions characterized only by insufficient development of hair and nails were grouped together, respectively. Before most of the genes underlying the diseases were known, another classification criterion was inheritance, i.e., whether a disease was inherited recessively, dominantly, or X-linked. Over the next decades, the number of reported ectodermal dysplasias continued to grow to more than 150 by the beginning of the new millennium. Freire-Maia's second wife, Eleidi Chautard-Freire-Maia, continued the work on the classification after his death and, together with Atila Visinoni, Toni Lisboa-Costa, and Nina Pagnan, published an update of the classification, in which also the first genetically determined ectodermal dysplasias were described [6]. After the publication of the human genome and with the widespread availability of DNA diagnostics, the focus of disease classifications shifted to the molecular causes of disease entities. This was discussed in a series of international conferences on the classification of ectodermal dysplasias in the following years, held under the auspices of Professor Carlos Salinas (Fig. 2.1) and sponsored by the National Foundation for Ectodermal Dysplasias of the U.S.A. [7–9]. In two follow-up publications on this matter, expert groups increasingly presented a molecular classification approach [10, 11], which will be outlined in the following sections.

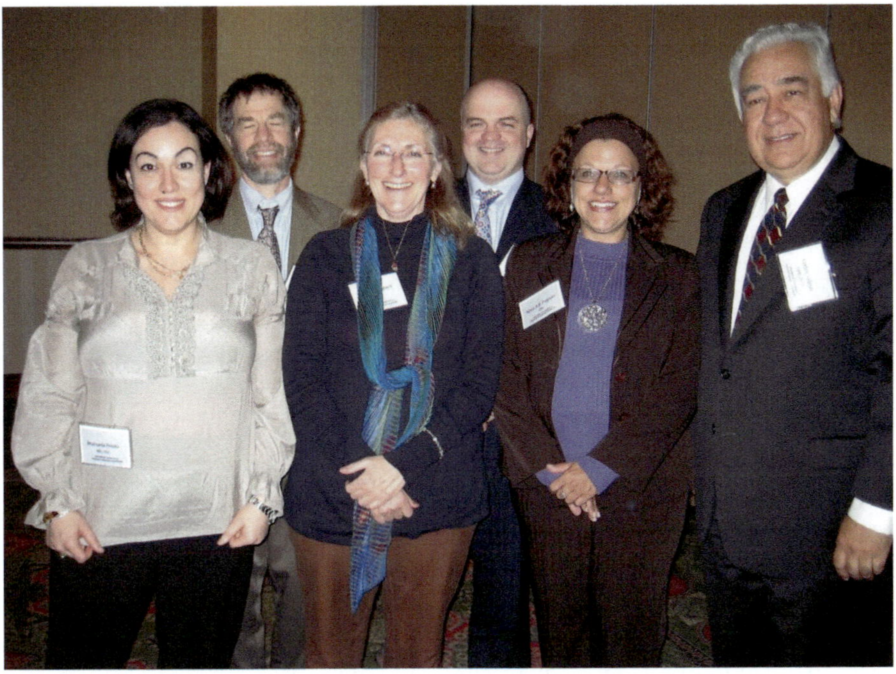

Fig. 2.1 A group of scientists who took part in the first international conference on the classification of ectodermal dysplasias chaired by Carlos Salinas (right)

2.2 Classification

Ectodermal dysplasias have been defined as congenital genetic conditions that affect the development of two or more ectodermal derivatives, including hair, teeth, nails, and certain glands. The individual disease entities are caused by pathogenic variants of genes involved in the formation of anatomical structures, which are (mainly) derived from the embryonic ectoderm. They have been grouped according to the molecular signaling pathway in which the affected gene is primarily active. Group 1 represents the ectodysplasin A (EDA)/nuclear factor kappa-B (NF-κB) signaling pathway, group 2 the Wnt/β-catenin signaling pathway, group 3 the p63 signaling cascade, group 4 includes genes that play an important role in the proper development of cell structure or keratinization, and group 5 comprises genes that play a role in other pathways such as Notch signaling. Group 6 is a collection of rare diseases with features of ectodermal dysplasia but caused by variants of genes that do not fit into any of the categories and signaling cascades described above, primarily affect organs of non-ectodermal origin or are classified elsewhere.

Table 2.1 The EDA/NF-κB signaling pathway (group 1)

Gene(s)	Disease(s)/syndrome(s) — previously suggested nomenclature	OMIM no.	References
EDA	Ectodermal dysplasia 1, hypohidrotic, X-linked (Christ-Siemens-Touraine syndrome, XLHED)	305100	Kere et al. [12]
EDAR	Ectodermal dysplasia 10A and 10B, AD and AR (ECTD10A, B)	129490, 224900	Monreal et al. [13]
EDARADD	Ectodermal dysplasia 11A and 11B, AD and AR (ECTD11A, B)	614940, 614941	Bal et al. [14], Munoz et al. [15]
IKBKG	Incontinentia pigmenti (IP)	308300	Smahi et al. [16]
IKBKG	Ectodermal dysplasia and immunodeficiency 1, AD and AR (EDAID1)	300291, 300301	Zonana et al. [17]
CHUK	Cocoon syndrome	613630	Lahtela et al. [18]
NFKBIA	Ectodermal dysplasia and immunodeficiency 2 (EDAID2)	612132	Courtois et al. [19]
PRKD1	Congenital heart defects and ectodermal dysplasia (CHDED)	617364	Sifrim et al. [20]
TRAF6	Hidrotic form of ectodermal dysplasia, not yet OMIM-listed	602355	Wisniewski und Trzeciak [21]

Pathogenic gene variants affecting the EDA/NF-κB pathway may lead to full-blown hypohidrotic ectodermal dysplasia, a milder disease phenotype, or non-syndromic oligodontia. Genes involved in the EDA/NF-κB pathway and the diseases caused by their known pathogenic variants are listed in Table 2.1. A graphical synopsis of the signaling pathway and the relationships between the different ectodermal dysplasias of this first group is shown in Fig. 2.2.

The released soluble part of EDA, a homotrimeric type II transmembrane protein cleaved by the protease furin, activates the signaling cascade. Interestingly, the mRNA transcribed from the X-chromosomal gene *EDA* that encodes EDA is spliced alternatively, resulting in several isoforms of the protein, the most important of which are EDA1 and EDA2 [22]. The binding of EDA1 to its cognate receptor (EDAR) [23] recruits the intracellular adaptor protein EDAR-associated death domain (EDARADD) [24], which activates downstream signaling. EDARADD further forms a complex with TNF receptor-associated factor 6 (TRAF6) [25], TAK1-binding protein 2 (TAB2) [26], and TGF-β-activated kinase 1 (TAK1) [27]. TAB2 is an adaptor protein that bridges the gap between TRAF6 and TAK1, allowing TAK1 activation and, subsequently, inhibitor of nuclear factor kappa-B kinase (IKK) complex activation [28]. Whether and to what extent EDA2 influences the development of ectodermal structures is currently being investigated. However, we already know that EDA2 interacts with the EDA2 receptor (EDA2R, formerly named XEDAR) [23]. Activation of the IKK complex, which consists of the conserved helix-loop-helix ubiquitous kinase (IKK-α, also referred to as CHUK) [29], IKK-β, and a

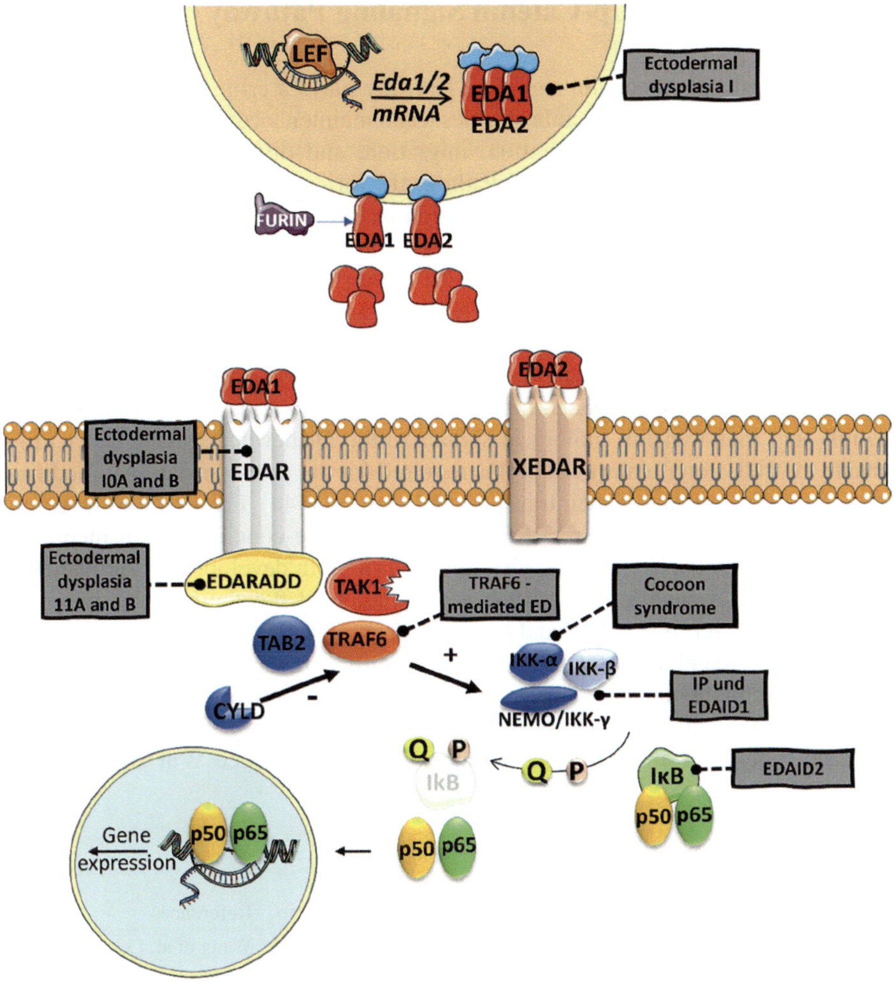

Fig. 2.2 The EDA/NF-κB signaling pathway and associated ectodermal dysplasias

structural component (IKK-γ, previously known as NEMO), leads to phosphorylation, ubiquitination, and proteasomal degradation of the NF-κB inhibitor (IkB) [30]. Now without inhibition, the transcription factor NF-κB is released into the cytosol and then translocated into the nucleus, where it activates the transcription of target genes involved in the development and morphogenesis of anatomical structures of ectodermal origin, such as hair, nails, teeth, and eccrine glands. Termination of signal transduction may be achieved by CYLD lysine-63 deubiquitinase, which deubiquitinates the TRAF6 protein [31].

2.3 Group 2: Wnt/β-Catenin Signaling Pathway

The canonical Wnt/β-catenin signaling pathway plays a critical role in many biological processes, including embryogenesis and maintenance of adult tissue homeostasis. It regulates cell proliferation, migration, and differentiation, e.g., during dental and orofacial development. Pathogenic variants of genes involved in this pathway may cause non-syndromic oligodontia, hypohidrotic (or hidrotic) ectodermal dysplasias, or Goltz syndrome [32].

Table 2.2 lists the ectodermal dysplasias associated with deficiencies of the Wnt/β-catenin pathway, which is named after its ligands, the proteins of the Wingless (Wnt) family. To date, 19 different Wnt family members have been described in humans, of which Wnt10A and Wnt10B have the greatest relevance to tooth development [42]. Both proteins can bind to a transmembrane receptor of the Frizzled family and thus transmit biological signals to the Disheveled protein (DVL) [43] inside the cell. Porcupine (PORCN) is required for the post-translational modification of all Wnts to enable their transport and secretion [44]. Frizzled's co-receptors, LDL receptor-related protein (LRP) [45] and Kringle-containing transmembrane protein 1 (KREMEN1) [46], are also involved in tooth development. Activation of canonical Wnt signaling leads to the accumulation of β-catenin in the cytoplasm [47] that can enter the nucleus and help transcription factors belonging to the T-cell factor/lymphoid enhancer factor (TCF/LEF) family to transcribe many genes important for developmental steps. LEF1 in turn activates the transcription of *EDA*, linking Wnt signaling to the EDA pathway [39]. There are a few other proteins involved in gene regulation at the transcriptional level that influence Wnt signaling: the

Table 2.2 Wnt pathway (group 2)

Gene(s)	Disease(s)/syndrome(s) — previously suggested nomenclature	OMIM no.	References
PORCN	Focal dermal hypoplasia (FDH) or Goltz-Gorlin syndrome	305600	Wang et al. [33]
TWIST2	Focal facial dermal dysplasia 3/ Ablepharon-macrostomia syndrome (AMS)	136500, 200110	Cervantes-Barragán et al. [34], Marchegiani et al. [35]
WNT10A	Odonto-onycho-dermal dysplasia (OODD)/Schöpf-Schulz-Passarge syndrome (SSPS)	257980, 224750	Adaimy et al. [36]
KREMEN1	Ectodermal dysplasia 13, hair/tooth type (ECTD13)	617392	Issa et al. [37]
TBX3	Ulnar-mammary syndrome (UMS)	181450	Bamshad et al. [38]
LEF1	Ectodermal dysplasia with or without hypohidrosis, not yet OMIM-listed	153245	Lévy et al. [39]
LRP6	Ectodermal dysplasia with or without hypohidrosis, not yet OMIM-listed	603507	Yu et al. [40], Peschel et al. [10]
MSX1	Ectodermal dysplasia 3, Witkop type (ECTD3 or Witkop syndrome)	189500	Jumlongras et al. [41]

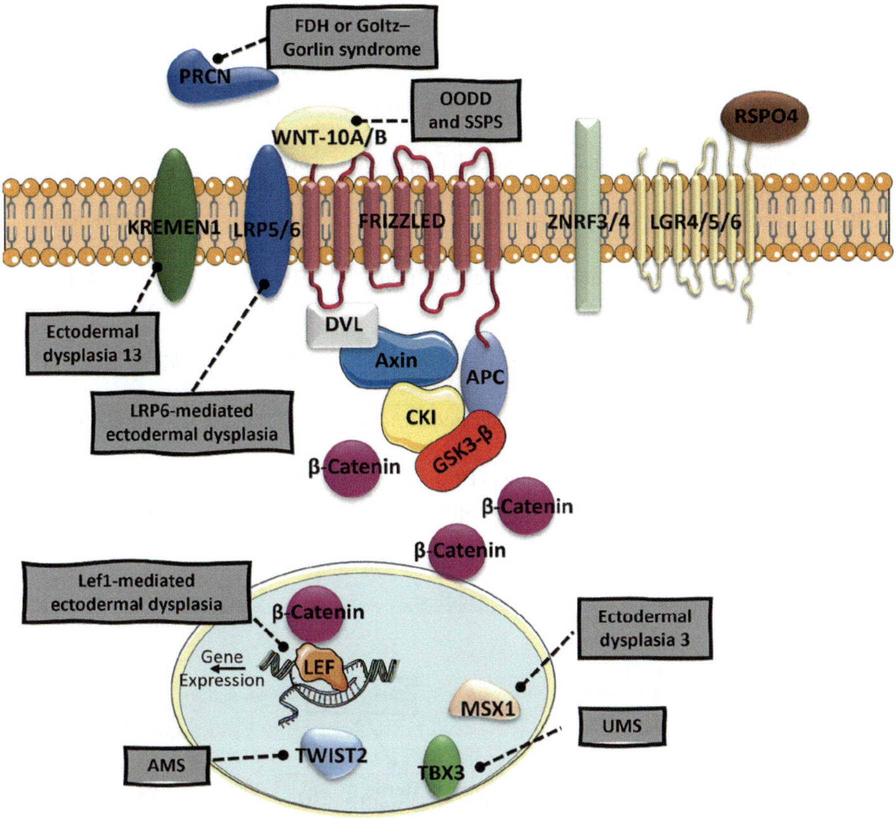

Fig. 2.3 The Wnt/β-catenin signaling pathway and associated ectodermal dysplasias

Twist-related protein 2 (TWIST2), known to act as a molecular switch activating or repressing target genes by binding to conserved E-boxes in the DNA sequence [35], T-box transcription factor 3 (TBX3) [48], which binds to T-boxes, and the transcriptional repressor msh homeobox 1 (MSX1) [49] (Fig. 2.3).

Table 2.3 gives an overview of ectodermal dysplasias caused by abnormalities of p63 or its target genes. The tumor protein p63 is an ancient member of the p53 family of transcription factors. It influences the expression of several hundred genes, including those relevant to the development of epithelial tissues. Therefore, various human disorders of the skin and its appendages are caused by alterations in p63 signaling [58]. Several protein isoforms with different N- and C-termini but identical DNA binding and oligomerization domains originate from the gene *TP63*. Depending on the domain of the protein that is altered by a distinct *TP63* mutation, the clinical picture may be quite different, which has been reflected in the classification of p63-associated ectodermal dysplasias (Fig. 2.4). While most C-terminal mutations cause ankyloblepharon-ectodermal defects-cleft lip/palate syndrome (AEC) and Rapp-Hodgkin syndrome (RHS), mutations in the DNA binding domain

Table 2.3 p63 pathway (group 3)

Gene(s)	Disease(s)/syndrome(s) — previously suggested nomenclature	OMIM no.	References
TP63	Acro-dermato-ungual-lacrimal-tooth syndrome (ADULT)	103285	Amiel et al. [50]
TP63	Ectrodactyly ectodermal dysplasia-cleft lip/palate syndrome (EEC)	604292	Celli et al. [51]
TP63	Limb-mammary syndrome (LMS)	603543	van Bokhoven et al. [52]
TP63	Ankyloblepharon-ectodermal defects-cleft lip/ palate (AEC/Rapp-Hodgkin syndrome)	106260, 129400	Bougeard et al. [53]
CDH3	Ectodermal dysplasia, ectrodactyly, macular dystrophy syndrome (EEMS)	225280	Kjaer et al. [54]
KDF1	Ectodermal dysplasia 12, hypohidrotic/hair/tooth/ nail type (ECTD12)	617337	Shamseldin et al. [55]
DLX3	Tricho-dento-osseous syndrome (TDO)	190320	Price et al. [56]
RIPK4	Curly hair-ankyloblepharon-nail dysplasia syndrome (CHANDS); complex lethal subtype known as Bartsocas-Papas syndrome 1 (BPS1)	214350, 263650	Gripp et al. [57]

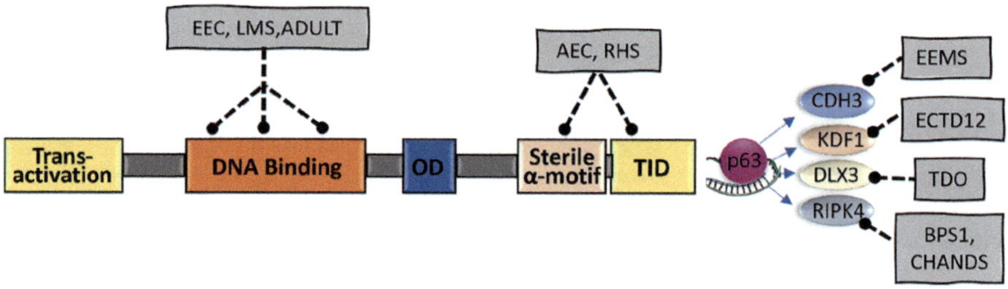

Fig. 2.4 Critical domains of *TP63*, target proteins of the gene product p63 and associated ectodermal dysplasias

cause ectrodactyly-ectodermal dysplasia-cleft lip/palate syndrome (EEC), limb-mammary syndrome (LMS), or acro-dermato-ungual-lacrimal-tooth syndrome (ADULT) [59]. In addition to the diseases caused by alterations of the p63 protein itself, the third group of ectodermal dysplasias also includes diseases due to pathogenic variants of p63 target genes leading to deficiencies in the respective proteins. Cadherin 3 deficiency (CDH3) [60] is linked to ectodermal dysplasia, ectrodactyly, macular dystrophy syndrome (EEMS), keratinocyte differentiation factor 1 deficiency (KDF1) [61] underlies ectodermal dysplasia 12 (ECTD12), distal reading homeobox 3 deficiency (DLX3) [62] causes tricho-dento-osseous syndrome (TDO), and receptor-interacting serine/threonine kinase 4 deficiency (RIPK4) [63] is associated with CHANDS syndrome and Bartsocas-Papas syndrome.

Group 4 (Table 2.4) comprises rare diseases that are related to proteins with similar functions for the epithel. They play important roles in the formation of cell

Table 2.4 Structure Group (group 4)

Gene(s)	Disease(s)/syndrome(s) — previously suggested nomenclature	OMIM no.	References
PKP1	Ectodermal dysplasia-skin fragility syndrome (EDSFS)	604536	McGrath et al. [64]
GRHL2	Ectodermal dysplasia-short stature syndrome (ECTDS)	616029	Petrof et al. [65]
PVRL1	Cleft lip/palate-ectodermal dysplasia syndrome (CLPED1)	225060	Suzuki et al. [66]
PVRL4	Ectodermal dysplasia-syndactyly syndrome 1 (EDSS1)	613573	Brancati et al. [67], Suzuki et al. [66]
KRT74	Ectodermal dysplasia 7, hair/nail type (ECTD7)	614929	Naeem et al. [68]
KRT85	Ectodermal dysplasia 4, hair/nail type (ECTD4)	602032	Calzavara-Pinton et al. [69]
GJB2	Keratitis-ichthyosis-deafness syndrome, AD (KID)	148210	van Steensel et al. [70]
GJA1	Oculo-dento-digital dysplasia (ODDD, ODDR)	164200, 257850	Paznekas et al. [71]
GJB6	Clouston syndrome or ectodermal dysplasia 2, Clouston type (ECTD2)	129500	Lamartine et al. [72]

structures, keratinization, or cell-cell interactions. Keratins are intermediate filament proteins and essential for providing structural stability to hair, epidermis, and nails [73]. Keratin 74 (KRT74) and keratin 85 (KRT85) belong to the type II keratin family; they act as heterodimers. The respective genes are expressed at the highest levels in the inner root sheath of hair follicles [74]. Pathogenetic *KRT74* or *KRT85* variants cause ectodermal dysplasias of the hair/nail type. Gap junctions, desmosomes, or adherens junctions (Fig. 2.5) represent structures that connect cells. Pathogenic variants of genes involved in cell-cell connection/communication may also underlie disorders of ectodermal development. For example, plakophilin (PKP1) [75] which is found in desmosomes participates in linking cadherins to intermediate filaments in the cytoskeleton. Its malfunction is associated with ectodermal dysplasia-skin fragility syndrome.

Grainyhead-like protein 2 (GRHL2) is a transcription factor required for epithelial development and morphogenesis [76]. Homozygous pathogenic variants of the respective gene impair tight junctions, leading to ectodermal dysplasia-short stature syndrome (ECTDS). Nectin-1 (PVRL1) and nectin-4 (PVRL4) are components of adherens junctions and tight junctions between epithelial cells [77]. Their deficiency causes cleft lip/palate-ectodermal dysplasia syndrome (CLPED1) and ectodermal dysplasia-syndactyly syndrome 1 (EDSS1), respectively. Pathogenic variants of genes encoding gap junction protein beta 2 (GJB2), gap junction protein beta 6 (GJB6), or gap junction protein alpha 1 (GJA1) are known to underlie keratitis-ichthyosis-deafness syndrome (KID), oculo-dento-digital dysplasia (ODDD or ODDR), and Clouston syndrome (Table 2.5).

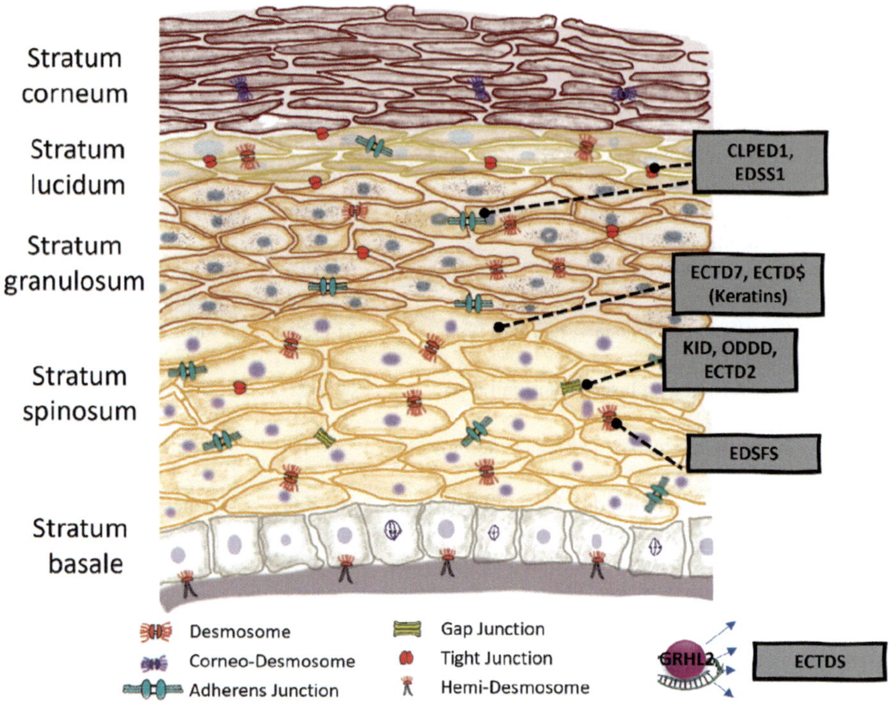

Fig. 2.5 Structure of the skin and associated ectodermal dysplasias

Table 2.5 Others (group 5)

Gene(s)	Disease(s)/syndrome(s) — previously suggested nomenclature	OMIM no.	References
TSPEAR	Ectodermal dysplasia 14, hair/tooth type with or without hypohidrosis (ECTD14)	618180	Peled et al. [78]
HOXC13	Ectodermal dysplasia 9, hair/nail type (ECTD9)	614931	Lin et al. [79]
CST6	Ectodermal dysplasia 15, hypohidrotic/hair type (ECTD15)	618535	van den Bogaard et al. [80]
AP1B1	Keratitis-ichthyosis-deafness syndrome, AR (KIDAR)	242150	Boyden et al. [81]
TRPS1	Trichorhinophalangeal syndrome, type I (TRPS1) or type III (TRPS3)	190350, 190351	Lüdecke et al. [82]
TRPS1 + *EXT1*	Trichorhinophalangeal syndrome, type II (TRPS2)	150230	Lüdecke et al. [83]

Some genes and the proteins they encode are linked to ectodermal dysplasias without being involved in the molecular signaling pathways described above or fulfilling the criteria for placement in the structure group. For example, thrombospondin-type laminin G domain and EAR repeats (TSPEAR) [84] is important for human tooth and hair follicle morphogenesis through regulation of the Notch signaling pathway, and its dysfunction can cause ectodermal dysplasia 14 (ECTD14). Homeobox transcription factor HOXC13 [85] plays a role in hair follicle differentiation and is associated with ectodermal dysplasia 9 (ECTD9). Cystatins are inhibitors of mammalian lysosomal cysteine proteinases, e.g., cathepsin B. The lack of cystatin E/M (CST6) [86] has been reported to cause ectodermal dysplasia 15 (ECTD15). Adaptins that contribute to the formation of adaptor complexes of clathrin-coated vesicles may also be essential for ectodermal development. The adaptor-related protein complex 1 subunit beta 1 (AP1B1) [87] is found at the cytoplasmic face of coated vesicles located at the Golgi complex. Pathogenic variants of the respective gene underlie the autosomal recessive keratitis-ichthyosis-deafness syndrome (KIDAR). Last but not least, the zinc finger transcriptional repressor GATA binding 1 (TRPS1) [88] was shown to be involved in the regulation of chondrocyte development and to be associated with trichorhinophalangeal syndromes (TRPS1, 2, 3).

2.4 Group 6: To Be Classified Elsewhere?

Table 2.6 lists syndromes with features of ectodermal dysplasia that are related to genes apparently not involved in the already known pathways and that mainly affect organs of non-ectodermal origin. Most if not all of these disorders could be classified elsewhere.

Table 2.6 Syndromes with a partial ectodermal dysplasia-like phenotype that may be classified elsewhere

Gene(s)	Syndrome(s)	OMIM no.	References
CDH1, *CTNND1*	Blepharocheilodontic syndrome 1/ Blepharocheilodontic syndrome 2 (BCDS1/BCDS2)	119580, 617681	Ghoumid et al. [89]
IFT43, −52, −122, −140, WDR19, −35	Cranioectodermal dysplasia, types 1–4 (CED) or Sensenbrenner syndrome	218330	Walczak-Sztulpa et al. [90]
EVC, EVC2	Ellis-van Creveld syndrome (EVC)	225500	Ruiz-Perez et al. [91]
EVC, EVC2	Weyers acrofacial dysostosis (WAD)	193530	Ye et al. [92]
KCTD1	Scalp-ear-nipple syndrome (SENS)	181270	Marneros et al. [93]
SOX9–CNJ2	Cooks syndrome	106995	Castori et al. [94]
ANTXR1	Growth retardation, alopecia, pseudoanodontia, and optic atrophy syndrome (GAPO)	230740	Stránecký et al. [95]

(continued)

Table 2.6 (continued)

Gene(s)	Syndrome(s)	OMIM no.	References
SMARCAD1	Huriez syndrome/Basan syndrome	181600, 129200	Günther et al. [96]
DSP	Carvajal syndrome (DCWHK)	605676	Norgett et al. [97]
KRT14	Dermatopathia pigmentosa reticularis (DPR)/Naegeli syndrome (NFJS)	125595, 161000	Lugassy et al. [98]
KRT16, −17	Pachyonychia congenita 1/Pachyonychia congenita 2 (PC1/PC2)	167200, 167210	McLean et al. [99]
ARID1A,−1B, SMARCA4, −B1, −E1	Coffin-Siris syndrome (CSS)	135900	Tsurusaki et al. [100]
ATP6V1B2	Deafness, congenital, and onychodystrophy, AD (DDOD)	124480	Yuan et al. [101]
TBC1D24	Deafness, onycho- and osteodystrophy, mental retardation, and seizures syndrome	220500	Campeau et al. [102]
SLC25A24	Gorlin-Chaudhry-Moss syndrome (FPS)	612289	Ehmke et al. [103]
PEX1, PEX6	Heimler syndrome 1 (HMLR1)/Heimler syndrome 2 (HMLR2)	234580, 616617	Ratbi et al. [104]
UBR1	Johanson–Blizzard syndrome (JBS)	243800	Zenker et al. [105]
FGFR3, −2, FGF10	Lacrimo-auriculo-dento-digital syndrome (LADD)	149730	Rohmann et al. [106]
SREBF1	Mucoepithelial dysplasia, hereditary (HMD)	158310	Morice-Picard et al. [107]
HEPHL1	Pili torti and developmental delay (HJDD)	261990	Sharma et al. [108]
KRT81, −83, −86, DSG4	Monilethrix (MNLIX)	158000	Winter et al. [109]
RODGI	Kohlschütter-Tönz syndrome	226750	Schossig et al. [110]
INSR	Pineal hyperplasia, insulin-resistant diabetes mellitus, and somatic abnormalities	262190	Kadowaki et al. [111]
CTSK	Pycnodysostosis (PKND)	265800	Gelb et al. [112]
SETBP1	Schinzel-Giedion midface retraction syndrome (SGS)	269150	Hoischen et al. [113]

2.5 Outlook

The current classification of ectodermal dysplasias as outlined in this chapter is just a snapshot of the year 2024. Disease classifications will always be in a state of flux, and the group of ectodermal dysplasias is likely to expand in the coming years. On the other hand, clinically separate disease entities may merge into a single one based on genetic findings. More sophisticated genetic diagnostics might reveal new links to genes associated with ectodermal development and to other molecular pathways, such as the Notch pathway affected by TSPEAR mutations.

References

1. Thurnam J. Two cases in which the skin, hair and teeth were very imperfectly developed. Med Chir Trans. 1848;31:71–82. https://doi.org/10.1177/095952874803100108.
2. Darwin C. The variations of animals and plants under domestication, vol. 2. London: John Murray; 1885.
3. Weech AA. Hereditary ectodermal dysplasia (congenital ectodermal defect). Am J Dis Child. 1929;37(4):766. https://doi.org/10.1001/archpedi.1929.01930040075005.
4. Freire-Maia N. Ectodermal dysplasias. Hum Hered. 1971;21(4):309–12. https://doi.org/10.1159/000152419.
5. Freire-Maia N. Nosologic groups. An overview. Hum Hered. 1977;27(4):251–6. https://doi.org/10.1159/000152876.
6. Visinoni AF, Lisboa-Costa T, Pagnan NAB, Chautard-Freire-Maia EA. Ectodermal dysplasias: clinical and molecular review. Am J Med Genet A. 2009;149A(9):1980–2002. https://doi.org/10.1002/ajmg.a.32864.
7. Pagnan NA, Visinoni ÁF. Update on ectodermal dysplasias clinical classification. Am J Med Genet A. 2014;164A(10):2415–23. https://doi.org/10.1002/ajmg.a.36616.
8. Salinas CF, Irvine AD, Itin PH, Giovanna D, John J, Schneider H, Clarke AJ, et al. Second International Conference on a classification of ectodermal dysplasias: development of a multiaxis model. Am J Med Genet A. 2014;164A(10):2482–9. https://doi.org/10.1002/ajmg.a.36507.
9. Salinas CF, Jorgenson RJ, Wright JT, DiGiovanna JJ, Fete MD. 2008 international conference on ectodermal dysplasias classification: conference report. Am J Med Genet A. 2009;149A(9):1958–69. https://doi.org/10.1002/ajmg.a.32882.
10. Peschel N, Wright JT, Koster MI, Clarke AJ, Tadini G, Fete M, et al. Molecular pathway-based classification of ectodermal dysplasias: first five-yearly update. Genes. 2022;13(12):–2327. https://doi.org/10.3390/genes13122327.
11. Wright JT, Fete M, Schneider H, Zinser M, Koster MI, Clarke AJ, et al. Ectodermal dysplasias: Classification and organization by phenotype, genotype and molecular pathway. Am J Med Genet A. 2019;179(3):442–7. https://doi.org/10.1002/ajmg.a.61045.
12. Kere J, Srivastava AK, Montonen O, Zonana J, Thomas N, Ferguson B, et al. X-linked anhidrotic (hypohidrotic) ectodermal dysplasia is caused by mutation in a novel transmembrane protein. Nat Genet. 1996;13(4):409–16. https://doi.org/10.1038/ng0895-409.
13. Monreal AW, Ferguson BM, Headon DJ, Street SL, Overbeek PA, Zonana J. Mutations in the human homologue of mouse dl cause autosomal recessive and dominant hypohidrotic ectodermal dysplasia. Nat Genet. 1999;22(4):366–9. https://doi.org/10.1038/11937.

14. Bal E, Baala L, Cluzeau C, El Kerch F, Ouldim K, Hadj-Rabia S, et al. Autosomal dominant anhidrotic ectodermal dysplasias at the EDARADD locus. Hum Mutat. 2007;28(7):703–9. https://doi.org/10.1002/humu.20500.
15. Munoz F, Lestringant G, Sybert V, Frydman M, Alswaini A, Frossard PM, et al. Definitive evidence for an autosomal recessive form of hypohidrotic ectodermal dysplasia clinically indistinguishable from the more common X-linked disorder. Am J Hum Genet. 1997;61(1):94–100. https://doi.org/10.1086/513905.
16. Smahi A, Courtois G, Vabres P, Yamaoka S, Heuertz S, Munnich A, et al. Genomic rearrangement in NEMO impairs NF-kappaB activation and is a cause of incontinentia pigmenti. The International Incontinentia Pigmenti (IP) Consortium. Nature. 2000;405(6785):466–72. https://doi.org/10.1038/35013114.
17. Zonana J, Elder ME, Schneider LC, Orlow SJ, Moss C, Golabi M, et al. A novel X-linked disorder of immune deficiency and hypohidrotic ectodermal dysplasia is allelic to incontinentia pigmenti and due to mutations in IKK-gamma (NEMO). Am J Hum Genet. 2000;67(6):1555–62. https://doi.org/10.1086/316914.
18. Lahtela J, Nousiainen HO, Stefanovic V, Tallila J, Viskari H, Karikoski R, et al. Mutant CHUK and severe fetal encasement malformation. N Engl J Med. 2010;363(17):1631–7. https://doi.org/10.1056/NEJMoa0911698.
19. Courtois G, Smahi A, Reichenbach J, Döffinger R, Cancrini C, Bonnet M, et al. A hypermorphic IkappaBalpha mutation is associated with autosomal dominant anhidrotic ectodermal dysplasia and T cell immunodeficiency. J Clin Invest. 2003;112(7):1108–15. https://doi.org/10.1172/JCI18714.
20. Sifrim A, Hitz M-P, Wilsdon A, Breckpot J, Al Turki SH, Thienpont B, et al. Distinct genetic architectures for syndromic and nonsyndromic congenital heart defects identified by exome sequencing. Nat Genet. 2016;48(9):1060–5. https://doi.org/10.1038/ng.3627.
21. Wisniewski SA, Trzeciak WH. A rare heterozygous TRAF6 variant is associated with hypohidrotic ectodermal dysplasia. Br J Dermatol. 2012;166(6):1353–6. https://doi.org/10.1111/j.1365-2133.2012.10871.x.
22. Ezer S, Bayés M, Elomaa O, Schlessinger D, Kere J. Ectodysplasin is a collagenous trimeric type II membrane protein with a tumor necrosis factor-like domain and co-localizes with cytoskeletal structures at lateral and apical surfaces of cells. Hum Mol Genet. 1999;8(11):2079–86. https://doi.org/10.1093/hmg/8.11.2079.
23. Yan M, Wang LC, Hymowitz SG, Schilbach S, Lee J, Goddard A, et al. Two-amino acid molecular switch in an epithelial morphogen that regulates binding to two distinct receptors. Science (New York, N.Y.). 2000;290(5491):523–7. https://doi.org/10.1126/science.290.5491.523.
24. Headon DJ, Emmal SA, Ferguson BM, Tucker AS, Justice MJ, Sharpe PT, et al. Gene defect in ectodermal dysplasia implicates a death domain adapter in development. Nature. 2001;414(6866):913–6. https://doi.org/10.1038/414913a.
25. Cao Z, Xiong J, Takeuchi M, Kurama T, Goeddel DV. TRAF6 is a signal transducer for interleukin-1. Nature. 1996;383(6599):443–6. https://doi.org/10.1038/383443a0.
26. Takaesu G, Kishida S, Hiyama A, Yamaguchi K, Shibuya H, Irie K, et al. TAB2, a novel adaptor protein, mediates activation of TAK1 MAPKKK by linking TAK1 to TRAF6 in the IL-1 signal transduction pathway. Mol Cell. 2000;5(4):649–58. https://doi.org/10.1016/s1097-2765(00)80244-0.
27. Shibuya H, Yamaguchi K, Shirakabe K, Tonegawa A, Gotoh Y, Ueno N, et al. TAB1: an activator of the TAK1 MAPKKK in TGF-beta signal transduction. Science (New York, N.Y.). 1996;272(5265):1179–82. https://doi.org/10.1126/science.272.5265.1179.
28. Morlon A, Munnich A, Smahi A. TAB2, TRAF6 and TAK1 are involved in NF-kappaB activation induced by the TNF-receptor, Edar and its adaptator Edaradd. Hum Mol Genet. 2005;14(23):3751–7. https://doi.org/10.1093/hmg/ddi405.
29. Delhase M, Hayakawa M, Chen Y, Karin M. Positive and negative regulation of IkappaB kinase activity through IKKbeta subunit phosphorylation. Science (New York, N.Y.). 1999;284(5412):309–13. https://doi.org/10.1126/science.284.5412.309.

30. Yamaoka S, Courtois G, Bessia C, Whiteside ST, Weil R, Agou F, et al. Complementation cloning of NEMO, a component of the IkappaB kinase complex essential for NF-kappaB activation. Cell. 1998;93(7):1231–40. https://doi.org/10.1016/s0092-8674(00)81466-x.
31. Brummelkamp TR, Nijman SMB, Dirac AMG, Bernards R. Loss of the cylindromatosis tumour suppressor inhibits apoptosis by activating NF-kappaB. Nature. 2003;424(6950):797–801. https://doi.org/10.1038/nature01811.
32. Yu M, Wong S-W, Han D, Cai T. Genetic analysis: Wnt and other pathways in nonsyndromic tooth agenesis. Oral Dis. 2019;25(3):646–51. https://doi.org/10.1111/odi.12931.
33. Wang X, Reid Sutton V, Omar Peraza-Llanes J, Yu Z, Rosetta R, Kou Y-C, et al. Mutations in X-linked PORCN, a putative regulator of Wnt signaling, cause focal dermal hypoplasia. Nat Genet. 2007;39(7):836–8. https://doi.org/10.1038/ng2057.
34. Cervantes-Barragán DE, Villarroel CE, Medrano-Hernández A, Durán-McKinster C, Bosch-Canto V, Del-Castillo V, et al. Setleis syndrome in Mexican-Nahua sibs due to a homozygous TWIST2 frameshift mutation and partial expression in heterozygotes: review of the focal facial dermal dysplasias and subtype reclassification. J Med Genet. 2011;48(10):716–20. https://doi.org/10.1136/jmedgenet-2011-100251.
35. Marchegiani S, Davis T, Tessadori F, van Haaften G, Brancati F, Hoischen A, et al. Recurrent mutations in the basic domain of TWIST2 cause ablepharon macrostomia and Barber-Say syndromes. Am J Hum Genet. 2015;97(1):99–110. https://doi.org/10.1016/j.ajhg.2015.05.017.
36. Adaimy L, Chouery E, Megarbane H, Mroueh S, Delague V, Nicolas E, et al. Mutation in WNT10A is associated with an autosomal recessive ectodermal dysplasia: the odonto-onychodermal dysplasia. Am J Hum Genet. 2007;81(4):821–8. https://doi.org/10.1086/520064.
37. Issa YA, Kamal L, Rayyan AA, Dweik D, Pierce S, Lee MK, et al. Mutation of KREMEN1, a modulator of Wnt signaling, is responsible for ectodermal dysplasia including oligodontia in Palestinian families. Eur J Hum Genet. 2016;24(10):1430–5. https://doi.org/10.1038/ejhg.2016.29.
38. Bamshad M, Lin RC, Law DJ, Watkins WC, Krakowiak PA, Moore ME, et al. Mutations in human TBX3 alter limb, apocrine and genital development in ulnar-mammary syndrome. Nat Genet. 1997;16(3):311–5. https://doi.org/10.1038/ng0797-311.
39. Lévy J, Capri Y, Rachid M, Dupont C, Vermeesch JR, Devriendt K, et al. LEF1 haploinsufficiency causes ectodermal dysplasia. Clin Genet. 2020;97(4):595–600. https://doi.org/10.1111/cge.13714.
40. Yu M, Fan Z, Wong SW, Sun K, Zhang L, Liu H, et al. Lrp6 dynamic expression in tooth development and mutations in oligodontia. J Dent Res. 2021;100(4):415–22. https://doi.org/10.1177/0022034520970459.
41. Jumlongras D, Bei M, Stimson JM, Wang WF, DePalma SR, Seidman CE, et al. A nonsense mutation in MSX1 causes Witkop syndrome. Am J Hum Genet. 2001;69(1):67–74. https://doi.org/10.1086/321271.
42. Doolan BJ, Onoufriadis A, Kantaputra P, McGrath JA. WNT10A, dermatology and dentistry. Br J Dermatol. 2021;185(6):1105–11. https://doi.org/10.1111/bjd.20601.
43. Wallingford JB, Rowning BA, Vogeli KM, Rothbächer U, Fraser SE, Harland RM. Dishevelled controls cell polarity during Xenopus gastrulation. Nature. 2000;405(6782):81–5. https://doi.org/10.1038/35011077.
44. Caricasole A, Ferraro T, Rimland JM, Terstappen GC. Molecular cloning and initial characterization of the MG61/PORC gene, the human homologue of the Drosophila segment polarity gene Porcupine. Gene. 2002;288(1–2):147–57. https://doi.org/10.1016/s0378-1119(02)00467-5.
45. Wehrli M, Dougan ST, Caldwell K, O'Keefe L, Schwartz S, Vaizel-Ohayon D, et al. arrow encodes an LDL-receptor-related protein essential for Wingless signalling. Nature. 2000;407(6803):527–30. https://doi.org/10.1038/35035110.
46. Nakamura T, Aoki S, Kitajima K, Takahashi T, Matsumoto K. Molecular cloning and characterization of Kremen, a novel kringle-containing transmembrane protein. Biochim Biophys Acta. 2001;1518(1–2):63–72. https://doi.org/10.1016/s0167-4781(01)00168-3.

47. Peifer M. Cancer, catenins, and cuticle pattern: a complex connection. Science (New York, N.Y.). 1993;262(5140):1667–8. https://doi.org/10.1126/science.8259511.
48. Meneghini V, Odent S, Platonova N, Egeo A, Merlo GR. Novel TBX3 mutation data in families with ulnar-mammary syndrome indicate a genotype-phenotype relationship: mutations that do not disrupt the T-domain are associated with less severe limb defects. Eur J Med Genet. 2006;49(2):151–8. https://doi.org/10.1016/j.ejmg.2005.04.021.
49. Odelberg SJ, Kollhoff A, Keating MT. Dedifferentiation of mammalian myotubes induced by msx1. Cell. 2000;103(7):1099–109. https://doi.org/10.1016/s0092-8674(00)00212-9.
50. Amiel J, Bougeard G, Francannet C, Raclin V, Munnich A, Lyonnet S, Frebourg T. TP63 gene mutation in ADULT syndrome. Eur J Hum Genet. 2001;9(8):642–5. https://doi.org/10.1038/sj.ejhg.5200676.
51. Celli J, Duijf P, Hamel BC, Bamshad M, Kramer B, Smits AP, et al. Heterozygous germline mutations in the p53 homolog p63 are the cause of EEC syndrome. Cell. 1999;99(2):143–53. https://doi.org/10.1016/s0092-8674(00)81646-3.
52. van Bokhoven H, Hamel BC, Bamshad M, Sangiorgi E, Gurrieri F, Duijf PH, et al. p63 Gene mutations in eec syndrome, limb-mammary syndrome, and isolated split hand-split foot malformation suggest a genotype-phenotype correlation. Am J Hum Genet. 2001;69(3):481–92. https://doi.org/10.1086/323123.
53. Bougeard G, Hadj-Rabia S, Faivre L, Sarafan-Vasseur N, Frébourg T. The Rapp-Hodgkin syndrome results from mutations of the TP63 gene. Eur J Hum Genet. 2003;11(9):700–4. https://doi.org/10.1038/sj.ejhg.5201004.
54. Kjaer KW, Hansen L, Schwabe GC, Marques-de-Faria AP, Eiberg H, Mundlos S, et al. Distinct CDH3 mutations cause ectodermal dysplasia, ectrodactyly, macular dystrophy (EEM syndrome). J Med Genet. 2005;42(4):292–8. https://doi.org/10.1136/jmg.2004.027821.
55. Shamseldin HE, Khalifa O, Binamer YM, Almutawa A, Arold ST, Zaidan H, Alkuraya FS. KDF1, encoding keratinocyte differentiation factor 1, is mutated in a multigenerational family with ectodermal dysplasia. Hum Genet. 2017;136(1):99–105. https://doi.org/10.1007/s00439-016-1741-z.
56. Price JA, Wright JT, Kula K, Bowden DW, Hart TC. A common DLX3 gene mutation is responsible for tricho-dento-osseous syndrome in Virginia and North Carolina families. J Med Genet. 1998;35(10):825–8. https://doi.org/10.1136/jmg.35.10.825.
57. Gripp KW, Ennis S, Napoli J. Exome analysis in clinical practice: expanding the phenotype of Bartsocas-Papas syndrome. Am J Med Genet A. 2013;161A(5):1058–63. https://doi.org/10.1002/ajmg.a.35913.
58. Koster MI. p63 in skin development and ectodermal dysplasias. J Invest Dermatol. 2010;130(10):2352–8. https://doi.org/10.1038/jid.2010.119.
59. Osterburg C, Osterburg S, Zhou H, Missero C, Dötsch V. Isoform-specific roles of mutant p63 in human diseases. Cancer. 2021;13:(3). https://doi.org/10.3390/cancers13030536.
60. Shimoyama Y, Yoshida T, Terada M, Shimosato Y, Abe O, Hirohashi S. Molecular cloning of a human Ca2+-dependent cell-cell adhesion molecule homologous to mouse placental cadherin: its low expression in human placental tissues. J Cell Biol. 1989;109(4 Pt 1):1787–94. https://doi.org/10.1083/jcb.109.4.1787.
61. Lee S, Kong Y, Weatherbee SD. Forward genetics identifies Kdf1/1810019J16Rik as an essential regulator of the proliferation-differentiation decision in epidermal progenitor cells. Dev Biol. 2013;383(2):201–13. https://doi.org/10.1016/j.ydbio.2013.09.022.
62. Hassan MQ, Javed A, Morasso MI, Karlin J, Montecino M, van Wijnen AJ, et al. Dlx3 transcriptional regulation of osteoblast differentiation: temporal recruitment of Msx2, Dlx3, and Dlx5 homeodomain proteins to chromatin of the osteocalcin gene. Mol Cell Biol. 2004;24(20):9248–61. https://doi.org/10.1128/MCB.24.20.9248-9261.2004.
63. Bähr C, Rohwer A, Stempka L, Rincke G, Marks F, Gschwendt M. DIK, a novel protein kinase that interacts with protein kinase Cdelta. Cloning, characterization, and gene analysis. J Biol Chem. 2000;275(46):36350–7. https://doi.org/10.1074/jbc.M004771200.
64. McGrath JA, McMillan JR, Shemanko CS, Runswick SK, Leigh IM, Lane EB, et al. Mutations in the plakophilin 1 gene result in ectodermal dysplasia/skin fragility syndrome. Nat Genet. 1997;17(2):240–4. https://doi.org/10.1038/ng1097-240.

65. Petrof G, Nanda A, Howden J, Takeichi T, McMillan JR, Aristodemou S, et al. Mutations in GRHL2 result in an autosomal-recessive ectodermal Dysplasia syndrome. Am J Hum Genet. 2014;95(3):308–14. https://doi.org/10.1016/j.ajhg.2014.08.001.
66. Suzuki K, Hu D, Bustos T, Zlotogora J, Richieri-Costa A, Helms JA, Spritz RA. Mutations of PVRL1, encoding a cell-cell adhesion molecule/herpesvirus receptor, in cleft lip/palate-ectodermal dysplasia. Nat Genet. 2000;25(4):427–30. https://doi.org/10.1038/78119.
67. Brancati F, Fortugno P, Bottillo I, Lopez M, Josselin E, Boudghene-Stambouli O, et al. Mutations in PVRL4, encoding cell adhesion molecule nectin-4, cause ectodermal dysplasia-syndactyly syndrome. Am J Hum Genet. 2010;87(2):265–73. https://doi.org/10.1016/j.ajhg.2010.07.003.
68. Naeem M, John P, Ali G, Ahmad W. Pure hair-nail ectodermal dysplasia maps to chromosome 12p11.1-q21.1 in a consanguineous Pakistani family. Clin Exp Dermatol. 2007;32(5):502–5. https://doi.org/10.1111/j.1365-2230.2007.02413.x.
69. Calzavara-Pinton P, Carlino A, Benetti A, de Panfilis G. Pili torti and onychodysplasia. Report of a previously undescribed hidrotic ectodermal dysplasia. Dermatologica. 1991;182(3):184–7.
70. van Steensel MAM, van Geel M, Nahuys M, Smitt JH, Sillevis; Steijlen, Peter M. A novel connexin 26 mutation in a patient diagnosed with keratitis-ichthyosis-deafness syndrome. J Invest Dermatol. 2002;118(4):724–7. https://doi.org/10.1046/j.1523-1747.2002.01735.x.
71. Paznekas WA, Boyadjiev SA, Shapiro RE, Daniels O, Wollnik B, Keegan CE, et al. Connexin 43 (GJA1) mutations cause the pleiotropic phenotype of oculodentodigital dysplasia. Am J Hum Genet. 2003;72(2):408–18. https://doi.org/10.1086/346090.
72. Lamartine J, Munhoz Essenfelder G, Kibar Z, Lanneluc I, Callouet E, Laoudj D, et al. Mutations in GJB6 cause hidrotic ectodermal dysplasia. Nat Genet. 2000;26(2):142–4. https://doi.org/10.1038/79851.
73. Ho M, Thompson B, Fisk JN, Nebert DW, Bruford EA, Vasiliou V, Bunick CG. Update of the keratin gene family: evolution, tissue-specific expression patterns, and relevance to clinical disorders. Hum Genomics. 2022;16(1):1. https://doi.org/10.1186/s40246-021-00374-9.
74. Rogers MA, Langbein L, Praetzel S, Moll I, Krieg T, Winter H, Schweizer J. Sequences and differential expression of three novel human type-II hair keratins. Differentiation. 1997;61(3):187–94. https://doi.org/10.1046/j.1432-0436.1997.6130187.x.
75. McMillan JR, Haftek M, Akiyama M, South AP, Perrot H, McGrath JA, et al. Alterations in desmosome size and number coincide with the loss of keratinocyte cohesion in skin with homozygous and heterozygous defects in the desmosomal protein plakophilin 1. J Invest Dermatol. 2003;121(1):96–103. https://doi.org/10.1046/j.1523-1747.2003.12324.x.
76. Chen W, Dong Q, Shin K-H, Kim RH, Oh J-E, Park N-H, Kang MK. Grainyhead-like 2 enhances the human telomerase reverse transcriptase gene expression by inhibiting DNA methylation at the 5'-CpG island in normal human keratinocytes. J Biol Chem. 2010;285(52):40852–63. https://doi.org/10.1074/jbc.M110.103812.
77. Takai Y, Irie K, Shimizu K, Sakisaka T, Ikeda W. Nectins and nectin-like molecules: roles in cell adhesion, migration, and polarization. Cancer Sci. 2003;94(8):655–67. https://doi.org/10.1111/j.1349-7006.2003.tb01499.x.
78. Peled A, Sarig O, Samuelov L, Bertolini M, Ziv L, Weissglas-Volkov D, et al. Mutations in TSPEAR, encoding a regulator of notch signaling, affect tooth and hair follicle morphogenesis. PLoS Genet. 2016;12(10):e1006369. https://doi.org/10.1371/journal.pgen.1006369.
79. Lin Z, Chen Q, Shi L, Lee M, Giehl KA, Tang Z, et al. Loss-of-function mutations in HOXC13 cause pure hair and nail ectodermal dysplasia. Am J Hum Genet. 2012;91(5):906–11. https://doi.org/10.1016/j.ajhg.2012.08.029.
80. van den Bogaard EHJ, van Geel M, van Vlijmen-Willems IMJJ, Jansen PAM, Peppelman M, van Erp PEJ, et al. Deficiency of the human cysteine protease inhibitor cystatin M/E causes hypotrichosis and dry skin. Genet Med. 2019;21(7):1559–67. https://doi.org/10.1038/s41436-018-0355-3.
81. Boyden LM, Atzmony L, Hamilton C, Zhou J, Lim YH, Hu R, et al. Recessive mutations in AP1B1 cause ichthyosis, deafness, and photophobia. Am J Hum Genet. 2019;105(5):1023–9. https://doi.org/10.1016/j.ajhg.2019.09.021.

82. Lüdecke HJ, Schaper J, Meinecke P, Momeni P, Gross S, von Holtum D, et al. Genotypic and phenotypic spectrum in tricho-rhino-phalangeal syndrome types I and III. Am J Hum Genet. 2001;68(1):81–91. https://doi.org/10.1086/316926.
83. Lüdecke HJ, Wagner MJ, Nardmann J, La Pillo B, Parrish JE, Willems PJ, et al. Molecular dissection of a contiguous gene syndrome: localization of the genes involved in the Langer-Giedion syndrome. Hum Mol Genet. 1995;4(1):31–6. https://doi.org/10.1093/hmg/4.1.31.
84. Delmaghani S, Aghaie A, Michalski N, Bonnet C, Weil D, Petit C. Defect in the gene encoding the EAR/EPTP domain-containing protein TSPEAR causes DFNB98 profound deafness. Hum Mol Genet. 2012;21(17):3835–44. https://doi.org/10.1093/hmg/dds212.
85. Godwin AR, Capecchi MR. Hoxc13 mutant mice lack external hair. Genes Dev. 1998;12(1):11–20. https://doi.org/10.1101/gad.12.1.11.
86. Zeeuwen PL, de Jongh GJ, van Vlijmen-Willems IM, Schalkwijk J, Dale BA, Fleckman P, Kimball JR, et al. The human cystatin M/E gene (CST6): exclusion candidate gene for harlequin ichthyosis. J Invest Dermatol. 2003;121(1):65–8. https://doi.org/10.1046/j.1523-1747.2003.12312.x.
87. Doray B, Ghosh P, Griffith J, Geuze HJ, Kornfeld S. Cooperation of GGAs and AP-1 in packaging MPRs at the trans-Golgi network. Science (New York, N.Y.). 2002;297(5587):1700–3. https://doi.org/10.1126/science.1075327.
88. Kaiser FJ, Tavassoli K, van den Bemd G-J, Chang GTG, Horsthemke B, Möröy T, Lüdecke H-J. Nuclear interaction of the dynein light chain LC8a with the TRPS1 transcription factor suppresses the transcriptional repression activity of TRPS1. Hum Mol Genet. 2003;12(11):1349–58. https://doi.org/10.1093/hmg/ddg145.
89. Ghoumid J, Stichelbout M, Jourdain A-S, Frenois F, Lejeune-Dumoulin S, Alex-Cordier M-P, et al. Blepharocheilodontic syndrome is a CDH1 pathway-related disorder due to mutations in CDH1 and CTNND1. Genet Med. 2017;19(9):1013–21. https://doi.org/10.1038/gim.2017.11.
90. Walczak-Sztulpa J, Eggenschwiler J, Osborn D, Brown DA, Emma F, Klingenberg C, et al. Cranioectodermal Dysplasia, Sensenbrenner syndrome, is a ciliopathy caused by mutations in the IFT122 gene. Am J Hum Genet. 2010;86(6):949–56. https://doi.org/10.1016/j.ajhg.2010.04.012.
91. Ruiz-Perez VL, Ide SE, Strom TM, Lorenz B, Wilson D, Woods K, et al. Mutations in a new gene in Ellis-van Creveld syndrome and Weyers acrodental dysostosis. Nat Genet. 2000;24(3):283–6. https://doi.org/10.1038/73508.
92. Ye X, Song G, Fan M, Shi L, Jabs EW, Huang S, et al. A novel heterozygous deletion in the EVC2 gene causes Weyers acrofacial dysostosis. Hum Genet. 2006;119(1–2):199–205. https://doi.org/10.1007/s00439-005-0129-2.
93. Marneros AG, Beck AE, Turner EH, McMillin MJ, Edwards MJ, Field M, et al. Mutations in KCTD1 cause scalp-ear-nipple syndrome. Am J Hum Genet. 2013;92(4):621–6. https://doi.org/10.1016/j.ajhg.2013.03.002.
94. Castori M, Brancati F, Mingarelli R, Mundlos S, Dallapiccola B. A novel patient with Cooks syndrome supports splitting from "classic" brachydactyly type B. Am J Med Genet A. 2007;143A(2):195–9. https://doi.org/10.1002/ajmg.a.31433.
95. Stránecký V, Hoischen A, Hartmannová H, Zaki MS, Chaudhary A, Zudaire E, et al. Mutations in ANTXR1 cause GAPO syndrome. Am J Hum Genet. 2013;92(5):792–9. https://doi.org/10.1016/j.ajhg.2013.03.023.
96. Günther C, Ae Lee-Kirsch M, Eckhard J, Matanovic A, Kerscher T, Rüschendorf F, et al. SMARCAD1 haploinsufficiency underlies huriez syndrome and associated skin cancer susceptibility. J Invest Dermatol. 2018;138(6):1428–31. https://doi.org/10.1016/j.jid.2018.01.015.
97. Norgett EE, Hatsell SJ, Carvajal-Huerta L, Cabezas JC, Common J, Purkis PE, et al. Recessive mutation in desmoplakin disrupts desmoplakin-intermediate filament interactions and causes dilated cardiomyopathy, woolly hair and keratoderma. Hum Mol Genet. 2000;9(18):2761–6. https://doi.org/10.1093/hmg/9.18.2761.

98. Lugassy J, Itin P, Ishida-Yamamoto A, Holland K, Huson S, Geiger D, et al. Naegeli-Franceschetti-Jadassohn syndrome and dermatopathia pigmentosa reticularis: two allelic ectodermal dysplasias caused by dominant mutations in KRT14. Am J Hum Genet. 2006;79(4):724–30. https://doi.org/10.1086/507792.
99. McLean WH, Rugg EL, Lunny DP, Morley SM, Lane EB, Swensson O, et al. Keratin 16 and keratin 17 mutations cause pachyonychia congenita. Nat Genet. 1995;9(3):273–8. https://doi.org/10.1038/ng0395-273.
100. Tsurusaki Y, Okamoto N, Ohashi H, Kosho T, Imai Y, Hibi-Ko Y, et al. Mutations affecting components of the SWI/SNF complex cause Coffin-Siris syndrome. Nat Genet. 2012;44(4):376–8. https://doi.org/10.1038/ng.2219.
101. Yuan Y, Zhang J, Chang Q, Zeng J, Xin F, Wang J, et al. De novo mutation in ATP6V1B2 impairs lysosome acidification and causes dominant deafness-onychodystrophy syndrome. Cell Res. 2014;24(11):1370–3. https://doi.org/10.1038/cr.2014.77.
102. Campeau PM, Kasperaviciute D, Lu JT, Burrage LC, Kim C, Hori M, et al. The genetic basis of DOORS syndrome: an exome-sequencing study. Lancet Neurol. 2014;13(1):44–58. https://doi.org/10.1016/S1474-4422(13)70265-5.
103. Ehmke N, Graul-Neumann L, Smorag L, Koenig R, Segebrecht L, Magoulas P, et al. De novo mutations in SLC25A24 cause a craniosynostosis syndrome with hypertrichosis, progeroid appearance, and mitochondrial dysfunction. Am J Hum Genet. 2017;101(5):833–43. https://doi.org/10.1016/j.ajhg.2017.09.016.
104. Ratbi I, Falkenberg KD, Sommen M, Al-Sheqaih N, Guaoua S, Vandeweyer G, et al. Heimler syndrome is caused by hypomorphic mutations in the peroxisome-biogenesis genes PEX1 and PEX6. Am J Hum Genet. 2015;97(4):535–45. https://doi.org/10.1016/j.ajhg.2015.08.011.
105. Zenker M, Mayerle J, Lerch MM, Tagariello A, Zerres K, Durie PR, et al. Deficiency of UBR1, a ubiquitin ligase of the N-end rule pathway, causes pancreatic dysfunction, malformations and mental retardation (Johanson-Blizzard syndrome). Nat Genet. 2005;37(12):1345–50. https://doi.org/10.1038/ng1681.
106. Rohmann E, Brunner HG, Kayserili H, Uyguner O, Nürnberg G, Lew ED, et al. Mutations in different components of FGF signaling in LADD syndrome. Nat Genet. 2006;38(4):414–7. https://doi.org/10.1038/ng1757.
107. Morice-Picard F, Michaud V, Lasseaux E, Rezvani HR, Plaisant C, Bessis D, et al. Hereditary mucoepithelial dysplasia results from heterozygous variants at p.Arg557 mutational hotspot in SREBF1, encoding a transcription factor involved in cholesterol homeostasis. J Invest Dermatol. 2020;140(6):1289–1292.e2. https://doi.org/10.1016/j.jid.2019.10.014.
108. Sharma P, Reichert M, Lu Y, Markello TC, Adams DR, Steinbach PJ, et al. Biallelic HEPHL1 variants impair ferroxidase activity and cause an abnormal hair phenotype. PLoS Genet. 2019;15(5):e1008143. https://doi.org/10.1371/journal.pgen.1008143.
109. Winter H, Rogers MA, Langbein L, Stevens HP, Leigh IM, Labrèze C, et al. Mutations in the hair cortex keratin hHb6 cause the inherited hair disease monilethrix. Nat Genet. 1997;16(4):372–4. https://doi.org/10.1038/ng0897-372.
110. Schossig A, Wolf NI, Fischer C, Fischer M, Stocker G, Pabinger S, et al. Mutations in ROGDI cause Kohlschütter-Tönz syndrome. Am J Hum Genet. 2012;90(4):701–7. https://doi.org/10.1016/j.ajhg.2012.02.012.
111. Kadowaki T, Kadowaki H, Accili D, Taylor SI. Substitution of lysine for asparagine at position 15 in the alpha-subunit of the human insulin receptor. A mutation that impairs transport of receptors to the cell surface and decreases the affinity of insulin binding. J Biol Chem. 1990;265(31):19143–50.
112. Gelb BD, Shi GP, Chapman HA, Desnick RJ. Pycnodysostosis, a lysosomal disease caused by cathepsin K deficiency. Science (New York, N.Y.). 1996;273(5279):1236–8. https://doi.org/10.1126/science.273.5279.1236.
113. Hoischen A, van Bon BWM, Gilissen C, Arts P, van Lier B, Steehouwer M, et al. De novo mutations of SETBP1 cause Schinzel-Giedion syndrome. Nat Genet. 2010;42(6):483–5. https://doi.org/10.1038/ng.581.

Chapter 3
X-Linked Hypohidrotic Ectodermal Dysplasia: The Pathogenic Role of the *EDA* Gene

Debora Vergani, Giulia Gori, and Giovanna Traficante

Keywords EDA1 pathway · Molecular diagnosis · Genotype

3.1 Introduction

The term ectodermal dysplasia (ED) describes a large group of clinically heterogeneous disorders characterized by developmental failure in two or more ectodermal structures involving alterations in hair, teeth, nails, or sweat glands.

With a lower frequency, other ectodermal structures could be involved in ED, such as mammary glands, thyroid glands, thymus, pituitary gland, adrenal medulla, melanocytes, external ear, lacrimal gland and duct, conjunctiva, cornea, and Meibomian glands [1].

To date, more than 200 types of ED have been described [2, 3], but the most common is the hypohidrotic ectodermal dysplasia (OMIM 305100), an X-linked hypohidrotic form of ectodermal dysplasia (XLHED), which has a frequency of one per 17,000 in the general population [4].

Interestingly, emerging studies have revealed the unexpected functions of the EDA pathway in multiple other diseases, including various types of carcinogenesis [5, 6], nonalcoholic fatty liver disease [7], and androgenetic alopecia [8].

D. Vergani · G. Gori · G. Traficante (✉)
Medical Genetics Unit, Meyer Children's Hospital IRCCS, Florence, Italy
e-mail: giovanna.traficante@meyer.it

G. Tadini et al. (eds.), *Multidisciplinary Approach to Ectodermal Dysplasia*,
https://doi.org/10.1007/978-3-031-75790-7_3

3.2 Ectodysplasin A (EDA): Molecular Aspects

3.2.1 Gene Structure

The ectodysplasin A gene (*EDA*; MIM*300451) is located on the long arm of chromosome X (Xq12-q13) and encodes for components of the tumor necrosis factor (TNF) superfamily. It plays a key role in the formation of ectodermal placodes, and it is involved in the differentiation of skin appendages [9].

The first *EDA* isoform was isolated in 1996 by Kere et al. using positional cloning, and it was represented by a single 858 bp cDNA, composed of two exons and producing a 135 amino acid protein (EDA-O form) [10].

A novel cDNA was then isolated from the homologous murine gene, called Tabby (Ta), allowing the identification of the longest and evolutionarily highly conserved EDA-A form [11], which shows an overall homology of 94.6% between human and mouse EDA protein [12].

Five other forms (EDA-B, -C, -D, -E, and -F), differentially expressed in several human tissues, are produced by complex splicing events, although their biological function is currently not well known [13].

EDA is a membrane protein and is composed of a short intracellular domain (ICD), a transmembrane domain (TMD), a stalk region of uncharacterized function, a consensus furin cleavage sequence responsible for proteolytic processing of EDA, a short positively charged sequence required for interactions with heparan-sulfate proteoglycans (PG binding), a bi-partite collagen-like domain and a 150 amino acid residue-long C-terminal TNF homology domain (THD), responsible for receptor binding (Fig. 3.1).

EDA-A1 (391 amino acids) and EDA-A2 (389 amino acids) are the two longest transcripts known to be biologically active, containing the THD, 19 repeats of Gly-X-Y, two putative N-glycosylation sites, and a cysteine-rich C-terminal domain.

The two forms of EDA-A differ from each other for two amino acids that are excluded or included dependent on the alternative usage of the splicing donor site in exon 8 [11]. EDA-A1/2 contain also two consensus sites for furin-like proteolytic processing by calcium-dependent serine endoprotease that cleaves most efficiently at the C-terminal side of an Arg(P4)-X-LysyArg-Arg(P1) sequence, where the basic residues at the P1 and P4 positions are critical for activity. This cleavage leads to the

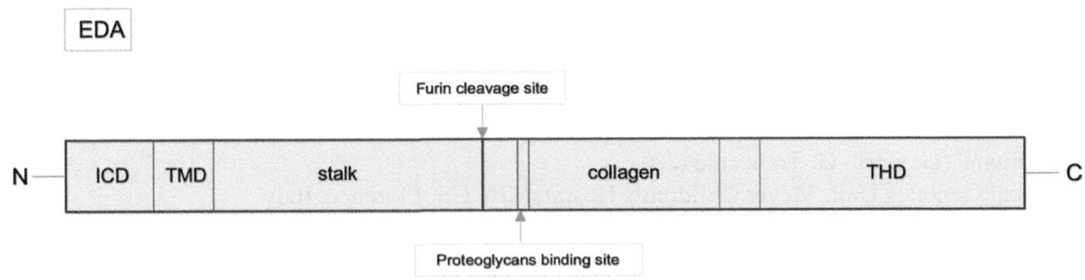

Fig. 3.1 EDA structural domains

formation of soluble extracellular molecules, which can interact with the corresponding receptors and mediate the signals [14].

EDA-A1 binds to the membrane ectodysplasin A receptor (EDAR), determining a complex with the intracellular EDAR-associated death domain (EDARADD) adaptor protein, which further builds a complex with TNF-receptor-associated factor 6 (TRAF6), TAK1-binding protein 2 (TAB2), and TGF-β-activated kinase 1 (TAK1). This complex activates IKK, the inhibitor of nuclear factor kappa-B kinase, composed of conserved helix–loop–helix ubiquitous kinase (CHUK, also known as IKK-α) and IKK-β, and a structural component (NEMO/IKK-γ) [15, 16].

IKK leads to phosphorylation, ubiquitination, and proteasomal degradation of the NF-κB inhibitor (IkB), allowing the transcription factor NF-κB to be released and translocated into the nucleus and to activate the transcription of different target genes involved in the development and morphogenesis of teeth, hair, nails, and eccrine glands [17]. Deubiquitination of TRAF6 protein by CYLD lysine-63 deubiquitinase leads to the termination of the signaling [18] (Fig. 3.2).

The crucial implication of NF-kB downstream of EDAR is demonstrated by studies of embryonic skin of wild-type mice, in which NF-kB is activated in primary hair placodes, contrary to EDA-deficient skin in which there are no placodes and there is no NF-kB activation. In these two conditions, the addition of ectopic recombinant EDA restores placodes and NF-kB signals in EDA-deficient skin, but

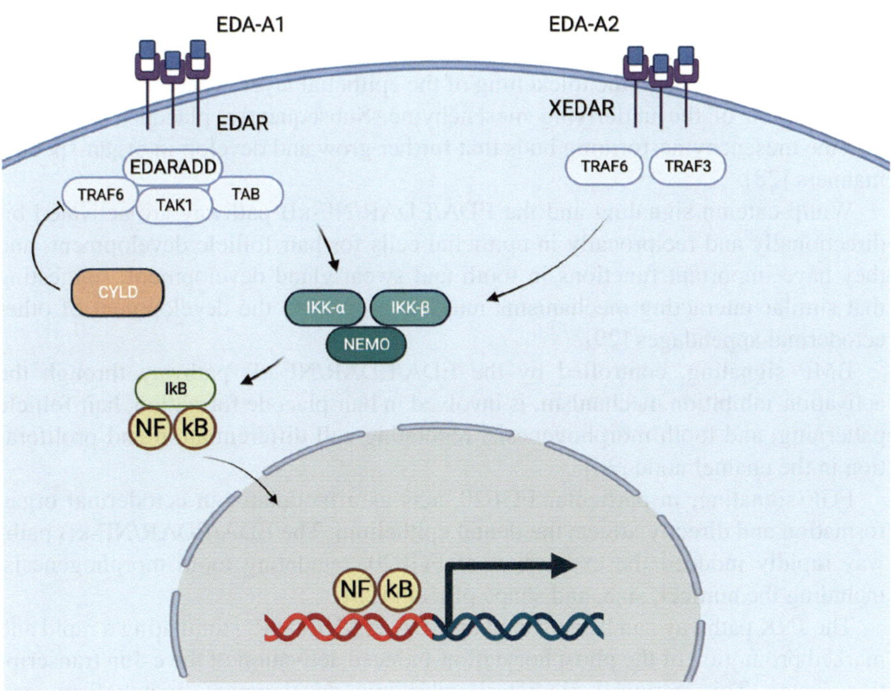

Fig. 3.2 Signaling transduction of EDA pathways. (Created with BioRender.com)

not in IkBaDN transgenic mice skin, that express a non-phosphorylable and therefore non-degradable form of an NF-kB inhibitor [19].

EDA-A2 binds to the X-linked ectodermal dysplasia receptor (XEDAR), also called EDA2R, leading to the interaction with TRAF3 and/or TRAF6, contributing to activation of the I-kappa-kinase (IKK) complex for translocation of NF-κB transcription factors into the nucleus [20, 21] (Fig. 3.2).

Intriguingly, a subtle difference of only two amino acids (Glu308 and Val309) between EDA-A1 and EDA-A2 determines the specificity, respectively, for EDAR and XEDAR receptors, although the mechanism still remains unknown.

3.2.2 The Role of EDA in Multiple Signaling Pathways

The variety of genes and pathways downstream of EDA further supports its role as a signal integrator or balancer that modulates simultaneously the Wnt/β-catenin [22], c-Jun N-terminal kinase (JNK) [23], bone morphogenetic protein (BMP)/ Smad [24], and fibroblast growth factor (FGF) signaling [25, 26], regulating a range of cellular functions, including proliferation, differentiation, and cell death [27].

These molecular signaling pathways are shared to a large extent among different organs and, in this specific context, are referable to organs with ectodermal dysplasias and developing as ectodermal appendages. This organ-specific morphogenesis is related to a sequence of inductive interactions between two adjacent tissue layers, the epithelium and the mesenchyme. In the first step of development, the formation of the placodes through the thickening of the epithelial layer is accompanied by the condensation of the underlying mesenchyme. Subsequently, placodes invaginate into the mesenchyme-forming buds that further grow and develop in organ-specific manners [28].

Wnt/β-catenin signaling and the EDA/EDAR/NF-κB pathway are activated bidirectionally and reciprocally in epithelial cells for hair follicle development, and they have important functions in tooth and sweat gland development, suggesting that similar interacting mechanisms may be relevant to the development of other ectodermal appendages [29].

BMP signaling, controlled by the EDA/EDAR/NF-κB pathway through the activation-inhibition mechanism, is involved in hair placode formation, hair follicle patterning, and tooth morphogenesis, regulating cell differentiation and proliferation in the enamel node [30].

FGF signaling, in particular FGF20, acts as a modulator in ectodermal organ formation and directly affects the dental epithelium. The EDA/EDAR/NF-κB pathway rapidly induced the expression of FGF20, regulating tooth morphogenesis, including the number, size, and shape of teeth [25].

The JNK pathway can be activated by EDA-A2/XEDAR, stimulating a rapid and marked promotion of the phosphorylation-induced activation of the c-Jun transcription factor. This pathway mediates embryonic development, metabolism, and growth and is involved in the regulation of many cellular events, including growth control, transformation, and programmed cell death [31], although its role in ectodermal differentiation is not well characterized.

3.2.3 Molecular Alterations in EDA

A variety of mutations in *EDA*, which include large deletions, insertions, and small in-frame deletions, as well as missense and nonsense mutations, have been identified over the years. The majority of *EDA* variants are known to cause an X-linked form of hypohidrotic ectodermal dysplasia (XLHED, MIM #305100), a clinical condition characterized by a triad of typical symptoms: missing or sparse hair (trichinosis or hypotrichosis), missing (anodontia or hypodontia) or misshapen teeth, and absent or reduced sweating (anhidrosis or hypohidrosis) [32]. Moreover, a few *EDA* variants are reported as being implicated in non-syndromic tooth agenesis [33, 34].

The *EDA* mutations identified in XLHED patients mainly affect three different regions of the protein, with distinctive functional significance: the collagen-like domain, the furin protease recognition sequence, and the C-terminal THD [35].

Missense mutations in conserved glycine residues in the collagenous domain appear to have a role in the multimerization of EDA trimers, thus serving to keep two or more EDA trimers in close proximity within the same molecule and therefore potentiate its ability to stimulate EDAR signaling [35].

Also, in-frame deletions removing either two or four of the Gly-X-Y repeats are identified; however, these mutations do not affect the ability of EDA to trimerize or to further multimerize, suggesting that the collagenous domain may serve additional functions [13].

EDA mutational hot spots, in which missense mutations cluster together, are represented by arginine residues in a CpG-rich sequence, coding for two overlapping consensus cleavage sites for the convertase furin protein. In XLHED patients with a mutation in the furin recognition sequence, the inhibition of the cleavage and the shedding of EDA from the cell surface occur, affecting the release of soluble signaling molecules [36, 37]. Thus, the proteolytic processing of EDA is required for proper EDA-EDAR signaling during development [28].

The THD contains the most important mutations that directly influence receptor binding. To date, about 100 pathogenic missense mutations in EDA·A1THD are registered in Human Gene Mutation Database (HGMD) (http://www.hgmd.cf.ac.uk/) [38].

Crystallographic structural analysis of EDA·$A1_{THD}$-$EDAR_{CRDS}$, by Yu et al. in 2023, enabled the study of the role and the mechanisms underlying the development of ectodermal tissues, providing structural insights into the pathogenesis of disease-related *EDA* variants [39].

According to these studies, the atomic details of ligand-receptor interaction are evaluated, allowing to classify mutations in EDA·$A1_{THD}$ into four distinct classes:

- Type I mutations involve the interior of EDA·A1_{THD} and lead to protein destabilization, resulting in the alteration of the local hydrophobicity or in the introduction of a bulky group or secondary structure disruption that determines the entire protein inactivation and severe clinical manifestations of XLHED.
- Type II mutations are localized at the promoter interface and affect the trimer formation of EDA-A1.
- Type III mutations involve the ligand-receptor interface, which perturbs the EDA·A1-EDAR interaction, essential in ectodermal organ development.
- Type IV mutations affect the region of EDA far from the EDAR binding interface, and their pathogenicity in developmental defects is still not well described.

Overall, mutations that result in only partial weakening of the interaction determine mild and non-syndromic manifestation, in contrast to mutations that involve and/or disrupt the EDA-EDAR interface that determine more severe phenotypes of XLHED.

3.3 Clinical Characteristics

Hypohidrotic/anhidrotic ectodermal dysplasia is characterized by three main clinical signs:

- Hypotrichosis (sparseness of scalp and body hair): scalp hair is thin and lightly pigmented. Beard, axillary, and pubic hair could be not involved.
- Hypohidrosis (reduced ability to sweat) that could lead to hyperthermia: this applies not only to hot weather but also to physical activities or febrile illness.
- Hypodontia (congenital absence/reduction of teeth). teeth are frequently smaller than common and feature an altered morphology (conic shape).

In addition to the classic triad of signs, XLHED can include the following:

- Phenotype variants: high forehead with bossing, sparse or absent eyebrows and eyelashes, ocular hypertelorism, periorbital hyperpigmentation, small nose with hypoplasic alae nasi, midface hypoplasia (linked to follicular tooth and gems absence/hypoplasia).
- Changes in nasal secretions from concretions in early infancy to large mucous clots after that.
- Reduction of sebaceous secretions.
- Abnormal meibomian gland secretions lead to dry eyes and sunlight intolerance.
- Fragile-appearing skin with a lack of dermal ridges.
- Abnormal bronchial glands with respiratory infection susceptibility.
- Raspy voice.

Physical growth and psychomotor development are generally within normal limits.

In XLHED patients, an issue that should not be underestimated is psychosocial discomfort, generally related to physical appearance and classic symptoms, mainly anhidrosis [40–43].

To date, no guidelines for hypohidrotic ectodermal dysplasia have been developed, and no proven treatment for XLHED is available, except for symptomatic therapies.

3.4 Diagnosis

At birth, XLHED may be recognized because of peeling skin and periorbital hyperpigmentation (Dennie-Morgan lines).

In infancy, heat intolerance could induce irritability, and hyperthermia is common and the commonest cause of the high mortality of the disease (2–30%) [44–46].

Diagnosis is generally difficult before the expected age of tooth eruption (6–9 months) or if the teeth show shape anomalies (mainly conical).

Multidisciplinary follow-up (dermatologist, geneticist, pneumologist, dentist, and otolaryngologist) is of fundamental importance to patient takeover.

Females with XLHED may exhibit milder clinical manifestations: tooth agenesis/hypodontia (60–80%), thinning hair, and sweat dysfunction. Also, agalattia/hypogalattia or underdeveloped nipples could be a minor sign of the condition.

Suggestive findings for XLHED in heterozygous females: mosaic patterns of sweat pore function and distribution (using an iodine solution to assess sweat gland function).

3.5 Genetic Counseling

XLHED is an X-linked condition: males with an EDA pathogenic variant will be affected; females with the pathogenic variant will be heterozygous and could show mild manifestations of ectodermal dysplasia.

Clinical symptoms generally allow for easier diagnosis in males, but clinical detection of mild symptomatic carriers is often imprecise, so females are generally identified after male diagnosis.

Rarely, female patients could show a severe XLHED phenotype, carrying heterozygous EDA pathogenic variants and skewed X-chromosome inactivation (XCI) [47]. XCI is the mechanism that assures dosage compensation in mammalian female cells to balance X-linked gene expression levels of the two sexes. This mechanism is random (generally 50%), so even pathogenic variants on an X-chromosome are balanced by the other. When the XCI is not balanced, it is called skewed inactivation, and it allows clinical manifestations of X-linked diseases in females.

Several studies have shown that skewed XCI can lead to severe XLHED in female probands [48, 49].

If the only affected family member is a male, the mother could be a carrier or he may have a de novo EDA pathogenic variant.

In a minority of cases, the mother may have somatic or germline mosaicism (the pathogenic variant is located only in a few cells).

So, to assess familial recurrence risk, molecular analysis of the mother DNA is recommended, even if the canonic tests may not detect mosaicism.

Clinical examination of the mother is mandatory to detect mild manifestations of XLHED.

In the case of a female proband, she may have inherited the EDA pathogenic variant from her affected father or from her carrier mother (who may be mildly affected) or may have a de novo variant, so DNA from both parents has to be analyzed.

If a woman is heterozygous for an EDA pathogenic variant, the chance of transmitting it in each pregnancy is 50%, and she should generate affected males and carrier females (except for XCI). If a male has an EDA pathogenic variant, he will transmit it to all his daughters (obligate carriers) but none of his sons.

3.6 Prenatal Perspectives

In an XLHED family, genetic counseling is essential to discuss the disease's natural history, perform any targeted genetic tests, and assess the familial risk of recurrence [50]. In a carrier, invasive prenatal diagnosis (villocentesis or amniocentesis) can be performed to search for the specific family variant on fetal DNA; in selected cases, non-invasive diagnosis can also be performed by tooth germ sonography [51].

Between 20 and 24 weeks of gestation, second-level ultrasound could also identify the hypoplasia of the jaw and/or sparse teeth and, at best, detect the average number of maxillary and mandibular teeth [52].

An accurate discussion of these issues may be helpful in planning the best prenatal management because of the different perspectives among medical professionals.

In XLHED, prenatal diagnosis of the disease may improve prognosis because hyperthermia can be avoided in affected infants.

To date, many carrier women avoid pregnancy or use medically assisted procreation; 30% of fertile women consider pre-implantation genetic diagnosis (during a medically assisted procreation pathway) to prevent XLHED in their children [53].

Moreover, the absence of possible treatment options leads to a higher rate of pregnancy termination in the case of an affected fetus.

3.7 Therapy Studies

To date, there is no treatment for XLHED, and the current therapy is based on treating symptoms and preventing complications.

Some studies in mouse models have shown that treatment with recombinant EDA protein across the placental barrier can partially recover the wild-type phenotype in the offspring [54].

EDI200, based on humanized recombinant EDA protein, seems to be a promising treatment for XLHED.

Although postnatal administration of EDI200 did not provide the expected improvement, prenatal administration in amniotic fluid appears to result in the proper development of sweat glands, recovering the ability to sweat [55]. Notably, in a case of prenatal diagnosis of XLHED, recombinant EDA protein was administrated with ultrasound-guided amniocentesis performed at 26 and 31 weeks of gestation, showing that sweat glands and tooth development were fully recovered after birth [56].

The EDELIFE trial (ClinicalTrials.gov Identifier: NCT04980638; https://edelife-clinicaltrial.com) provides an innovative therapeutic concept with the aim of a complete correction of XLHED. This trial would assess the safety and efficacy of ER004, a high-affinity protein that binds the EDA1 receptor (EDAR).

A prenatal XLHED therapy option could positively influence the reproductive choices of affected/carrier individuals.

References

1. Visinoni AF, Lisboa-Costa T, Pagnan NAB, et al. Ectodermal dysplasias: clinical and molecular review. Am J Med Genet A. 2009;149:1980–2002.
2. Priolo M, Lagana C. Ectodermal dysplasias: a new clinical-genetic classification. J Med Genet. 2001;38:579–85.
3. Wohlfart S, Hammersen J, Schneider H. Mutational spectrum in 101 patients with hypohidrotic ectodermal dysplasia and breakpoint mapping in independent cases of rare genomic rearrangements. J Hum Genet. 2016;61:891–7.
4. Trzeciak WH, Koczorowski R. Molecular basis of hypohidrotic ectodermal dysplasia: an update. J Appl Genet. 2016;57:51–61.
5. Vial J, Royet A, Cassier P, Tortereau A, Dinvaut S, Maillet D, Gratadou-Hupon L, Creveaux M, Sadier A, Tondeur G, et al. The ectodysplasin receptor EDAR acts as a tumor suppressor in melanoma by conditionally inducing cell death. Cell Death Differ. 2019;26:443–54.
6. Wang X, Zhang Z, Yuan S, et al. A novel EDA1 missense mutation in X-linked hypohidrotic ectodermal dysplasia. Medicine (Baltimore). 2020b;99(11):e19244.
7. Bayliss J, Ooi GJ, De Nardo W, Shah YJH, Montgomery MK, McLean C, Kemp W, Roberts SK, Brown WA, Burton PR, et al. Ectodysplasin a is increased in non-alcoholic fatty liver disease, but is not associated with type 2 diabetes. Front Endocrinol. 2021;12:642432.

8. Kwack MH, Jun MS, Sung YK, Kim JC, Kim MK. Ectodysplasin-A2 induces dickkopf 1 expression in human balding dermal papilla cells overexpressing the ectodysplasin A2 receptor. Biochem Biophys Res Commun. 2020;529:766–72.
9. Yang R, Mei Y, Jiang Y, et al. Ectodysplasin a (EDA) signaling: from skin appendage to multiple diseases. Int J Mol Sci. 2022;23(16):8911.
10. Kere J, Srivastava AK, Montonen O, et al. X-linked anhidrotic (hypohidrotic) ectodermal dysplasia is caused by mutation in a novel transmembrane protein. Nat Genet. 1996;13(4):409–16.
11. Monreal AW, Zonana J, Ferguson B. Identification of a new splice form of the EDA1 gene permits detection of nearly all X-linked hypohidrotic ectodermal dysplasia mutations. Am J Hum Genet. 1998;63(2):380–9.
12. Srivastava AK, Pispa J, Hartung AJ, et al. The Tabby phenotype is caused by mutation in a mouse homologue of the EDA gene that reveals novel mouse and human exons and encodes a protein (ectodysplasin-A) with collagenous domains. Proc Natl Acad Sci USA. 1997;94(24):13069–74.
13. Bayés M, Hartung AJ, Ezer S, et al. The anhidrotic ectodermal dysplasia gene (EDA) undergoes alternative splicing and encodes ectodysplasin-A with deletion mutations in collagenous repeats. Hum Mol Genet. 1998;7(11):1661–9.
14. Botchkarev VA, Fessing MY. Edar signaling in the control of hair follicle development. J Investig Dermatol Symp Proc. 2005;10(3):247–51.
15. Cui CY, Schlessinger D. EDA signaling and skin appendage development. Cell Cycle. 2006;5(21):2477–83.
16. Kumar A, Eby MT, Sinha S, Jasmin A, Chaudhary PM. The ectodermal dysplasia receptor activates the nuclear factor-kappaB, JNK, and cell death pathways and binds to ectodysplasin a. J Biol Chem. 2001;276(4):2668–77.
17. Morlon A, Munnich A, Smahi A. TAB2, TRAF6 and TAK1 are involved in NF-kappaB activation induced by the TNF-receptor, Edar and its adaptator Edaradd. Hum Mol Genet. 2005;14(23):3751–7.
18. Trompouki E, Hatzivassiliou E, Tsichritzis T, Farmer H, Ashworth A, Mosialos G. CYLD is a deubiquitinating enzyme that negatively regulates NF-kappaB activation by TNFR family members. Nature. 2003;424(6950):793–6.
19. Schmidt-Ullrich R, Aebischer T, Hülsken J, Birchmeier W, Klemm U, Scheidereit C. Requirement of NF-kappaB/Rel for the development of hair follicles and other epidermal appendices. Development. 2001;128(19):3843–53.
20. Reyes-Reali J, Mendoza-Ramos MI, Garrido-Guerrero E, Méndez-Catalá CF, Méndez-Cruz AR, Pozo-Molina G. Hypohidrotic ectodermal dysplasia: clinical and molecular review. Int J Dermatol. 2018;57(8):965–72.
21. Yan M, Wang LC, Hymowitz SG, et al. Two-amino acid molecular switch in an epithelial morphogen that regulates binding to two distinct receptors. Science. 2000;290(5491):523–7.
22. Wang B, Liang Y, Chai X, Chen S, Ye Z, Li R, Li X, Kong G, Li Y, Zhang X, et al. Ectodysplasin A receptor (EDAR) promotes colorectal cancer cell proliferation via regulation of the Wnt/β--catenin signaling pathway. Exp Cell Res. 2020a;395:112170.
23. Sinha SK, Zachariah S, Quiñones HI, Shindo M, Chaudhary PM. Role of TRAF3 and −6 in the activation of the NF-kappa B and JNK pathways by X-linked ectodermal dysplasia receptor. J Biol Chem. 2002;277(47):44953–61.
24. Han X, Yoshizaki K, Miyazaki K, et al. The transcription factor NKX2-3 mediates p21 expression and ectodysplasin-A signaling in the enamel knot for cusp formation in tooth development. J Biol Chem. 2018;293(38):14572–84.
25. Häärä O, Harjunmaa E, Lindfors PH, et al. Ectodysplasin regulates activator-inhibitor balance in murine tooth development through Fgf20 signaling. Development. 2012;139(17):3189–99.
26. Huh SH, Närhi K, Lindfors PH, et al. Fgf20 governs formation of primary and secondary dermal condensations in developing hair follicles. Genes Dev. 2013;27(4):450–8.
27. Mikkola ML, Thesleff I. Ectodysplasin signaling in development. Cytokine Growth Factor Rev. 2003;14(3–4):211–24.

28. Kowalczyk-Quintas C, Schneider P. Ectodysplasin A (EDA)—EDA receptor signalling and its pharmacological modulation. Cytokine Growth Factor Rev. 2014;25(2):195–203.
29. Zhang Y, Tomann P, Andl T, et al. Reciprocal requirements for EDA/EDAR/NF-kappaB and Wnt/beta-catenin signaling pathways in hair follicle induction. Dev Cell. 2009;17(1):49–61.
30. Mou C, Jackson B, Schneider P, Overbeek PA, Headon DJ. Generation of the primary hair follicle pattern. Proc Natl Acad Sci USA. 2006;103(24):9075–80.
31. de Los Reyes Corrales T, Losada-Pérez M, Casas-Tintó S. JNK pathway in CNS pathologies. Int J Mol Sci. 2021;22(8):3883.
32. Pinheiro M, Freire-Maia N. Ectodermal dysplasias: a clinical classification and a causal review. Am J Med Genet. 1994;53(2):153–62.
33. Nikopensius T, Annilo T, Jagomägi T, et al. Non-syndromic tooth agenesis associated with a nonsense mutation in ectodysplasin-A (EDA). J Dent Res. 2013;92(6):507–11.
34. Yu M, Wong SW, Han D, Cai T. Genetic analysis: Wnt and other pathways in nonsyndromic tooth agenesis. Oral Dis. 2019;25(3):646–51.
35. Schneider P, Street SL, Gaide O, et al. Mutations leading to X-linked hypohidrotic ectodermal dysplasia affect three major functional domains in the tumor necrosis factor family member ectodysplasin-a. J Biol Chem. 2001;276(22):18819–27.
36. Chen Y, Molloy SS, Thomas L, et al. Mutations within a furin consensus sequence block proteolytic release of ectodysplasin-A and cause X-linked hypohidrotic ectodermal dysplasia. Proc Natl Acad Sci USA. 2001;98(13):7218–23.
37. Elomaa O, Pulkkinen K, Hannelius U, Mikkola M, Saarialho-Kere U, Kere J. Ectodysplasin is released by proteolytic shedding and binds to the EDAR protein. Hum Mol Genet. 2001;10(9):953–62.
38. The Human Gene Mutation Database. http://www.hgmd.cf.ac.uk/
39. Yu K, Huang C, Wan F. et al. Structural insights into pathogenic mechanism of hypohidrotic ectodermal dysplasia caused by ectodysplasin A variants. Nat Commun 2023;14:767.
40. Hummel P, Guddack S. Psychosocial stress and adaptive functioning in children and adolescents suffering from hypohidrotic ectodermal dysplasia. Pediatr Dermatol. 1997;14:180–5.
41. Pavlis MB, Rice ZP, Veledar E, et al. Quality of life of cutaneous disease in the ectodermal dysplasias. Pediatr Dermatol. 2010;27:260–5.
42. Saltnes SS, Jensen JL, Sæves R, et al. Associations between ectodermal dysplasia, psychological distress and quality of life in a group of adults with oligodontia. Acta Odontol Scand. 2017;75:564–72.
43. Tanner BA. Psychological aspects of hypohidrotic ectodermal dysplasia. Birth Defects Orig Artic Ser. 1988;24:263–75.
44. Dietz J, Kaercher T, Schneider AT, et al. Early respiratory and ocular involvement in X-linked hypohidrotic ectodermal dysplasia. Eur J Pediatr. 2013;172:1023–31.
45. Fete M, Hermann J, Behrens J, Huttner KM. X-linked hypohidrotic ectodermal dysplasia (XLHED): clinical and diagnostic insights from an international patient registry. Am J Med Genet A. 2014;164:2437–42.
46. Schneider H, Hammersen J, Preisler-Adams S, et al. Sweating ability and genotype in individuals with X-linked hypohidrotic ectodermal dysplasia. J Med Genet. 2011;48:426–32.
47. Belmont JW. Genetic control of X inactivation and processes leading to X-inactivation skewing. Am J Hum Genet. 1996;58:1101–8.
48. Cantone I, Fisher AG. Human X chromosome inactivation and reactivation: implications for cell reprogramming and disease. Philos Trans R Soc B Biol Sci. 2017;372:20160358.
49. Lei K, Zhang Y, Dong Z, Sun Y, Yi Z, Chen Z. A novel 1-bp deletion mutation and extremely skewed X-chromosome inactivation causing severe X-linked hypohidrotic ectodermal dysplasia in a Chinese girl. Clin Exp Dermatol. 2018;43:60–2.
50. Han Y, Wang X, Zheng L, Zhu T, Li Y, Hong J, Xu C, Wang P, Gao M. EDA pathogenic mutations in Chinese Han families with hypohidrotic ectodermal dysplasia and genotype-phenotype: a correlation analysis. Front Genet. 2020;11:21.

51. Hammersen J, Wohlfart S, Goecke TW, et al. Reliability of prenatal detection of X-linked hypohidrotic ectodermal dysplasia by tooth germ sonography. Prenat Diagn. 2019;39:796–805.
52. Wünsche S, Jüngert J, Faschingbauer F, Mommsen H, Goecke T, Schwanitz K, Stepan H, Schneider H. Noninvasive prenatal diagnosis of hypohidrotic ectodermal dysplasia by tooth germ sonography. Ultraschall Der Med. 2015;36:381–5.
53. Leo B, Schneider H, Hammersen J. Reproductive decision-making by women with X-linked hypohidrotic ectodermal dysplasia. J Eur Acad Dermatol Venereol. 2022;36(10):1863–70.
54. Wahlbuhl M, Schuepbach-Mallepell S, Kowalczyk-Quintas C, Dick A, Fahlbusch F, Schneider P, Schneider H. Attenuation of mammary gland dysplasia and feeding difficulties in Tabby mice by fetal therapy. J Mammary Gland Biol Neoplasia. 2018;23:125–38.
55. Körber I, Klein O, Morhart P, Faschingbauer F, Grange D, Clarke A, Bodemer C, Maitz S, Huttner K, Kirby N, et al. Safety and immunogenicity of Fc-EDA, a recombinant ectodysplasin A1 replacement protein, in human subjects. Br J Clin Pharmacol. 2020;86:2063–9.
56. Schneider H, Faschingbauer F, Schuepbach-Mallepell S, Körber I, Wohlfart S, Dick A, Wahlbuhl M, Kowalczyk-Quintas C, Vigolo M, Kirby N, et al. Prenatal correction of X-linked hypohidrotic ectodermal dysplasia. N Engl J Med. 2018;378:1604–10.

Chapter 4
X-Linked Hypohidrotic Ectodermal Dysplasia: Clinical Features

Átila Visinoni and Nina Pagnan

Keywords Hypohidrotic ectodermal dysplasia · X-linked · Clinical features
Hypohidrosis · Hypotrichosis · Hypodontia

4.1 Historical Considerations

Ectodermal dysplasias constitute a heterogeneous group of conditions whose common denominator is the occurrence of anomalies of the structures derived from the ectoderm. Among the conditions classified as ectodermal dysplasia, the best-known and most common is undoubtedly X-linked hypohidrotic ectodermal dysplasia (XLHED). It is estimated that XLHED affects one in 5,000–10,000 newborns [1, 2]. Another estimate, which included only individuals whose diagnosis was confirmed by molecular analysis, is a frequency of 1.6/100,000 [3, 4].

The first known report of patients with ectodermal dysplasia was published in 1792 by Danz in a treatise entitled "Concerning Men Without Teeth" [5]. The author describes two men of Jewish origin with the absence of hair and teeth, or in his own words, "two adult sons which neither have, or ever had hair or teeth."

Forty-six years later, in a letter to Charles Darwin, Wedderburn referred to a Hindu family with ten affected males with anhidrosis, hypotrichosis, and hypodontia. Later, in 1848, Thurnam published a detailed description of the clinical picture of two related individuals (a 58-year-old man and his cousin). In a postscript from the same publication, Thurnam [6] comments that similar cases might not be so rare and comments on the case of a 15-year-old woman with the same clinical condition.

Á. Visinoni
School of Health Sciences, Positivo University, Curitiba, Brazil

N. Pagnan (✉)
Department of Genetics, Federal University of Paraná, Curitiba, Brazil

G. Tadini et al. (eds.), *Multidisciplinary Approach to Ectodermal Dysplasia*,
https://doi.org/10.1007/978-3-031-75790-7_4

In 1875, Charles Darwin, in his book entitled "The Variation of Animals and Plants Under Domestication," mentions the Hindu family reported by Wedderburn, noting that there were affected men in four generations and that the mothers of those affected did not present the phenotype but transmitted the tendency to their children [7]. In a sense, he described the X-linked recessive inheritance. This family was reviewed by Thadani in 1921, who describes the characteristics of the mode of inheritance and mentions that the affected individuals were known as Budhas, which literally means toothless [8].

The denomination "ectodermal dysplasia" was created in 1929 by Weech, who also suggested the term "anhidrotic" since sweating seemed absent in affected individuals [9]. Felsher (1944) suggested that the term anhidrotic should be replaced by the more accurate "hypohidrotic," since there was not an absence but a relevant decrease in sweating [10]. Before this report, several patients with hypotrichosis, hypodontia, anhidrosis, and onychodystrophy were described under different designations as "imperfect development of skin, hair, and teeth" or "congenital ectodermal defect," among others. Weech highlighted the involvement of the ectoderm and the genetic character of the phenotype.

Christ (1913) had already emphasized that the clinical signs present in the patients were due to a congenital ectodermal defect; Siemens's observations (1921) left no doubt regarding the inheritance pattern of this increasingly well-known form of ectodermal dysplasia; and Touraine (1936) gave a more detailed description of the phenotypic characteristics and suggested the term "ectodermal polydysplasia" to describe these conditions [11–13]. In this way, XLHED became known as Christ-Siemens-Touraine syndrome (CST syndrome) [14–16]. Over time, many other similar cases were described, leading to the inclusion of phenotypes unrelated to XLHED, thus creating a heterogeneous group of conditions.

4.2 Etiology and Genetic Counseling

XLHED, being the most common and well-known disorder related to abnormal development of the structures derived from the ectoderm, has inappropriately ended up becoming synonymous with ectodermal dysplasia for those not familiar with the large number of disorders classified as such. The clinical picture of XLHED, however, may be related to mutations in two different autosomal loci in addition to the locus (*ED1, EDA1, Ectodysplasin A*) located on the X chromosome and have an autosomal dominant or recessive inheritance. This can be understood by knowing that the product of the X-linked gene (ectodysplasin-A), its receptor, and an adapter protein interact in the same metabolic pathway. The binding of ectodysplasin to the receptor (Ectodysplasin A receptor, EDAR, *EDAR autosomal gene.*) and adapter protein (Ectodysplasin A receptor associated adapter protein, EDARADD, *EDARADD autosomal gene*) triggers a signal transduction that results in activation of the NF-kB pathway [17–19].

Considering the X-linked form, which is the most frequent, with the woman being heterozygous, there is a 50% chance that the disease allele will be transmitted to a child. A boy who receives this allele will manifest XLHED, whereas the phenotype of a girl who receives the allele is quite variable; however, it can be said that it is very likely that the girl will show signs. If a child is confirmed to have the recessive form of ectodermal dysplasia, the probability of recurrence is 25%. Finally, if there is evidence of autosomal dominant inheritance (for instance, an affected father with an affected male child), there is a 50% risk of recurrence in a future child. The confirmation of which gene is responsible for the phenotype of an affected person/family can be done by molecular analysis. In addition, if it is in the interest of the family, there is the possibility of prenatal diagnosis as well as intrauterine treatment.

4.3 Clinical Features

The cardinal signs of XLHED are hypotrichosis, hypodontia and tooth malformation, hypohidrosis, and characteristic facies with frontal bossing, saddle nose, thick and prominent lips, and hyperpigmented wrinkles around eyes and mouth (Fig. 4.1). These features are often conspicuous during childhood, especially in boys who present the phenotype more intensely [1, 20]. Sometimes the diagnosis is suspected when the first teeth appear with anomalous morphology (conical, peg shaped, or knife edged) or due to delayed eruption [21]. Hypohidrosis due to the lack of sweat glands causes the occurrence of febrile episodes that can be recurrent. This may be

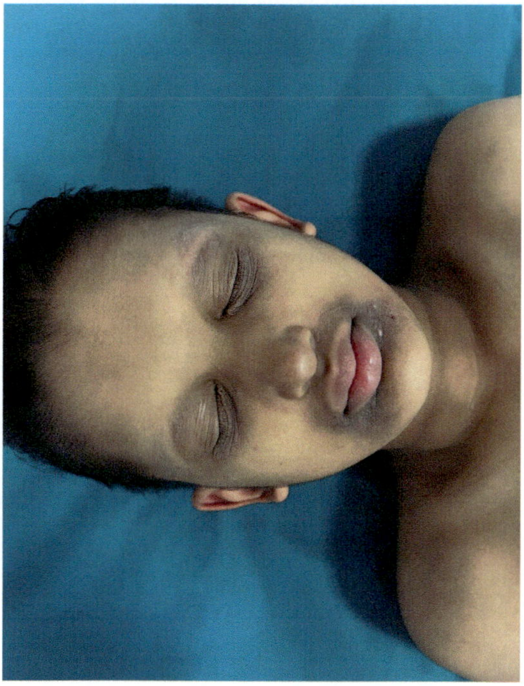

Fig. 4.1 Characteristic facies of a male patient with the EDA1 mutation: frontal bossing, saddle nose, thick and prominent lips, hyperpigmented and wrinkled eyelids. (Image Credit: Dr Gianluca Tadini)

the first indication of a diagnosis of XLHED. Neuropsychomotor development is usually normal.

4.3.1 *Craniofacial Aspects*

Facies is quite characteristic, although facial signs may not be obvious in the newborn [22]. In affected boys, there is frontal skull bossing, a prominent supraorbital ridge, thick and prominent lips, malar flattening with sunken cheeks, a saddle nose with a flattened base and short philtrum, everted nostrils, protruding chin and mandible, and midfacial hypoplasia. According to Goodwing et al. (2014), affected individuals have an overall reduction in the size of the face, and prominent lips are related to the decrease in the vertical dimension of the oral cavity as a result of dental anomalies [23–26]. Ears can be prominent, low-set, and pointed (Fig. 4.2) [22, 27]. Periorbital skin hyperpigmentation and wrinkling are striking characteristics, along with wrinkles around the mouth, which contribute to an aged appearance.

4.3.2 *Hair*

In a systematic review, Anbouba, Carmany, and Natoli (2020) comment that although hair alterations are considered cardinal signs, data analysis does not allow for establishing a key characteristic considering hair changes. They also point out that diagnosis should not be ruled out in the absence of hypotrichosis, especially if

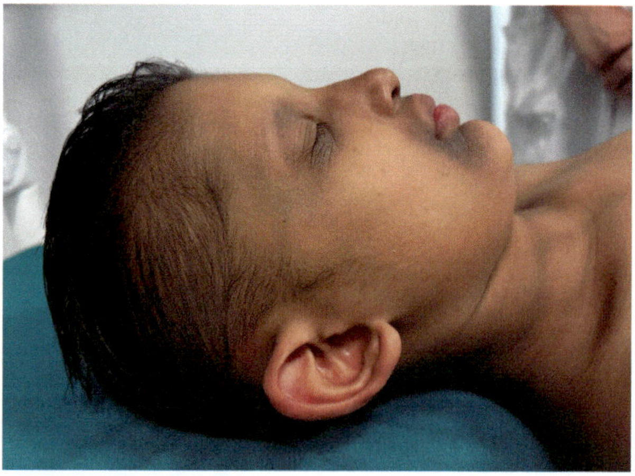

Fig. 4.2 EDA1 mutated patient with malar hypoplasia, protruding chin, and low-set ears. (Image Credit: Dr Gianluca Tadini)

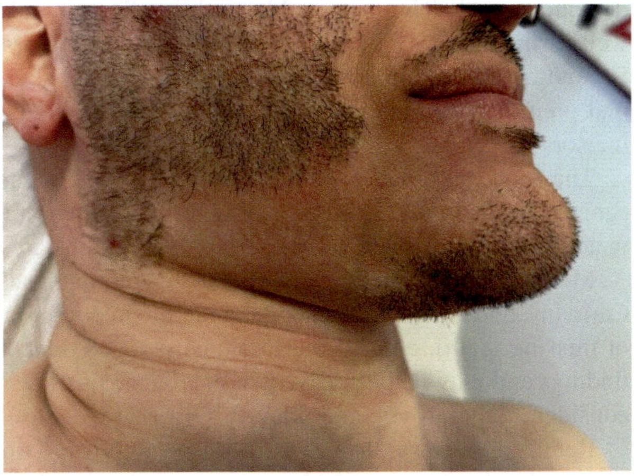

Fig. 4.3 Young adult with a peculiar distribution of beard hair. (Image Credit: Dr Gianluca Tadini)

other signs are present [28]. The hair is sparse and lightly pigmented, with slow growth and brittleness in the shafts [29]. Body hair, eyebrows, and eyelashes are also scarce and thin. Adult men tend to have early baldness. Interestingly, the beard and mustache can be normal, although pubic and axillary hair may be sparse (Fig. 4.3) [1, 15].

Hennig et al. (2021) compared the effects of SARS-CoV-2 infection in individuals with XLHED and normal controls and noted that there was a greater number of people with post-infection hair loss in the affected group. The hair loss started suddenly—about 2 months after COVID-19 infection—and lasted about 6 months [30].

4.3.3 *Teeth and Salivary Glands*

Dental anomalies are a regular feature of XLHED and are expected in both males and heterozygous females. In affected men, hypodontia of the primary and/or permanent teeth is generally severe. On the other hand, anodontia is not a frequent finding.

The presence of few teeth, poorly positioned and with morphological changes, in the oral cavity often makes it impossible to precisely identify which teeth are present in the mouth. The identification of teeth is based on position in the alveolar bone, time of eruption, and general tooth morphology. The development of the alveolar process in early fetal life depends on the development of teeth; therefore, it is absent in edentulous areas and underdeveloped in dentate regions [25, 26].

Lexner et al. (2007) conducted a study in Denmark and concluded that "generally, affected males have agenesis of most of the primary and permanent teeth, while heterozygous females have an increased frequency of agenesis of permanent teeth, but to a much lesser degree than the affected males." The average number of missing permanent teeth was 22 in males [31]. This number has been corroborated by other authors [28, 32]. Clauss et al. (2010) also indicated an average agenesis of 14 deciduous teeth. The most stable teeth in affected males are the central incisors as well as the canines in the maxilla and the first molars in both dental arches [31]. Second molars and deciduous canines may be impacted due to agenesis of the second premolars or ectopic eruption of the deciduous canine teeth where the lateral incisors should be.

The most frequent morphological alterations of teeth are conical incisors and canines, molars with hooked cusps and fused or pyramidal roots, and taurodontism, in addition to decreased tooth size. Both dentitions are affected [29, 31, 33].

Most heterozygous females have dental anomalies (73% according to Anbouba, Carmany, and Natoli, 2020 [28]). Moderate hypodontia (four is the average number of missing teeth), conical incisors, and delayed dental eruption are not infrequent findings and may be indicative that the diagnosis of ectodermal dysplasia should be considered, therefore being relevant for genetic counseling [34, 35].

Reduced salivary flow with reduced amylase concentration and activity are observed in both males and heterozygous females. Inorganic constituents (sodium, potassium, calcium, chloride, phosphate) and proteins (except amylase) are present in greater quantities [36]. The decreased salivary flow leads to complaints of dry mouth, swallowing difficulties, throat hoarseness, decreased sense of taste and/or smell, respiratory difficulties, and predisposition to pharyngo-laryngitis [15, 37].

4.3.4 Sweating

Reduced sweating ability with varying degrees of severity occurs in almost all affected men and in more than 70% of heterozygous women [28]. The decreased sweat production leads to episodes of hyperthermia in early childhood and infancy that can be severe. Febrile seizures can occur in young children and may be associated with developmental abnormalities [38]. In adult life, heat hypersensitivity causes discomfort and affects activities of daily living, while episodes of hyperthermia may also occur after sun exposure or physical exercise [39, 40]. The drastic reduction in sweating relates to sparse or absent eccrine sweat glands [1, 29].

4.3.5 Skin

The skin is usually thin, smooth, and fragile appearing since childhood. The dryness of the skin is due to hypoplasia, or the absence of sweat and sebaceous glands. Curiously, there are reports of hyperplasia of the sebaceous glands on the face [27, 41, 42]. In newborns, there may be peeling of the skin that can be confused with the colloidal membrane [22, 43]. The skin is hyperpigmented and wrinkled in the periorbital region, and wrinkling of the skin is also seen in the perioral region, signs characterizing the typical facies of the syndrome. Eczematous dermatitis is common, preferably in flexion areas [22]. Several authors reported the occurrence of milia-like lesions on the affected's face [44–46].

Nipple abnormalities may be seen in affected males, such as absent, simple, or supernumerary [15, 22, 47].

Palmoplantar hyperkeratosis (PPK) is not a frequent finding in XLHED-affected patients, but its occurrence has been reported by several authors [1, 48, 49].

The occurrence of dermatoglyphic alterations is observed in affected males and heterozygous women. These include hypoplasia of the dermal ridges, digital patterns with a higher incidence of arches, and ridge dissociation [50, 51]. There is a significant decrease or even absence of sweat pores.

4.3.6 *Nails*

The literature shows contradictory data regarding XLHED and nails. Most reports refer to normal nails, but there are observations of dystrophic, hypoplastic, or spoon-shaped nails [22, 52]. An interesting observation was made by Fete et al. (2014), who analyzed data from the Ectodermal Dysplasia International Registry (EDIR), which was provided by patients themselves, and found that 47% of affected men reported nail problems [20]. According to Maier-Wohlfart et al. (2022), this contradiction may be related to subjectivity regarding the interpretation of nail defects, especially in mild cases. Although the authors did not find nail abnormalities in their patients, they consider it important to have a greater awareness about this issue as it can lead to more and better information on patients' nails, whether children or adults (Fig. 4.4) [53].

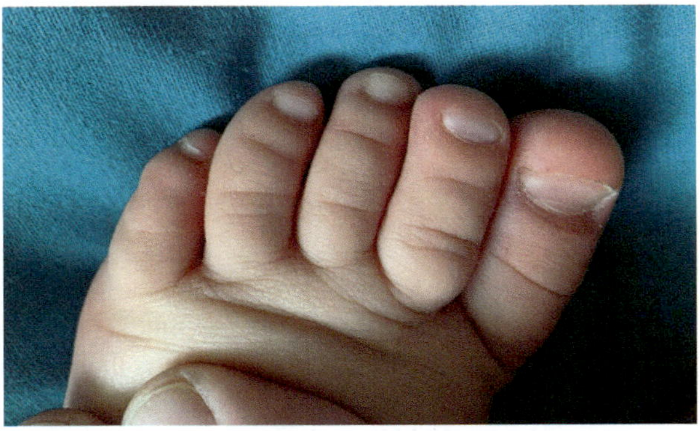

Fig. 4.4 An example of very mild nail dystrophy in an EDA1 male patient. (Image Credit: Dr Gianluca Tadini)

4.3.7 Nose and Throat

Dryness of the nose cavity with concretion of nasal secretions is a very common feature in XLHED patients. This is related to impaired development of the serous mucous glands and reduced ciliary function in the sinonasal tract. Similar changes are found in the auditory tracts [37, 54, 55]. These alterations contribute to complications such as chronic atrophic rhinitis, epistaxis, sore throat, and upper respiratory tract infections, which may be recurrent [38, 56]. Atrophic rhinitis, sometimes with ozena (related to secretion retention) and concretions, can trouble the patient throughout their lifetime [29, 57, 58]. Hoarseness or dysphonia is not uncommon and, according to Myer (1986), may be secondary to chronic laryngitis and inadequate lubrication of the vocal folds [59]. Pharyngeal symptoms may also be related to the decrease in the amount of saliva [56]. The absence of seromucous glands in the airways also predisposes patients to bronchial disease. Compared to the general population, XLHED-affected people are more likely to have airway infections due to the lack of seromucous glands in the respiratory tract [60]. The thick consistency of the mucus, as well as the enzymes present in it, play a key role in defending against irritant particles existing in the air by preventing them from reaching the lungs. The lack of glands makes the barrier ineffective, which makes affected people prone to infections and allergen exposure.

4.3.8 Eyes

Ocular anomalies are not rare and may involve the eyelids, eyelashes, conjunctiva, corneal epithelium, lens, and lacrimal glands. In some patients, there may be hypertelorism and epicanthal folds. Eyelashes are usually sparse, and growth may be inward toward the eye (trichiasis) causing irritation. A chronic problem of the surface of the eye may be related to dry eye syndrome, which irritates the eye, leading to itching, redness, and photophobia. Dry eye syndrome is related to the decreased number of Meibomian glands, which compromises the lipidic layer of the tear film. Furthermore, patients also show a reduction of aqueous secretion of the lacrimal glands. Corneal ulceration, perforation, and neovascularization may occur on the ocular surface [20, 21, 61].

4.3.9 Heterozygous Females

As in cases of other X-linked conditions, the phenotype of heterozygous females can range from normal to manifesting a clinical picture similar to that of the affected man. According to García-Delgado (2020), the vast majority of carriers show at least one clinical manifestation. Characteristics observed most frequently in heterozygous females are mild hypodontia, hypohidrosis, and hypotrichosis [62]. It should be noted that, in the case of women who present many signs, it may be difficult to differentiate XLHED from the form of HED with autosomal inheritance [63].

An interesting observation is that the distribution of body hair and functional sweat glands in the skin can occur with different patterns, sometimes following the Blaschko lines or showing laterality [64]. Impaired breast development is also observed in heterozygous women, which causes problems with breastfeeding. Difficulties can also be due to hypothelia and low production of milk. Breasts can be of different sizes, or there may be uni- or bilateral amastia. Additional signs are supernumerary nipples and fewer or absent Montgomery glands [22, 64–66].

4.4 Treatment

The treatment of patients with XLHED is symptomatic and, at first, aims to protect against hyperthermia. Whatever the season, patients may have a significant increase in body temperature, which is particularly dangerous for babies and children with a greater risk of heat-related or life-threatening illness. In fact, mortality from XLHED is most significant during the first year and remains elevated in early childhood [39]. Care must be taken regarding the practice of exercise, which also increases body temperature. Heat loss can be achieved through evaporative, conductive, or convective methods [67]. Easy access to water and cold drinks throughout the day is recommended. In addition, whenever possible, it is useful to splash fresh water and wear wet clothes. Other simple solutions are the use of a fan (including portable models) or air conditioning.

Parents should be alerted about the possibility of respiratory symptoms so that any problem can be detected early. Saline irrigation can prevent the formation of nasal concretions and is quite efficient when associated with the use of room humidifiers. If concretions are present, they should be removed by the pediatrician. The early detection of asthma-like symptoms allows for an immediate drug intervention [60].

Dry eye syndrome related to deficient tear production can be treated with drops of artificial tears and prescription eye drop medicines.

From birth, children have pale, thin, dry, and sometimes flaky skin. Such skin characteristics increase susceptibility to infections, irritation, and mechanical trauma [68]. Skincare can be done with creams with a moisturizing function, which can also be useful for eczema and rashes. Dermatological findings are important enough to warrant follow-up by a dermatologist [69, 70].

Patients with XLHED usually have severe hypodontia and must undergo prosthetic treatments in order to improve masticatory and phonetic efficiency, as well as to provide a more harmonic appearance, raising their self-esteem. Although prosthetic treatment in children is recommended, it can be complicated by the need for periodic replacement (every 2 or 3 years since the dental arches are in development) [47, 71–73]. Oral rehabilitation for children includes treatment for conoid teeth, which can be restored with composite resin or crowns. Missing teeth are replaced with the use of a removable prosthesis. Such procedures require considerable time in the clinic, which can be a complicating factor when dealing with children who may not be cooperative [74]. Fixed or mobile orthodontic appliances, palatal expanders, and traction on impacted teeth are often required. In some cases, orthognathic surgery may be indicated [75].

In adults, composite restorations or crowns and implant-supported prostheses are used, usually preceded by pre-implant bone augmentation in atrophic alveolar regions [74]. Monitoring and maintenance must be constant regardless of patient age. Fluoride treatments and other caries-preventive approaches are indicated.

Successful dental treatments are usually carried out by a team that includes a pediatric dentist, an orthodontist, a prosthodontist, and an oral-maxillofacial surgeon [73]. It should be noted that, in addition to hypodontia, patients present severely underdeveloped maxilla and mandible and poorly positioned teeth. Consequently, there is speech impairment, which indicates follow-up by a speech therapist.

Children with XLHED face difficulties with chewing, swallowing, and decreased taste since they have hypodontia and low production of saliva. Dry mouth (xerostomia) can be treated with the use of salivary stimulants, topical agents, saliva substitutes, and systemic sialogogues [76]. Guidance by a nutritionist can help parents with regard to feeding difficulties related to hypodontia and impaired salivation.

Facial features, missing teeth, and speech problems can lead to low self-esteem and social isolation. Thus, the sooner the aesthetic and dental procedures begin, the better for the patient. Therefore, it is essential that the XLHED patient is accompanied by a multidisciplinary team composed of a pediatrician and other medical specialists, a dentist, a speech therapist, a nutritionist, and a psychologist, and the indispensable genetic counseling for the family.

4.4.1 Prenatal Diagnosis and In-Utero Treatment

Non-invasive prenatal diagnosis is possible by tooth germ counting sonography, a highly trustworthy way to identify fetuses with XLHED for women who have already had a child with this condition [77]. Early diagnosis can also be done by amniocentesis or chorionic villus sampling, which allows obtaining fetal DNA for molecular analysis [66].

Intra-amniotic administration of EDA1 recombinant protein (Fc-EDA) with the aim of prenatal treatment has already been carried out with encouraging results. A long-term follow-up of six treated boys evidenced the restoration of the ability to sweat, and there was no occurrence of hyperthermia. The correction of hypotrichosis was not observed, and results for dental anomalies were unsatisfactory in treated patients, although it is too early to say that these results are conclusive. Studies with larger samples are planned, which may give a better overview of the subject. Treatment with the EDA protein is possible for pregnant women with male fetuses diagnosed with XLHED in the twenty-sixth week of pregnancy [78, 79].

References

1. Wright JT, Grange DK, Fete M. Hypohidrotic ectodermal dysplasia. In: Adam MP, Mirzaa GM, Pagon RA, Wallace SE, LJH B, Gripp KW, Amemiya A, editors. GeneReviews Seattle. University of Washington; 2003. (Updated 2022).
2. Tuna EB, Guven Y, Bozdogan E, Aktoren O. Assessment of dental features in 16 children with hypohidrotic ectodermal dysplasia. Pediatr Dent J. 2009;19(1):106–11.
3. Nguyen-Nielsen M, Skovbo S, Svaneby D, Pedersen L, Fryzek J. The prevalence of X-linked hypohidrotic ectodermal dysplasia (XLHED) in Denmark, 1995–2010. Eur J Med Genet. 2013;56(5):236–42.
4. Guazzarotti L, Tadini G, Mancini GE, Giglio S, Willoughby CE, Callea M, Sani I, Nannini P, Mameli C, Tenconi AA, Mauri S, Bottero A, Caimi A, Morelli M, Zuccotti GV. Phenotypic heterogeneity and mutational spectrum in a cohort of 45 Italian males subjects with X-linked ectodermal dysplasia. Clin Genet. 2015;87(4):338–42.
5. Danz DFG. Sechste Bemerkung. Von Menschen ohne Haare und Zähne. Stark Arch Geburtsh Frauenz Neugeb Kinderkr. 1792;4:684.
6. Thurnam J. Two cases in which the skin, hair and teeth were very imperfectly developed. Proc R M Chirurg Soc. 1848;31:71–82.
7. Darwin C. The variation of animals and plants under domestication. 2nd ed. London: John Murray; 1875.
8. Thadani KI. A toothless type of man: the "Bhudas" of India—a case of sex-linked inheritance. J Hered. 1921;12:87–8.
9. Weech AA. Hereditary ectodermal dysplasia (congenital ectodermal defect). A report of two cases. Am J Dis Child. 1929;37:766–90.
10. Felsher Z. Hereditary ectodermal dysplasia. Arch Dermatol Syphilol. 1944;49:410–4.
11. Christ J. Über die kongenitalen ektodermalen Defekte und ihre Beziehungen zueinander. Arch F Derinat Syph. 1913;116:685.
12. Siemens HW. Über rezessiv-geschlechtsgebundene Vererbung bei Hautkrankheiten. Arch F Dermat. 1921;136:69–88.
13. Touraine A. L' "anidrose avec hypotrichose et anodontie" (polydysplasie ectodermique héréditaire). Presse Méd. 1936;44:145–9.
14. Freire-Maia N. Ectodermal dysplasias revisited. Acta Genet Med Gemellol. 1977;26:121–31.
15. Freire-Maia N, Pinheiro M. Ectodermal dysplasias: a clinical and genetic study. New York, NY: Alan R. Liss Inc; 1984.
16. More CB, Bhavsar K, Joshi J, Varma SN, Tailor M. Hereditary ectodermal dysplasia: a retrospective study. J Nat Sci Biol Med. 2013;4(2):445–50.
17. Visinoni AF, Lisboa-Costa T, Pagnan NA, Chautard-Freire-Maia EA. Ectodermal dysplasias: clinical and molecular review. Am J Med Genet A. 2009;149A(9):1980–2002.
18. Pagnan NA, Visinoni ÁF. Update on ectodermal dysplasias clinical classification. Am J Med Genet A. 2014;164A(10):2415–23.
19. Wright JT, Fete M, Schneider H, Zinser M, Koster MI, Clarke AJ, Hadj-Rabia S, Tadini G, Pagnan N, Visinoni AF, Bergendal B, Abbott B, Fete T, Stanford C, Butcher C, D'Souza RN, Sybert VP, Morasso MI. Ectodermal dysplasias: classification and organization by phenotype, genotype and molecular pathway. Am J Med Genet A. 2019;179(3):442–7.
20. Fete M, Hermann J, Behrens J, Huttner KM. X-linked hypohidrotic ectodermal dysplasia (XLHED): clinical and diagnostic insights from an international patient registry. Am J Med Genet A. 2014;164A:2437–42.
21. Callea M, Bignotti S, Semeraro F, Cammarata-Scalisi F, El-Feghaly J, Morabito A, Romano V, Willoughby CE. Extended overview of ocular phenotype with recent advances in hypohidrotic ectodermal dysplasia. Children (Basel). 2022;9(9):1357.
22. Asai Y, Irvine AD. Ectodermal dysplasias. In: Irvine AD, Hoeger PH, Yan AC, editors. Harper's textbook of pediatric dermatology; 2011. https://doi.org/10.1002/9781444345384.ch127.

23. Goodwin AF, Larson JR, Jones KB, Liberton DK, Landan M, Wang Z, Boekelheide A, Langham M, Mushegyan V, Oberoi S, Brao R, Wen T, Johnson R, Huttner K, Grange DK, Spritz RA, Hallgrímsson B, Jheon AH, Klein OD. Craniofacial morphometric analysis of individuals with X-linked hypohidrotic ectodermal dysplasia. Mol Genet Genomic Med. 2014;2(5):422–9.
24. Saksena SS, Bixler D. Facial morphometrics in the identification of gene carriers of X-linked hypohidrotic ectodermal dysplasia. Am J Med Genet. 1990;35(1):105–14.
25. Kupietzky A, Houpt M. Hypohidrotic ectodermal dysplasia: characteristics and treatment. Quintessence Int. 1995;26(4):285–91.
26. Tape MW, Tye E. Ectodermal dysplasia: literature review and a case report. Compend Contin Educ Dent. 1995;16(5):524–8.
27. Paller AS, Mancini AJ. Hurwitz clinical pediatric dermatology: a textbook of skin disorders of childhood and adolescence. 6th ed. St. Louis, MO: Elsevier; 2022.
28. Anbouba GM, Carmany EP, Natoli JL. The characterization of hypodontia, hypohidrosis, and hypotrichosis associated with X-linked hypohidrotic ectodermal dysplasia: a systematic review. Am J Med Genet A. 2020;182(4):831–41.
29. Grange DK. Ectodermal dysplasias. In: Emery and Rimoin's principles and practice of medical genetics. Elsevier; 2013. https://doi.org/10.1016/B978-0-12-383834-6.00157-9.
30. Hennig V, Schuh W, Neubert A, Mielenz D, Jäck HM, Schneider H. Increased risk of chronic fatigue and hair loss following COVID-19 in individuals with hypohidrotic ectodermal dysplasia. Orphanet J Rare Dis. 2021;16(1):373.
31. Lexner MO, Bardow A, Hertz JM, Nielsen LA, Kreiborg S. Anomalies of tooth formation in hypohidrotic ectodermal dysplasia. Int J Paediatr Dent. 2007;17(1):10–8.
32. Clauss F, Chassaing N, Smahi A, Vincent MC, Calvas P, Molla M, Lesot H, Alembik Y, Hadj-Rabia S, Bodemer C, Manière MC, Schmittbuhl M. X-linked and autosomal recessive Hypohidrotic Ectodermal Dysplasia: genotypic-dental phenotypic findings. Clin Genet. 2010;78(3):257–66.
33. Bergendal B. Orodental manifestations in ectodermal dysplasia-a review. Am J Med Genet A. 2014;164A(10):2465–71.
34. Sybert VP. Ectodermal dysplasias. In: Wolff K, Goldsmith LA, Katz SI, Gilchrest BA, Paller AS, Leffell DJ, editors. Fitzpatrick's dermatology in general medicine. 7th ed. New York, NY: McGraw-Hill; 2008.
35. Clauss F, Manière MC, Obry F, Waltmann E, Hadj-Rabia S, Bodemer C, Alembik Y, Lesot H, Schmittbuhl M. Dento-craniofacial phenotypes and underlying molecular mechanisms in hypohidrotic ectodermal dysplasia (HED): a review. J Dent Res. 2008;87(12):1089–99.
36. Lexner MO, Bardow A, Hertz JM, Almer L, Nauntofte B, Kreiborg S. Whole saliva in X-linked hypohidrotic ectodermal dysplasia. Int J Paediatr Dent. 2007;17(3):155–62.
37. Callea M, Teggi R, Yavuz I, Tadini G, Priolo M, Crovella S, Clarich G, Grasso DL. Ear nose throat manifestations in hypoidrotic ectodermal dysplasia. Int J Pediatr Otorhinolaryngol. 2013;77(11):1801–4.
38. Blüschke G, Nüsken KD, Schneider H. Prevalence and prevention of severe complications of hypohidrotic ectodermal dysplasia in infancy. Early Hum Dev. 2010;86(7):397–9.
39. Hammersen JE, Neukam V, Nüsken KD, Schneider H. Systematic evaluation of exertional hyperthermia in children and adolescents with hypohidrotic ectodermal dysplasia: an observational study. Pediatr Res. 2011;70(3):297–301.
40. Jones KB, Goodwin AF, Landan M, Seidel K, Tran DK, Hogue J, Chavez M, Fete M, Yu W, Hussein T, Johnson R, Huttner K, Jheon AH, Klein OD. Characterization of X-linked hypohidrotic ectodermal dysplasia (XL-HED) hair and sweat gland phenotypes using phototrichogram analysis and live confocal imaging. Am J Med Genet A. 2013;161A(7):1585–93.
41. Sato K, Kang WH, Saga K, Sato KT. Biology of sweat glands and their disorders. II. Disorders of sweat gland function. J Am Acad Dermatol. 1989;20(5):713–26.
42. Xu XG, Lv Y, Yan H, Qu L, Xiao T, Geng L, He CD, Liu CX, Gao XH, Li YH, Chen HD. Next-generation sequencing identified a novel EDA mutation in a Chinese pedigree of hypohi-

drotic ectodermal dysplasia with hyperplasia of the sebaceous glands. Acta Derm Venereol. 2017;97(8):984–5.
43. Thomas C, Suranyi E, Pride H, Tyler W. A child with hypohidrotic ectodermal dysplasia with features of a collodion membrane. Pediatr Dermatol. 2006;23(3):251–4.
44. Martin-Pascual A, de Unamuno P, Aparicio M, Herreros V. Anhidrotic (or hypohidrotic) ectodermal dysplasia. Dermatology. 1977;154:235–43.
45. Berk DR, Bayliss SJ. Milia: a review and classification. J Am Acad Dermatol. 2008;59(6):1050–63.
46. Mehta S, Agarwal N, Khare AK, Kuldeep CM, Mittal A, Gupta LK. Hypohidrotic ectodermal dysplasia in association with milia. Indian J Dermatol Venereol Leprol. 2014;80(5):483.
47. Clarke A, Phillips DI, Brown R, Harper PS. Clinical aspects of X-linked hypohidrotic ectodermal dysplasia. Arch Dis Child. 1987;62(10):989–96.
48. García-Martín P, Hernández-Martín A, Torrelo A. Ectodermal dysplasias: a clinical and molecular review. Actas Dermosifiliogr. 2013;104(6):451–70.
49. Haghighi A, Nikuei P, Haghighi-Kakhki H, Saleh-Gohari N, Baghestani S, Krawitz PM, Hecht J, Mundlos S. Whole-exome sequencing identifies a novel missense mutation in EDAR causing autosomal recessive hypohidrotic ectodermal dysplasia with bilateral amastia and palmoplantar hyperkeratosis. Br J Dermatol. 2013;168(6):1353–6.
50. Pinheiro M, Freire-Maia N. Christ-Siemens-Touraine syndrome—a clinical and genetic analysis of a large Brazilian kindred: I. Affected females. II. Affected males. III. Carrier detection. Am J Med Genet. 1979;4(2):113–34.
51. Rodewald A, Zahn-Messow K. Dermatoglyphics findings in families with X-linked hypohidrotic(or anhidrotic) ectodermal dysplasia(HED). Prog Clin Biol Res. 1982;84:451–8.
52. Sedano HO, Sauk JJ, Gorlin RJ. Oral manifestations of inherited disorders. Boston, MA: Butterworth; 1977.
53. Maier-Wohlfart S, Aicher C, Willershausen I, Peschel N, Meißner U, Gölz L, Schneider H. Congenital nail disorders among children with suspected ectodermal dysplasias. Genes (Basel). 2022;13(11):2119.
54. Azar A, Piccinelli C, Brown H, Headon D, Cheeseman M. Ectodysplasin signalling deficiency in mouse models of hypohidrotic ectodermal dysplasia leads to middle ear and nasal pathology. Hum Mol Genet. 2016;25(16):3564–77.
55. Del-Pozo J, MacIntyre N, Azar A, Headon D, Schneider P, Cheeseman M. Role of ectodysplasin signalling in middle ear and nasal pathology in rat and mouse models of hypohidrotic ectodermal dysplasia. Dis Model Mech. 2019;12(4):dmm037804.
56. Daniel E, McCurdy EA, Shashi V, McGuirt WF Jr. Ectodermal dysplasia: otolaryngologic manifestations and management. Laryngoscope. 2002;112(6):962–7.
57. Ibañes Cárcamo E. Displasia ectodérmica anhidrótica: ozena congénita [Anhidrotic ectodermal dysplasia: congenital ozena]. Acta Otorrinolaringol Esp. 1990;41(2):107–9.
58. Koerner HN, Bettega S, Mocellin M, Soccol AT, Adriano CF, Moccellin L, Pilotto RF, Mair A. Atrophic rhinits: a case report related to ectodermal dysplasia. Arq Int Otorrinolaringol. 2006;10:249–53.
59. Myer CM 3rd. Otolaryngologic manifestations of the ectodermal dysplasias—clinical note. Int J Pediatr Otorhinolaryngol. 1986;11(3):307–10.
60. Dietz J, Kaercher T, Schneider AT, Zimmermann T, Huttner K, Johnson R, Schneider H. Early respiratory and ocular involvement in X-linked hypohidrotic ectodermal dysplasia. Eur J Pediatr. 2013;172(8):1023–31.
61. Tyagi P, Tyagi V, Hashim AA. Ocular and non-ocular manifestations of hypohidrotic ectodermal dysplasia. Case Rep. 2011;2011:bcr0120113731.
62. García-Delgado C, Noriega-Juárez MA, Cervantes A, Abad-Flores JD, Toledo-Bahena M, Valencia-Herrera A, et al. High penetrance of EDA pathogenic variants in Mexican female carriers with hypohidrotic ectodermal dysplasia. Dermatol Sin. 2020;38:172–5.
63. Levi SS, Molho-Pessach V. Gender and genodermatoses. In: Tur E, Maibach H, editors. Gender and dermatology. Cham: Springer; 2018. https://doi.org/10.1007/978-3-319-72156-9_9.

64. Körber L, Schneider H, Fleischer N, Maier-Wohlfart S. No evidence for preferential X-chromosome inactivation as the main cause of divergent phenotypes in sisters with X-linked hypohidrotic ectodermal dysplasia. Orphanet J Rare Dis. 2021;16:1–8.
65. Wahlbuhl-Becker M, Faschingbauer F, Beckmann MW, Schneider H. Hypohidrotic ectodermal dysplasia: breastfeeding complications due to impaired breast development. Geburtshilfe Frauenheilkd. 2017;77(04):377–82.
66. Leo B, Schneider H, Hammersen J. Reproductive decision-making by women with X-linked hypohidrotic ectodermal dysplasia. J Eur Acad Dermatol Venereol. 2022;36(10):1863–70.
67. Massey H, House J, Tipton M. Thermoregulation in ectodermal dysplasia: a case series. Int J Environ Res Public Health. 2019;16(22):4514.
68. Trzeciak WH, Koczorowski R. Molecular basis of hypohidrotic ectodermal dysplasia: an update. J Appl Genet. 2016;57(1):51–61.
69. Pavlis MB, Rice ZP, Veledar E, Bradley BR, Spraker MK, Chen SC. Quality of life of cutaneous disease in the ectodermal dysplasias. Pediatr Dermatol. 2010;27(3):260–5.
70. Reyes-Reali J, Mendoza-Ramos MI, Garrido-Guerrero E, Méndez-Catalá CF, Méndez-Cruz AR, Pozo-Molina G. Hypohidrotic ectodermal dysplasia: clinical and molecular review. Int J Dermatol. 2018;57(8):965–72.
71. Itthagarun A, King NM. Oral rehabilitation of a hypohidrotic ectodermal dysplasia patient: a 6-year follow-up. Quintessence Int. 2000;31(9):642–8.
72. Visinoni AF. Displasias ectodérmicas—Revisão do grupo A, atualização de banco de dados informatizado e análise de variantes do gene *ED1*, Ph.D. thesis, Universidade Federal do Paraná, 2009
73. Montanari M, Callea M, Battelli F, Piana G. Oral rehabilitation of children with ectodermal dysplasia. BMJ Case Rep. 2012;2012:bcr0120125652.
74. Schnabl D, Grunert I, Schmuth M, Kapferer-Seebacher I. Prosthetic rehabilitation of patients with hypohidrotic ectodermal dysplasia: a systematic review. J Oral Rehabil. 2018;45(7):555–70.
75. Cerezo-Cayuelas M, Pérez-Silva A, Serna-Muñoz C, Vicente A, Martínez-Beneyto Y, Cabello-Malagón I, Ortiz-Ruiz AJ. Orthodontic and dentofacial orthopedic treatments in patients with ectodermal dysplasia: a systematic review. Orphanet J Rare Dis. 2022;17(1):376.
76. Alhejoury HA, Mogharbel LF, Al-Qadhi MA, Shamlan SS, Alturki AF, Babatin WM, Mohammed Alaishan RA, Pullishery F. Artificial saliva for therapeutic management of xerostomia: a narrative review. J Pharm Bioallied Sci. 2021;13(Suppl 2):S903–7.
77. Hammersen J, Wohlfart S, Goecke TW, Köninger A, Stepan H, Gallinat R, Morris S, Bücher K, Clarke A, Wünsche S, Beckmann MW, Schneider H, Faschingbauer F. Reliability of prenatal detection of X-linked hypohidrotic ectodermal dysplasia by tooth germ sonography. Prenat Diagn. 2019;39(9):796–805.
78. Schneider H. Ectodermal dysplasias: new perspectives on the treatment of so far immedicable genetic disorders. Front Genet. 2022;13:1000744.
79. Schneider H, Schweikl C, Faschingbauer F, Hadj-Rabia S, Schneider PA. Causal treatment for X-linked hypohidrotic ectodermal dysplasia: long-term results of short-term perinatal ectodysplasin A1 replacement. Int J Mol Sci. 2023;24:7155.

Chapter 5
Incontinentia Pigmenti

Alessandra Pescatore, Matilde Valeria Ursini, and Francesca Fusco

Keyword Incontinentia pigmenti · *IKBKG/NEMO* · NF-κB

5.1 Clinical Features

Incontinentia pigmenti (IP) (OMIM#308300) is neuroectodermal dysplasia with typical skin abnormalities combined with anomalies of the teeth, eyes, and central nervous system (CNS) [1, 2].

Skin: The cutaneous lesions are major criteria for IP clinical diagnosis. They occur as a severe dermatosis that usually starts within 2 weeks after birth and follows four stages. First, patients exhibit skin blisters and an inflammatory response, accompanied by massive eosinophilic granulocytes' infiltration into the epidermis (Stage I/*vesicular stage*). Subsequently, verrucous hyperkeratotic lesions develop (Stage II/*verrucous stage*) that disappear over time, leaving behind areas of hyperpigmentation due to melanin accumulation (Stage III/*hyperpigmented stage*). These areas that follow the lines of Blaschko usually vanish by the second decade (Stage IV/*atrophic stage*), but adults may still exhibit areas of dermal scarring with a lack of hair follicles. In most patients, the successive or combined Stages I and II outbreaks occurring during the first months of life regress spontaneously [3].

Teeth: Odonatological problems are characterized by delayed eruption, oligodontia, agenesis, peg-shaped or malformed teeth, supernumerary teeth, and supplementary cusps and affect more than 80% of IP patients [4]. The main anomalies are the following: multiple dental agenesis in temporary and permanent dentition (prevalence of approximately 60% and 90%, respectively), coronary morphological abnormalities (in approximately 70% of cases), delayed dentition, and various types

A. Pescatore · M. V. Ursini · F. Fusco (✉)
Institute of Genetics and Biophysics 'Adriano Buzzati-Traverso' (CNR), Naples, Italy
e-mail: francesca.fusco@igb.cnr.it

G. Tadini et al. (eds.), *Multidisciplinary Approach to Ectodermal Dysplasia*,
https://doi.org/10.1007/978-3-031-75790-7_5

of dental-maxillary dysmorphia (class II in 40% of cases, class III in 30% of cases, and/or transverse maxillo-mandibular hypodevelopment) and an arched palate or an orofacial cleft [5–7].

Eyes: Ophthalmological problems that affect approximately between 35 and 70% of IP patients, including early active retinal vasculopathy (the most common abnormality, which may lead to retinal detachment and blindness), optic nerve damage, or asymptomatic corneal abnormalities (*cornea verticillate*) [7]. Retinal detachment can be observed as a consequence of neovascularization following retinal ischemia caused by abnormal peripheral retinal vessels. In the most severe cases, blindness can occur [8–11]. Strabismus, cataracts, conjunctival pigmentation, optic atrophy, retinal pigment abnormalities, foveal hypoplasia, foveal disorganization, and microphthalmia are less common eye findings [12].

Breast: The presence of abnormalities of mammary tissue, ranging from aplasia of the breast, breast hypoplasia, and nipple hypoplasia to excessive nipples, may occur, and it is more common than in the general population [1, 2, 12].

Central Nervous System (CNS): Neurological abnormalities, found in approximately 30% of IP cases, start during the first weeks of life, which may concord with the neonatal cutaneous eruption, and include epilepsy, mental retardation, hemiparesis, spasticity, microcephaly, and cerebellar ataxia [13]. In very rare instances, CNS abnormalities can be fatal, when seizures lead to death due to severe vascular cerebral damage resulting in thalamic hemorrhage, ischemia, and necrosis of both hemispheres. Neurologic involvement is often present along with retinal vasculopathy and may result from ischemia/vaso-occlusive events [13, 14].

Among the most frequent CNS abnormalities found in IP using magnetic resonance imaging (MRI) are corpus callosum abnormalities [15].

Cognitive impairments, when present, can range from severe intellectual deficiency to learning disorders without intellectual disability (particularly dyslexia and dyscalculia). It is not yet known whether certain cognitive functions are more likely to be affected than others. In addition, cognitive impairments were observed without any motor disorders [16, 17].

Hair: In roughly 38% of IP patients, vertex alopecia occurs most commonly in a mild manner and often goes unnoticed. Alopecia is often associated with inflammation, vesiculation, and scarring. A rare manifestation of IP is agenesis of the eyebrows and eyelashes. Hair, eyelashes, and eyebrows are usually thin and sparse. Scalp hair may also present with a "woolly" texture (without characteristic abnormalities of the hair shaft). Mild to severe nail abnormalities may also be observed, such as striations or thickening, but these are non-pathognomonic signs for IP [7].

Nails: Ridging, pitting, or nail disruption may occur intermittently and can affect all or most of the fingernails and toenails. These changes tend to regress and disappear with age. Subungual and periungual keratotic tumors are usually present between puberty and the third decade. The lesions sometimes spontaneously regress but often cause pain, nail dystrophy, and, most importantly, destruction of the bone underneath [1, 2, 12].

5.2 Genetic Features

IP is due to mutations of the *IKBKG/NEMO* gene (Inhibitor of Kappa polypeptide gene enhancer in B-cells, Kinase Gamma/Nuclear Factor κB, Essential Modulator) located in the Xq28 region. A recurrent deletion (*IKBKG/NEMOdel*4–10), removing the exon 4–10 and causing a loss-of-function (LoF) of *IKBKG,* is frequently associated with IP (78% of cases); 2% have non-recurrent genomic deletions in the IP *locus*; 17% have point mutations in the coding region. Most *IKBKG* mutations are de novo; indeed, the IP syndrome is typically a sporadic condition (>70% of cases) [18–27].

IKBKG maps in a region with a unique genomic organization, called "IP *locus*" (Fig. 5.1a). In the centromeric direction, it partially overlaps with the *glucose-6-phosphate dehydrogenase* (*G6PD*) gene. It is worth noting that *G6PD* is a disease gene causing the X-linked *G6PD* deficiency (OMIM#305900), the most common enzymopathy in humans. The two overlapping genes share a conserved promoter region (called Promoter B), which has a housekeeping bidirectional activity and it is distinct from the specific *IKBKG* promoter (Promoter A) exclusive for *IKBKG* transcription. In the telomeric direction, *IKBKG* is part of a 35.7-kb segmental duplication (Low Copy Repeats, LCRs) containing also its nonfunctional truncated copy, *pseudoNEMO* [28] (Fig. 5.1a). The presence of highly homologous regions (LCR1 and LCR2) and the high density of repetitive sequences cause a genomic structure-destabilizing effect and predispose the IP *locus* to generate novel pathologic alleles by various different aberrant mechanisms (Non-Allelic Homologous Recombination-NAHR, Gene Conversion). The two LCRs, covering the functional gene (LCR1) and its pseudogene copy (LCR2), are arranged in opposite orientations and are highly homologous and prone to recombination by sequence exchange between the LCR1 and LCR2 copies [29]. Moreover, it has been observed that recombination events produced by NAHR between the two LCRs repositioned into the *IKBKG* gene, the polymorphic alterations arising in the pseudogene (i.e., *pseudoNEMOdel* and point mutation), causing de novo IP pathogenic mutations [30–32]. In addition to the recurrent event driven by MER67B sequences causing *NEMOdel4–10* in most patients, a high density of repetitive sequences, located in each LCR, gives a genome structure-destabilizing effect, predisposing the IP *locus* to generate novel rearrangements that eliminate *IKBKG* and sometimes also *G6PD* and *pseudoNEMO*. In several instances, NAHR, causing both benign and pathological alleles [31, 32], and non-homologous end-joining (NHEJ) and *Alu-Alu*-mediated recombination events, producing either recurrent or non-recurrent deletions, have been reported [33, 34]. Indeed, the local architecture of the locus with a high frequency of micro–/macro-homologies, tandem repeats, and repeat/repetitive sequences increases its vulnerability to the production of de novo genomic rearrangements through different mechanisms [30–32]. Non-pathological variants into the pseudogene, including segmental duplication/deletion, do not interfere with the function of *IKBKG* but are considered to be structural variations of the human genome or small Copy Number Variations (CNVs), with low frequencies in the

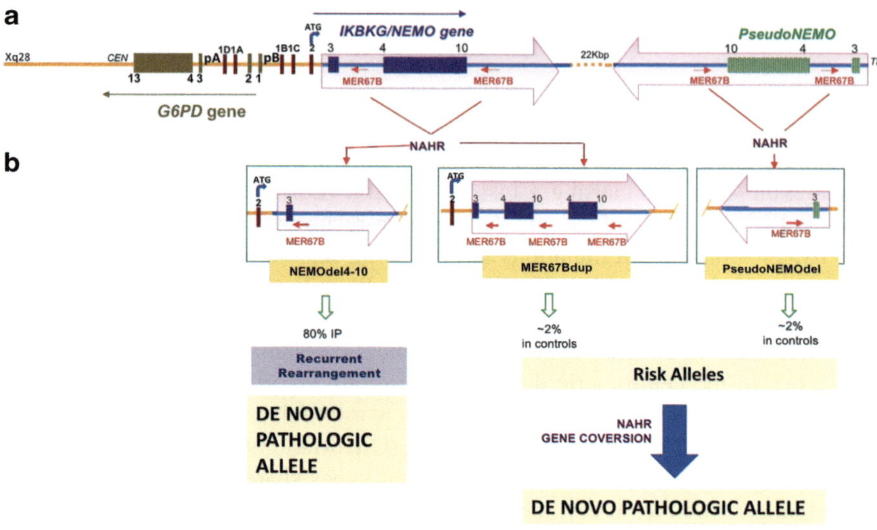

Fig. 5.1 (**a**) Schematic representation of the IP *locus* in Xq28 (chrX:153, 740–153, 900 kb, UCSC Genome Browser on Human February 2009, GRCh37/hg19). Promoter B (pB) is bidirectional and maps in the region between *G6PD* exon1 and *IKBKG* exon1B. *IKBKG* Promoter A (pA) maps in the region between exon3 of the *G6PD* gene and exon1D of the *IKBKG* gene. The transcriptional direction of each gene is indicated by arrows. The square arrows represent LCRs. *G6PD* exons, *IKBKG/NEMO* exons, and *pseudoNEMO* exons are shown. (**b**) Rearrangements in the IP *locus*. A schematic representation of the recurrent pathogenic *NEMOdel4–10* deletion and the benign CNVs, *MER67Bdup,* and *pseudoNEMOdel*, produced by NAHR. The frequency of each rearrangement is also shown

control population (1%). Genetic evidences have demonstrated that *pseudoNEMOdel* and *MER67Bdup* variants should be considered as risk alleles for sporadic IP cases [30] (Fig. 5.1b).

A wide spectrum of point mutations in the coding *IKBKG* have been identified so far, and, on the basis of the activity of the NEMO mutated protein that is essential for the NF-κB activation, they are considered hypomorphic or amorphic (LoF) mutations. The LoF or amorphic mutations of *IKBKG*, abolishing NF-κB activation in the cells, are embryonically lethal in hemizygous males (Fig. 5.2a1_II:1), while heterozygous females survive affected by IP because of unbalanced X-inactivation profile due to survival of cells expressing NEMO wild type (Fig. 5.2a1_I:2, II:2). The few surviving IP males carrying *IKBKG* amorphic mutations have turned out to be obligatory somatic mosaics of the mutation (Fig. 5.2a3_ I:1 and b1_II:1). Indeed, the IP pathogenesis in the females and most likely also in the male somatic mosaics is based on the cellular effects of impaired NEMO activity, but in the context of the interaction of genetically different cells in the affected tissue, which might underline the inflammatory status [35–37]. Recently, it has been reported in 2 families a father-to-daughter transmission of IP where the combination of somatic and germline mosaicism for *IKBKG* LoF mutations, p.Gln132X mutation or the

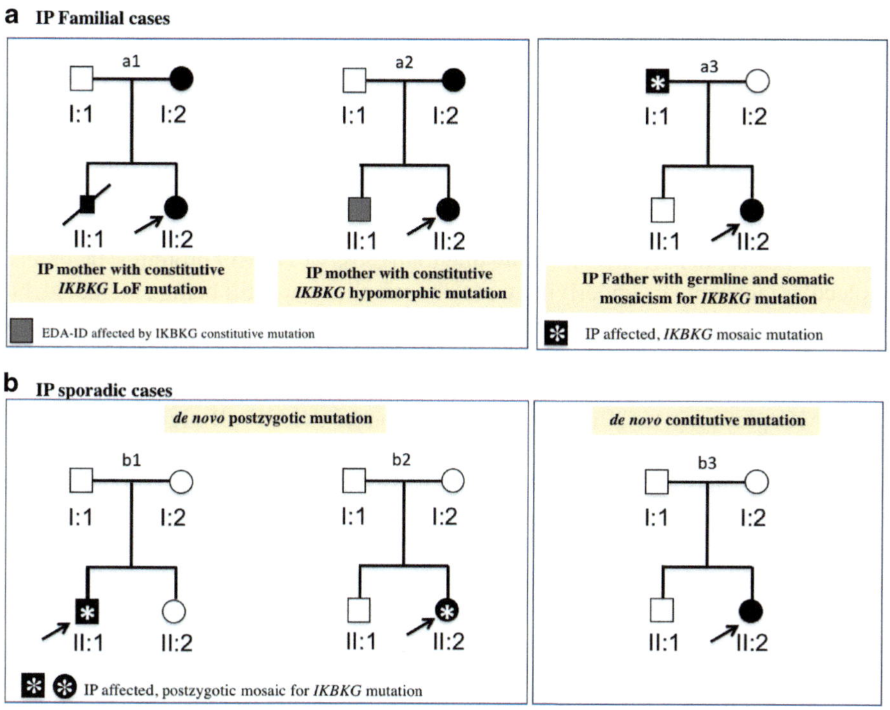

Fig. 5.2 (**a**) A schematic representation of IP familial cases. (**a1**) IP mother (I:2) has *IKBKG* LoF mutation that is lethal in hemizygous son (II:1) and causes IP in heterozygous daughter (II:2); (**a2**) IP mother (I:2) has *IKBKG* hypomorphic mutation that causes EDA-ID in hemizygous son (II:1) and IP in heterozygous daughter (II:2). (**a3**) IP father is a somatic and germline mosaic for the *IKBKG* mutation that can pass only to the IP heterozygous daughter (II:2). (**b**) A schematic representation of IP sporadic cases. (**b1** and **b2**) the onset of mutation is a postzygotic event; **b3**) the *IKBKG* mutation is constitutive IP heterozygous daughter (II:2)

NEMOdel4–10, in IP males-father resulted in the transmission of the mutated allele to a female child (Fig. 5.2a3_II:2 IP). The *IKBKG* mutant allele was found in blood, urine, skin, and sperm DNA, demonstrating that fathers were somatic and germline mosaics [36].

IKBKG hypomorphic mutations, reducing but not abolishing NF-κB activation, are not lethal in hemizygous males that survive affected by anhidrotic ectodermal dysplasia with immunodeficiency (EDA-ID) (OMIM#300291) and they have been identified in female IP and in male EDA-ID patients [26] (Fig. 5.2a2_II:1 and II:2, respectively).

While the IP familial cases represent 22%, occurring when the IP female daughter has inherited the *IKBKG* mutation from one of her affected parents (Fig. 5.2a), about 78% of cases are a sporadic condition (Fig. 5.2b), including constitutive de novo mutation in heterozygous IP females (Fig. 5.2b3_II:2) and somatic mosaicisms in rare IP males (Fig. 5.2b1_II:1) and IP females (Fig. 5.2b2_II:2) [36–39].

5.3 The Role of NEMO Protein Loss in the Pathogenesis of IP

IP is primarily caused by mutations in the inhibitor of kappaB kinase gamma (*IKBKG*)/NF-kB essential modulator (*NEMO*) gene, which encodes the NEMO protein. The pathogenesis of IP is linked to the loss or dysfunction of the NEMO protein due to genetic mutations. The clinical manifestations seen in IP are a consequence of disrupted NF-κB signaling due to the loss of NEMO protein. The precise molecular mechanisms underlying these abnormalities are still being elucidated, but it is clear that NF-κB-mediated regulation of development and differentiation processes during embryogenesis is perturbed in IP, leading to the observed features in affected individuals.

NEMO plays a crucial role in the regulation of the NF-κB signaling pathway, which is involved in various cellular processes, including immune responses, inflammation, and cell survival. NEMO serves as the regulatory subunit of the inhibitor of κB kinase (IKK) complex, which also includes the catalytic subunits IKK-1 and IKK-2. NEMO acts as the bridge between the catalytic subunits (IKK1 and IKK2) and upstream signaling molecules, facilitating the activation of the IKK complex in response to different stimuli. The IKK complex is responsible for the canonical activation of the NF-κB pathway. The transcriptional program of NF-κB can be specifically adapted and modulated depending on the tissue context [40]. Different cell types and tissues have unique requirements and responses to various stimuli, and NF-κB signaling can be tailored to meet these specific needs. The exact mechanisms by which NEMO deficiency leads to the characteristic features of IP are still under investigation, but several key aspects have been identified, including dysregulated cell death processes.

NEMO deficiency has been extensively studied in the context of inflammatory cytokine signaling, particularly the tumor necrosis factor (TNF) receptor-1 (TNFR1) pathway. TNFR1 is a major receptor involved in initiating the canonical NF-kB activation pathway.

In physiologic conditions, TNF-R triggering induces recruitment and full activation of IKK at the level of the membrane in a multiprotein complex called TNF-R Complex I. The subsequent phosphorylation of the inhibitor of NF-κB (IκB) and NF-κB. In the presence of NEMO, IKK is recruited to TNF receptor complexes, leading to the activation of NF-κB and cell survival signaling pathways. However, in the absence of NEMO, the signaling balance shifts toward cell death pathways [18, 41, 42].

In male mice, NEMO ablation (NEMO-KO) caused lethality during embryo development due to cell death in multiple tissues, while heterozygous females manifested a skin IP-like phenotype [18, 43–45]. TNF-induced cell death mediated by receptor-interacting protein kinase-1 (RIPK1) kinase activity is a significant factor contributing to the embryonic lethality observed in male embryos lacking functional NEMO [46]. During embryo development, IKK and NF-κB signaling act at multiple levels in the inhibition of cell death, both by directly modulating upstream components of the cell death machinery, such as RIPK1, but also by inducing pro-survival gene expression [47]. An inflammatory response requiring TNFR1 has been shown to be essential also for the pathogenesis of skin lesions in IP female mice, suggesting that TNF-mediated inflammation is an obligatory component of the disease [18, 48]. Indeed, it has been observed that chimeras generated from NEMO-KO ES cells develop IP-like skin lesions, mimicking the cutaneous manifestations seen in human IP patients. However, an interesting observation is that chimeric mice derived from NEMO-KO ES cells do not possess any lymphocytes derived from the NEMO-deficient ES cells. This finding suggests that NEMO-KO lymphocytes are selectively eliminated during development, potentially due to defects in lymphocyte survival and proliferation caused by NEMO deficiency [45]. The latter condition is very similar to the one observed in mosaic human males, where a counterselection against NEMO-deficient cells is necessary for sustaining and complete embryo development in some tissues, such as the fetal liver. Whether or not an equivalent mechanism operates also in other IP-affected tissues (CNS or retina) is an open question. Ultimately, a greater appreciation of the effects of cell death in a specific context will improve our understanding of the altered processes, which are on the basis of symptoms of the most severe IP cases, with global developmental delay, seizures, and blindness [37] to develop tailored therapies.

References

1. Landy SJ, Donnai D. Incontinentia pigmenti (Bloch-Sulzberger syndrome). J Med Genet. 1993;30:53–9.
2. Scheuerle AE, Ursini MV. Incontinentia pigmenti. In: Adam MP, Mirzaa GM, Pagon RA, et al., editors. GeneReviews® [Internet]. Seattle, WA: University of Washington, Seattle; 1999, Updated 2017. p. 1993–2023. https://www.ncbi.nlm.nih.gov/books/NBK1472/
3. Minic S, Trpinac D, Obradovic M. Incontinentia pigmenti diagnostic criteria update. Clin Genet. 2014;85:536–42.
4. Minic S, Trpinac D, Gabriel H, Gencik M, Obradovic M. Dental and oral anomalies in incontinentia pigmenti: a systematic review. Clin Oral Investig. 2013;17:1–8.
5. Chen AY, Chen K. Dental treatment considerations for a pediatric patient with incontinentia pigmenti (Bloch-Sulzberger syndrome). Eur J Dent. 2017;11:264–7.
6. Santa-Maria FD, Mariath LM, Poziomczyk CS, et al. Dental anomalies in 14 patients with IP: clinical and radiological analysis and review. Clin Oral Investig. 2017;21:1845–52.
7. Bodemer C, Diociaiuti A, Hadj-Rabia S, Robert MP, Desguerre I, Manière MC, de la Dure-Molla M, De Liso P, Federici M, Galeotti A, Fusco F, Fraitag S, Demily C, Taieb C, Valeria Ursini M, El Hachem M, Steffann J. Multidisciplinary consensus recommendations from a European network for the diagnosis and practical management of patients with incontinentia pigmenti. J Eur Acad Dermatol Venereol. 2020;34:1415–24. https://doi.org/10.1111/jdv.16403.
8. Minic S, Obradovic M, Kovacevic I, Trpinac D. Ocular anomalies in incontinentia pigmenti: literature review and meta-analysis. Srp Arh Celok Lek. 2010;138:408–13.
9. O'Doherty M, Mc Creery K, Green AJ, Tuwir I, Brosnahan D. Incontinentia pigmenti ophthalmological observation of a series of cases and review of the literature. Br J Ophthalmol. 2011;95:11–6.

10. Swinney CC, Han DP, Karth PA. Incontinentia pigmenti: a comprehensive review and update. Ophthalmic Surg Lasers Imaging Retina. 2015;46:650–7. https://doi.org/10.3928/23258160-20150610-09.
11. Bryan J, Issa R, Bakall B, Welch M, Bryan JS. Retinal manifestations of incontinentia pigmenti: a case series of 14 patients highlighting the importance of intravenous fluorescein angiography and the benefits of early laser photocoagulation. J Vitreoretin Dis. 2021;5:60–5. https://doi.org/10.1177/2474126420962645.
12. Yadlapati S, Tripathy K. Incontinentia pigmenti (Bloch-Sulzberger syndrome). In: StatPearls [Internet]. Treasure Island, FL: StatPearls Publishing; 2023. https://www.ncbi.nlm.nih.gov/books/NBK578194/.
13. Meuwissen ME, Mancini GM. Neurological findings in incontinentia pigmenti; a review. Eur J Med Genet. 2012;55:323–31.
14. Minic S, Trpinac D, Obradovic M. Systematic review of central nervous system anomalies in incontinentia pigmenti. Orphanet J Rare Dis. 2013;8:25.
15. Minić S, Cerovac N, Novaković I, Gazikalović S, Popadić S, Trpinac D. The impact of the IKBKG gene on the appearance of the corpus callosum abnormalities in incontinentia pigmenti. Diagnostics (Basel). 2023;13:1300. https://doi.org/10.3390/diagnostics13071300.
16. Pizzamiglio MR, Piccardi L, Bianchini F, et al. Incontinentia pigmenti: learning disabilities are a fundamental hallmark of the disease. PLoS One. 2014;9:e87771.
17. Pizzamiglio MR, Piccardi L, Bianchini F, et al. Cognitive-behavioural phenotype in a group of girls from 1.2 to 12 years old with the incontinentia pigmenti syndrome: recommendations for clinical management. Appl Neuropsychol Child. 2017;6:327–34.
18. Smahi A, Courtois G, Vabres P, et al. Genomic rearrangement in NEMO impairs NF-kappa B activation and is a cause of incontinentia pigmenti. The international incontinentia pigmenti (IP) consortium. Nature. 2000;405:466–72.
19. Aradhya S, Woffendin H, Jakins T, et al. A recurrent deletion in the ubiquitously expressed NEMO (IKK-gamma) gene accounts for the vast majority of incontinentia pigmenti mutations. Hum Mol Genet. 2001c;10:2171–9.
20. Fusco F, Bardaro T, Fimiani G, et al. Molecular analysis of the genetic defect in a large cohort of IP patients and identification of novel NEMO mutations interfering with NF-kappaB activation. Hum Mol Genet. 2004;13:1763–73.
21. Nelson DL. NEMO, NFkappaB signaling and incontinentia pigmenti. Curr Opin Genet Dev. 2006;16:282–8.
22. Fusco F, Pescatore A, Bal E, Ghoul A, Paciolla M, Lioi MB, D'Urso M, Rabia SH, Bodemer C, Bonnefont JP, Munnich A, Miano MG, Smahi A, Ursini MV. Alterations of the IKBKG locus and diseases: an update and a report of 13 novel mutations. Hum Mutat. 2008;29:595–604. https://doi.org/10.1002/humu.20739. PMID: 18350553
23. Fusco F, Paciolla M, Conte MI, et al. Incontinentia pigmenti: report on data from 2000 to 2013. Orphanet J Rare Dis. 2014;9:93. https://doi.org/10.1186/1750-1172-9-93.
24. Fusco F, Paciolla M, Napolitano F, et al. Genomic architecture at the incontinentia pigmenti locus favours de novo pathological alleles through different mechanisms. Hum Mol Genet. 2012;21:1260–71.
25. Conte MI, Pescatore A, Paciolla M, Esposito E, Miano MG, Lioi MB, McAleer MA, Giardino G, Pignata C, Irvine AD, et al. Insight into IKBKG/NEMO locus: report of new mutations and complex genomic rearrangements leading to incontinentia pigmenti disease. Hum Mutat. 2014;35:165–77.
26. Fusco F, Pescatore A, Conte MI, Mirabelli P, Paciolla M, Esposito E, Lioi MB, Ursini MV. EDA-ID and IP, two faces of the same coin: how the same IKBKG/NEMO mutation affecting the NF-κB pathway can cause immunodeficiency and/or inflammation. Int Rev Immunol. 2015;34:445–59. https://doi.org/10.3109/08830185.2015.1055331.
27. Fusco F, Valente V, Fergola D, Pescatore A, Lioi MB, Ursini MV. The incontinentia pigmenti genetic biobank: study design and cohort profile to facilitate research into a rare disease worldwide. Eur J Hum Genet. 2019;27:1509–18.

28. Fusco F, Mercadante V, Miano MG, Ursini MV. Multiple regulatory regions and tissue-specific transcription initiation mediate the expression of NEMO/IKKgamma gene. Gene. 2006;383:99–107.
29. Aradhya S, Bardaro T, Galgoczy P, et al. Multiple pathogenic and benign genomic rearrangements occur at a 35kb duplication involving the NEMO and LAGE2 genes. Hum Mol Genet. 2001a;10:2557–67.
30. Fusco F, Paciolla M, Pescatore A, et al. Microdeletion/duplication at the Xq28 IP locus causes a de novo IKBKG/NEMO/IKKgamma exon4_10 deletion in families with Incontinentia pigmenti. Hum Mutat. 2009;30:1284–91.
31. Fusco F, D'Urso M, Miano MG, Ursini MV. The LCR at the IKBKG locus is prone to recombine. Am J Hum Genet. 2010;86:650–2.
32. Fusco F, Paciolla M, Napolitano F, Pescatore A, D'Addario I, Bal E, Lioi MB, Smahi A, Miano MG, Ursini MV. Genomic architecture at the incontinentia pigmenti locus favours de novo pathological alleles through different mechanisms. Hum Mol Genet. 2012a;21:1260–71.
33. Fusco F, Pescatore A, Steffann J, Royer G, Bonnefont JP, Ursini MV. Clinical utility gene card for: Incontinentia pigmenti. Eur J Hum Genet. 2012b;21:792.
34. Fusco F, Pescatore A, Steffann J, Bonnefont JP, De Oliveira J, Lioi MB, Ursini MV. Clinical utility gene card: for incontinentia pigmenti. Eur J Hum Genet. 2019;27(12):1894–900. https://doi.org/10.1038/s41431-019-0463-9.
35. Fusco F, Fimiani G, Tadini G, Michele D, Ursini MV. Clinical diagnosis of incontinentia pigmenti in a cohort of male patients. J Am Acad Dermatol. 2007;56:264–7. https://doi.org/10.1016/j.jaad.2006.09.019.
36. Fusco F, Conte MI, Diociaiuti A, Bigoni S, Branda MF, Ferlini A, El Hachem M, Ursini MV. Unusual father-to-daughter transmission of incontinentia pigmenti due to mosaicism in IP males. Pediatrics. 2017;140:e20162950. https://doi.org/10.1542/peds.2016-2950.
37. Pescatore A, Spinosa E, Casale C, Lioi MB, Ursini MV, Fusco F. Human genetic diseases linked to the absence of NEMO: an obligatory somatic mosaic disorder in male. Int J Mol Sci. 2022;23:1179. https://doi.org/10.3390/ijms23031179. PMID: 35163099; PMCID: PMC8835834
38. Kawai M, Kato T, Tsutsumi M, et al. Molecular analysis of low-level mosaicism of the IKBKG mutation using the X Chromosome inactivation pattern in incontinentia pigmenti. Mol Genet Genomic Med. 2020;8:e1531. https://doi.org/10.1002/mgg3.1531. Epub 2020 Oct 21. PMID: 33085210; PMCID: PMC7767561
39. Shibata K, Kunisada M, Miyai S, et al. Incontinentia pigmenti in a female infant with somatic mosaicism due to the IKBKG variant. J Dermatol. 2021;48:e577–8. https://doi.org/10.1111/1346-8138.16141.
40. Hayden MS, Ghosh S. NF-κB, the first quarter-century: remarkable progress and outstanding questions. Genes Dev. 2012;26:203–34. https://doi.org/10.1101/gad.183434.111. PMID: 22302935; PMCID: PMC3278889
41. Maubach G, Schmädicke AC, Naumann M. NEMO links nuclear factor-κB to human diseases. Trends Mol Med. 2017;23:1138–55.
42. Pescatore A, Esposito E, Draber P, Walczak H, Ursini MV. NEMO regulates a cell death switch in TNF signaling by inhibiting recruitment of RIPK3 to the cell death-inducing complex II. Cell Death Dis. 2016;7:e2346.
43. Rudolph D, Yeh WC, Wakeham A, Rudolph B, Nallainathan D, Potter J, Elia AJ, Mak TW. Severe liver degeneration and lack of NF-kappaB activation in NEMO/IKKgamma-deficient mice. Genes Dev. 2000;14:854–62.
44. Makris C, Godfrey VL, Krähn-Senftleben G, et al. Female mice heterozygous for IKK gamma/NEMO deficiencies develop a dermatopathy similar to the human X-linked disorder incontinentia pigmenti. Mol Cell. 2000;5:969–79.
45. Schmidt-Supprian M, Bloch W, Courtois G, et al. NEMO/IKK gamma-deficient mice model incontinentia pigmenti. Mol Cell. 2000;5:981–92.

46. Vlantis K, Wullaert A, Polykratis A, et al. NEMO prevents RIP kinase 1-mediated epithelial cell death and chronic intestinal inflammation by NF-κB-dependent and independent functions. Immunity. 2016;15:553–67.
47. Delanghe T, Dondelinger Y, Bertrand MJM. RIPK1 kinase-dependent death: a symphony of phosphorylation events. Trends Cell Biol. 2020;30:189–200.
48. Nenci A, Huth M, Funteh A, et al. Skin lesion development in a mouse model of incontinentia pigmenti is triggered by NEMO deficiency in epidermal keratinocytes and requires TNF signaling. Hum Mol Genet. 2006;15:531–42.

Chapter 6
Genetic Basis and Molecular Diagnosis of p63-Associated Ectodermal Dysplasia

Daniela Di Girolamo and Caterina Missero

Keywords Cleft palate · Ectrodactyly · Skin erosions · Epidermal development · Phenotype-genotype

6.1 Introduction

Since its identification, the p63 protein, a paralog of the p53 tumor suppressor, has been shown to play a pivotal role as a master regulator of several ectodermal derivatives. In this chapter, we will describe the structure and function of the human TP63 gene and its corresponding p63 proteins. In addition, we will describe the molecular and phenotypic alterations that occur in p63-associated disorders and the differential genetic diagnosis of these syndromes. Finally, we will discuss the potential therapeutic strategies under development for the most severe manifestations.

6.2 Architecture of p63 Gene and Its Protein Products

In humans, the *TP63* gene is composed of 17 exons and is located on chromosome 3q28. The generation of the 13 annotated transcripts is the result of the action of different alternative promoters and splicing sites [1, 2] (Fig. 6.1a). Transcription initiation from exon 1 generates a long transcript encoding the TAp63 variant, which

---

D. Di Girolamo · C. Missero (✉)
CEINGE Biotecnologie Avanzate Franco Salvatore, Naples, Italy

Biology Department, University of Naples Federico II, Naples, Italy
e-mail: missero@ceinge.unina.it

G. Tadini et al. (eds.), *Multidisciplinary Approach to Ectodermal Dysplasia*,
https://doi.org/10.1007/978-3-031-75790-7_6

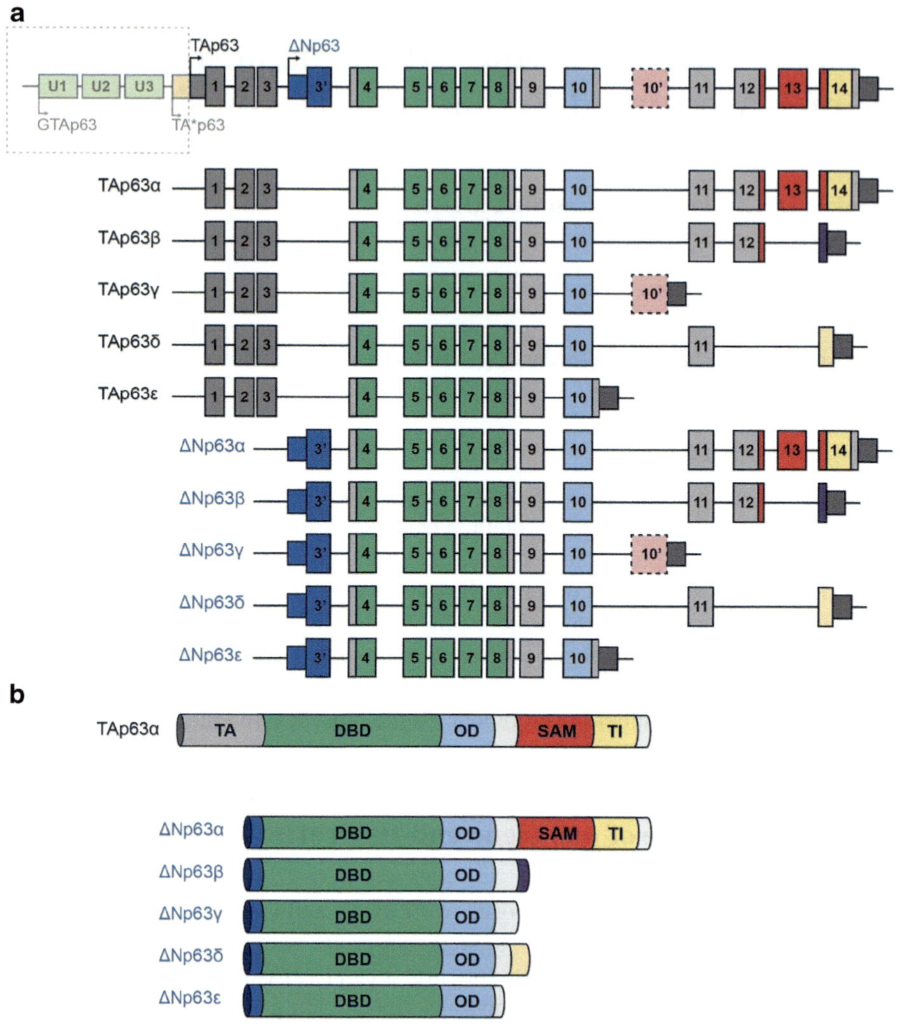

Fig. 6.1 Human *TP63* gene and protein. (**a**) Human *TP63* gene structure. Promoters are indicated by the arrows. Isoforms generated by alternative splicing are indicated. The color code reflects the protein domains. (**b**) Summary of the main p63 protein isoforms found in ectodermal tissues and their domains. Transactivation domain (TA, in gray), alternative transactivation domain (ΔN, in blue), DNA-binding domain (DBD, in green), oligomerization domain (OD, in light blue), sterile alpha motif domain (SAM, in red), and transactivation inhibitory domain (TI, in yellow)

contains an acidic transactivation domain (TA) at the amino-terminal end. A promoter within intron 3 instead directs the transcription from an alternative exon (exon 3′), resulting in a truncated protein, ΔNp63, lacking the TA domain but containing 14 unique amino acid residues with an alternative trans-activating function [3]. At the 3′ end of the gene, several isoforms arise from alternative splicing. The longest isoform, p63α, includes all exons at the 3′ end and is predominantly expressed in ectodermal structures. Alternative splicing events generate shorter protein isoforms, such as p63β, which lacks exon 13, p63γ, which lacks exons 11–14 but contains a γ-specific exon 10′, and p63δ, which lacks exon 12 and 13 [3, 4]. An additional ε isoform results from intron 10 retention and premature transcription termination in the 5′ portion of the intron [4]. In humans, two additional TAp63 isoforms have been identified: the TA*p63α, that has a longer N-terminal domain, and the GATp63α (germ cell-encoded trans-activating p63), generated by fusion of an endogenous retrovirus with exon 2.Previous findings, together with more recent RNA-seq data, demonstrated a selective expression of p63 and its isoforms [2]. ΔNp63α is expressed at high levels (83% on average) in several stratified epithelia, including skin, esophageal mucosa, and vagina, and to a lesser extent in the ectocervix, bladder, salivary gland, prostate, and mammary gland. The second most abundant isoform is ΔNp63β (15% on average). Because of its critical function in epidermal development and its involvement in ectodermal dysplasia (ED)-associated disorders, ΔNp63α will be extensively discussed in detail below, while the relevant function of the TAp63α in the DNA damage response in the ovary is outside of the scope of this chapter and will not be discussed [5, 6]. All p63 isoforms are characterized by an identical zinc-finger DNA-binding domain (DBD) and oligomerization domain (OD) that are similar to those found in p53 (65% and 25% homology, respectively). DNA binding induces protein dimerization mediated by the p63 OD: p63 dimer of dimers (tetramers) forms in the presence of the two half-binding sites on the DNA. Consequently, two p63 DBD dimers interact with each other when the two hemi-sites are adjacent [7]. The DBD contains a loop-sheet-helix motif that consists of the L1 loop, a three-stranded β-sheet (S2, S2′, and S10), and the H2 α-helix [8]. The residues that contact the DNA are R311, A307, C308, R304, and A307, whereas positions H208, C269, and C273 are essential for zinc coordination [7, 9]. Mutations in most of these amino acids are causative of p63-associated syndromes (see below).

At the C-terminal, the longest isoform p63α includes a sterile alpha motif (SAM) and a transactivation inhibitory domain (TID) (Fig. 6.1b). The p63 SAM domain is a compact structure consisting of five helices present only in the p63α isoform [10]. The compact hydrophobic core of the SAM domain is highly conserved and is formed by aliphatic isoleucine and leucine residues [11]. In eukaryotes, the SAM domain is a highly abundant protein interaction domain consisting of ~70 residues that fold into a five-helix bundle. The SAM domain performs multiple functions, acting as a protein-protein interaction domain as well as binding to a variety of substrates, including RNA and lipids [12, 13]. This domain allows head-to-tail closed oligomerization or polymerization, resulting in homo- and/or heterocomplexes that are important for proper protein localization and function. The precise function of the SAM domain in the p63 protein is still unknown; however, the presence of the SAM domain in the p63/p73 orthologous gene in nematodes, mollusks, echinoderms, and urochordates indicates its functional relevance. Structural studies in the p63 orthologous gene (CEP-1) in *C. elegans* have revealed the presence of the SAM domain that contacts the OD domain and may play a role in its stabilization [14].

The last 25 C-terminal amino acids (the C-terminal subdomain) contain classical sumoylation sequences, which regulate the protein concentration [15, 16]. Importantly, mutations in the sumoylation consensus sites (such as Q634X) have been associated with split hand/foot malformation (SHFM) [16].

6.3 p63 Biological Function in Stratified Epithelium Development

Several studies in humans and mice have demonstrated the crucial role of p63 in the commitment of cells from the ectoderm to a keratinocyte cell fate. In mouse embryonic development, at embryonic day 9–9.5 (E9–9.5), the ΔNp63 protein is the first specific keratinocyte-specific marker in the simple epithelium of the surface ectoderm [17, 18]. Starting at E10.5, the expression of the simple epithelial keratins is progressively silenced and the basal layer epithelial keratin 5 (Krt5) and keratin 14 (Krt14) are turned on in a p63-dependent manner [17, 19, 20]. As the surface epithelium undergoes progressive stratification at E14.5, p63 expression is progressively restricted to the proliferative layers.

Studies in p63-deleted mouse models have contributed greatly to our understanding of p63 function and are critical to gaining insight into p63-associated disorders. In p63 null (p63-/-) mice, severe malformations of all stratified epithelia result in neonatal lethality. The absence of p63 leads to the formation of a disorganized epithelium due to the loss of proliferative capacity of epidermal progenitor cells [21, 22] and their inability to undergo proper stratification and differentiation [19, 23]. Consistent with the disorganized epidermis, p63-/- ectodermal derivatives such as mammary glands, hair follicles, and teeth are absent. Other developmental abnormalities include severe craniofacial abnormalities due to aberrant morphogenesis of the medial nasal, lateral nasal, and maxillary processes [22–24]. In addition, p63-/- mice are characterized by severely underdeveloped hind limbs and truncated forelimbs. Defective limb formation is dependent on the inability to properly form the apical ectodermal ridge (AER), a stratified epithelium at the tip of the growing limb that is essential for limb morphogenesis [22, 23]. In particular, the AER fails to stratify in homozygous p63-/- mice due to the downregulation of AER-specific target genes such as the Dlx5 and Dlx6 genes [25]. Similar defects are observed in homozygous ΔNp63-/- mice, including poorly developed stratified epidermis, craniofacial malformations, truncated forelimbs, and absence of hindlimbs [26], strongly suggesting that ΔNp63 is the predominant isoform required for the formation of stratified epithelia.A similar maturation of ectodermal cells into keratinocytes is observed in embryonic stem cells (ESCs) [20, 27, 28]. Studies in mouse ESCs have shown that epidermal (and corneal) lineage commitment occurs through a retinoic acid- and BMP4-dependent initiation step that turns on p63 expression, which in turn is essential for the maturation steps [27–30]. In human ESCs, the transcription factor AP-2 gamma (TFAP2C) initially drives chromatin dynamics and activates the expression of epithelial genes, including p63 itself and the simple epithelial keratins Krt8/Krt18 during the initiation phase [31]. Subsequently, p63 activates transcription of epidermal genes, including Krt5 and Krt14, as well as its own transcription through an autoregulatory loop [31–33]. Consistent with these observations, organotypic cultures of postnatal human epidermal keratinocytes lacking p63 form hypoplastic and hypoproliferative epithelium, characterized by ectopic expression of simple keratins and loss of basal Krt5/Krt14 and terminal differentiation markers [34].

6.4 Causative Mutations in the *TP63* Gene in Syndromic and Non-syndromic Diseases

Syndromic disorders associated with *TP63* mutations follow an autosomal dominant pattern and are associated with abnormal development of stratified epithelia. A variety of manifestations characterize these conditions, the most common being ED, orofacial clefts (OFC), and limb malformations. However, defects in genitourinary development, lacrimal and meibomian glands, cornea, and ear have been associated with all p63-related syndromes. p63-associated disorders include ectrodactyly, ectodermal dysplasia and cleft lip/palate syndrome (EEC) (OMIM 604292), ankyloblepharon-ectodermal defects cleft lip/palate syndrome (AEC) (OMIM 106260), Rapp-Hodgkin syndrome (RHS) (OMIM 129400), limb-mammary syndrome (LMS) (OMIM 603543), and acro-dermato-ungual-lacrimal-tooth syndrome (ADULT) (OMIM 103285) [35]. Notably, these syndromes exhibit substantial phenotypic differences, with specific mutations clustering in regions of the *TP63* gene that encode specific domains of the protein (Figs. 6.2a and 6.3). This indicates a correlation between genotype and phenotype and suggests specific pathogenic mechanisms for each syndrome. In addition, specific mutations in the TP63 gene have been associated with non-syndromic conditions such as SHFM4 (OMIM 605289) and OFC8 (OMIM 618149).In this section, we provide a brief description of the p63-associated syndromes and their corresponding mutations.

6.4.1 Ankyloblepharon-Ectodermal Defects Cleft Lip/Palate Syndrome (AEC) Syndrome

AEC syndrome is a rare severe disorder with fewer than 100 affected individuals described in the medical literature. Mutations associated with AEC syndrome are mainly found in exons 13 and 14, which encode the C-terminal domain of the p63α isoform [36]. They typically manifest as missense mutations that occur predominantly in the SAM domain. However, missense or single nucleotide frameshift mutations have also been found in the TI domain, the latter resulting in an extension

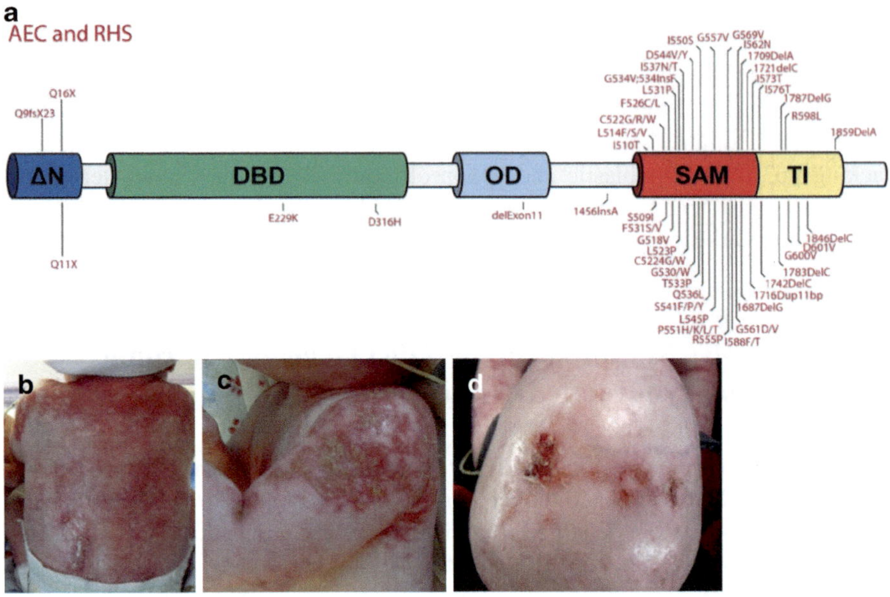

Fig. 6.2 AEC syndrome mutations and phenotype. (**a**) AEC and RHS mutations are mainly clustered in the SAM and TI domains of the *TP63* gene. Mutations in individuals affected by AEC and RHS syndromes are indicated. *DBD* DNA-binding domain, *OD* oligomerization domain, *SAM* sterile alpha motif domain, *TI* transactivation inhibitory domain. (**b**) Reticulated scarring is typically seen in infants affected by AEC syndrome as a result of skin erosions. A bulla (a large blister) is also present in the lower portion of the back. (**c**) Residual hemorrhagic crusting and scarring. (**d**) Scarring alopecia and residual erosion of the scalp. Photos courtesy of V.P. Sybert, M.D. University of Washington, Seattle (USA)

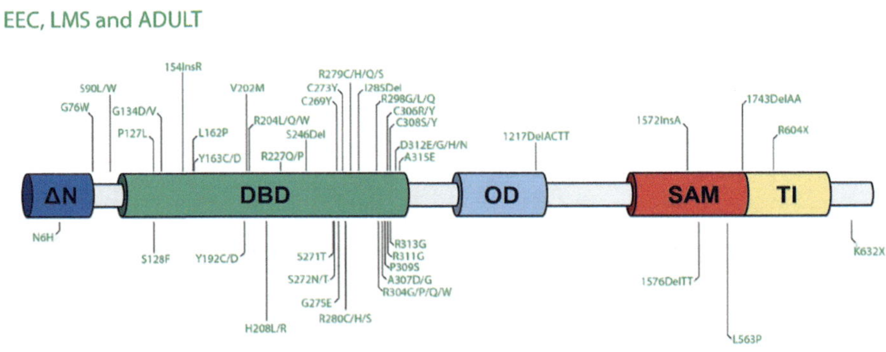

Fig. 6.3 *TP63* mutations in ELA syndromes (including EEC, LMS, and ADULT syndromes) are mainly but not exclusively clustered in the DBD domain

of the amino acid sequence [36]. Both types of mutations lead to thermodynamic protein destabilization, misfolding, and aggregation [37]. In turn, these mutant proteins exhibit reduced DNA binding and impaired transcriptional activity, leading to dominant-negative effects due to co-aggregation with wild-type p63 and the cognate protein p73. Aggregation of the p63 protein in AEC syndrome results in severe epidermal defects, contributing to the skin fragility observed in affected individuals [37].

AEC syndrome was first documented in 1976 by Hay and Wells, who found the same phenotypic abnormalities in seven affected individuals from four families; consequently, it was initially named Hay-Wells syndrome [38]. To date, a condition previously annotated as RHS syndrome is considered a phenotypic variant of AEC syndrome, not only because of the overlap in clinical manifestations but also because of the presence of mutations in the same p63 region [39]. RHS/AEC syndrome can also result from mutations that introduce a premature termination in the N-terminal region of the p63 protein (e.g., p.Gln9fsX23, p.Gln11X, and p.Gln16X) [40]. A second start codon in exon 4 is used in order to produce an ΔΔNp63 isoform, which exerts a dominant-negative effect on the wild-type protein.

Clinical manifestations: Individuals with AEC syndrome typically present with several distinctive features [38, 41–44], as detailed below.

1. **Craniofacial anomalies**, which include:

   - Cleft palate is observed in almost all patients and is characterized by a cleft of the soft palate with or without a cleft of the hard palate and lip; the cleft may be bilateral or unilateral;
   - Nasal septum deviation and chronic sinusitis;
   - Chronic ear inflammation and infection, scarring of the tympanic membrane, otitis media, stenosis of the external auditory canal, and hearing loss [45];
   - Distinctive facial appearance with short philtrum length, small ears, and decreased canthal distance;
   - High incidence of maxillary hypoplasia and missing permanent maxillary incisors and canines compared to other ED syndrome; hypodontia in both primary and/or permanent teeth; conical-shaped incisors and narrow occlusal table in molars are typical [46].

2. **Skin fragility** is associated with erosions, blisters, or bullae in areas of friction or trauma. Skin erosions are the most severe manifestation of this disorder and can vary in intensity and location [47]. They frequently affect the scalp, head and neck, skin folds, palms, and/or soles and are often associated with crusting, granulation tissue, and secondary infection (Fig. 6.2b–d). They occur at birth or in infancy and may recur and/or persist for a very long time, leading to secondary infections and affecting the patient's quality of life. Healing results in scarring alopecia on the scalp or reticular scarring on the rest of the body. In adults, skin erosions are rare and may occur on friction points such as the palms or soles. A colloidal skin manifestation and frequent extensive erosions at birth may lead to an initial misdiagnosis of epidermolysis bullosa (EB). The most severe erosions

involve the scalp, whereas erosions elsewhere tend to be more superficial than the bullae and erosions of EB. Atrophy, erythema, hyperkeratosis, ichthyosiform scale, skin hypopigmentation, or hyperpigmentation are typical of giving the skin a mottled appearance. Keratoderma of the palms and soles is also typical [47].

Histology reveals relatively subtle changes in non-affected areas, including mild hyperkeratosis, epidermal atrophy, hypo- and hyperpigmentation and/or pigment incontinence, and dermal edema with mild perivascular lymphocytic infiltrate [48–51].

3. **Phenotypes associated with ED**:
   - Scalp hair is sparse, thin, wiry, and brittle, and in people of Caucasian origin of fair color; sparse or absent eyebrows, eyelashes, and body hair; microscopically the hair shafts are irregular including pili torti and focal grooved contours;
   - Nails are absent or dystrophic;
   - Decreased function of sweat glands (hypohidrosis) [52].
4. **Ankyloblepharon filiforme adnatum and ocular manifestations**: the presence of single or multiple thin bands of connective tissue between the upper and lower eyelids, preventing full opening of the eye, which can lead to eye complications if left untreated [38, 41, 42]; lacrimal duct obstruction; blepharitis; absence of Meibomian glands; and corneal erosions (see EEC syndrome for further details).
5. **Limb defects**: frequent syndactyly (fusion of fingers or toes); split hand and foot malformation has been rarely observed in AEC syndrome [53–55].
6. **Difficulty with feeding** and gastrostomy placement is often necessary and is not a mere consequence of cleft palate [56, 57].
7. **Hypoplastic or absent nipples**
8. **Genitourinary abnormalities**, such as hypospadias and rare renal involvement;
9. **Alteration of the immune system**: one child was diagnosed with autoimmune lymphoproliferative syndrome (ALPS) [58], in the other two cases T-cell lymphopenia was observed [55, 59]. This latter phenotype may be linked to the expression of p63 in the thymic epithelial cells. In support of this possibility, studies in mice have shown that deletion of p63 specifically in thymic epithelial cells causes severe thymic and peripheral T-cell lymphopenia [60].

Although symptoms vary from person to person, the most serious aspect of this condition is skin erosion, which often causes severe pain, interferes with daily activities, and requires extensive care. Currently, there are no effective treatments for skin erosion, and the primary care of AEC patients is to prevent skin infection.The skin fragility observed in AEC syndrome has led researchers to focus on the critical role of p63 in cell-cell and cell-matrix adhesion. In normal skin, p63 binds to enhancer regions of desmosomal genes and regulates their expression. Desmocollin 3 (Dsc3), desmoplakin (Dsp), and desmoglein 1 (Dsg1) were severely reduced in p63 mutant mice mimicking AEC syndrome [61]. Similarly, another component of the desmosome, PERP1, was downregulated in the skin of individuals with AEC syndrome [62]. In addition, there was a reduction in the expression of the Pvrl1 and Pvrl4 genes, which encode components of adherens junctions, observed both in patients and in a conditional mouse model of AEC syndrome [63]. Reduced expression was also observed for genes encoding the basement membrane proteins Fraser extracellular matrix complex subunit 1 (FRAS1) and collagen VII (COL7A1) [48, 64]. In addition, defective proliferation of epidermal progenitor cells associated with reduced expression of the Fgfr2 and Fgfr3 genes has been observed in heterozygous AEC mutant mice and in skin from AEC patients, which may at least partially explain the epidermal atrophy observed at the histologic level [65, 66].

In conclusion, p63-mediated skin fragility in AEC syndrome is a complex phenotype that likely results from multiple defects, including desmosome alterations and cell-matrix adhesion defects. Understanding the molecular mechanisms underlying these defects is critical to developing effective treatments for the skin erosions observed in AEC patients.

6.4.2 Ectrodactyly, Ectodermal Dysplasia and Cleft Lip/Palate Syndrome (EEC) Syndrome

EEC syndrome is the most common of the ectodermal-associated disorders caused by p63 mutations. It is characterized by the triad of ectrodactyly, ectodermal dysplasia, and facial clefts (cleft lip/palate) and is caused predominantly by missense mutations in the DBD, which is critical for direct interactions with DNA target sequences. The most frequent mutations are in arginine residues R204, R227, R279, R280, R298, and R304, accounting for 75% of all EEC syndrome cases, with the most reported aminoacidic alterations being R204W/Q, R279C/H/Q, R280C/H/S, and R304W/Q (Fig. 6.3) [67]. Interestingly, mutations of these residues may affect in a different way the phenotypic manifestation [68]. For example, a mutation in the arginine R304 is associated with severe cleft lip/palate phenotype, while patients with a mutation in the arginine R227 rarely present this malformation [68], further indicating that different impairing mechanisms are in place.

Some mutations in the p63 DBD affect direct DNA contacts, while others target the zinc coordinating residues and induce the extrusion of the zinc ion [69]. In addition, mutations in the H2 helix disrupt the folding and/or the position of the DNA-contacting residues. Finally, some scattered mutations in the DBD cause defects in the DBD/DBD interface affecting dimerization or tetramerization; for example, R227Q and R298Q bind to incomplete p63 consensus sequences [69].

As in all other p63-associated disorders, mutations occur in heterozygosity and have a dominant-negative function by inactivating tetramers composed of mutant and wild-type proteins. In addition, the EEC mutant p63 has a longer half-life than its wild-type counterpart, leading to an accumulation of tetramers composed predominantly of the mutant proteins [70].

6.5 Clinical Manifestations

1. **Craniofacial abnormalities:** cleft lip and palate, depending on the mutation, facial maxillary hypoplasia (Fig. 6.4).
2. **Ectodermal dysplasia:** skin is thin and dry, with hypokeratosis, hypopigmentation, and/or increased freckles; dystrophic nails with pits, hypotrichosis, microdontia, and hypodontia.
3. **Limb abnormalities:** ectrodactyly also known as split hand/split foot malformation and syndactyly (Fig. 6.5).
4. **Ocular manifestations:** similar to AEC syndrome, associated with the absence of meibomian glands resulting in faster tear evaporation, lacrimal duct abnormalities and reduced aqueous tear production, and defects in the tear drainage system (absence, occlusion, or stenosis); corneal scarring and conjunctivalization (cornea covered by a dense vascularized corneal pannus), thought to be caused by limbal stem cell deficiency and ultimately leading to visual impairment [71–73].
5. **Other defects:** hypospadias, malformation of the kidney, ureters, or bladder, which are most frequently seen in association with mutation in R227. In addition, diffuse large B-cell type non-Hodgkin lymphoma [74, 75] and arrhythmogenic right ventricular cardiomyopathy [76, 77] have been described.

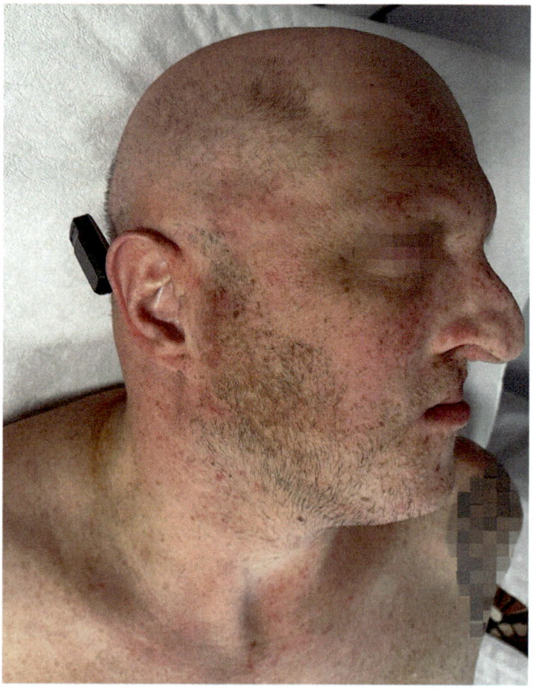

Fig. 6.4 Facies of an adult patient with EEC syndrome

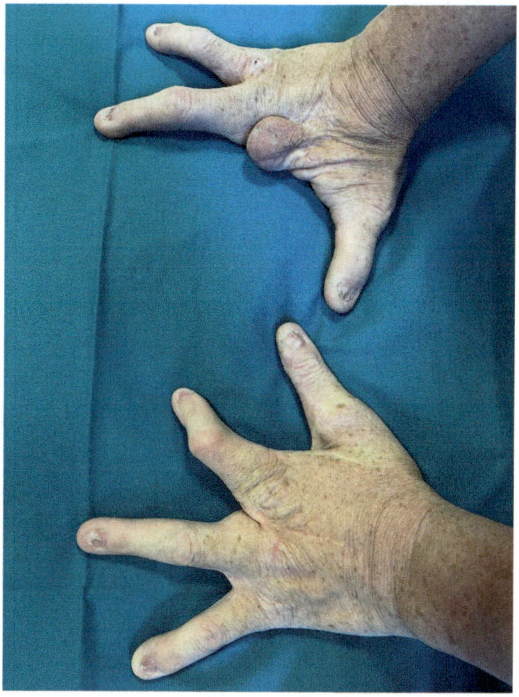

Fig. 6.5 Ectrodactyly in EEC syndrome

6.5.1 Limb-Mammary (LMS) and Acro-Dermato-Ungual-Lacrimal-Tooth (ADULT) Syndromes

LMS is a rare autosomal dominant disorder characterized by variable expressivity of severe hand and/or foot anomalies, hypoplasia/aplasia of the mammary gland and nipple, and other less common findings such as lacrimal duct atresia, nail dysplasia, hypohidrosis, hypodontia, and cleft palate, usually involving only the palate and not the lip. LMS is caused by missense variants in the DBD, such as R204Q and R227Q, found in LSM patients and have been identified also in patients with EEC (Fig. 6.3). In addition, SAM domain truncating variants have been observed in exon 13 or in exon 14 (1693-1694DelTT and 1860-1861DelAA), which lead to premature termination of the protein in contrast to the deletions and insertions found in AEC syndrome that lead to a frameshift and an extension of the protein [78].

ADULT syndrome causes ED, primary hypodontia and early loss of permanent teeth, excessive freckling and dry skin, frontal alopecia, dysplastic nails, lacrimal duct atresia, breast hypoplasia, and ectrodactyly [79, 80] and differs from LMS syndrome mainly by the absence of a cleft palate. Urinary retention, vesicoureteral reflux, prominent ears, and conductive hearing loss have also been described [81]. The pathogenic variants typically associated with this condition reside mainly in the DBD, with the hotspot mutation in residue R298 (R298G/Q). Mutations in this residue moderately affect the DNA-binding ability of the p63 protein [68, 69, 79].

Not only are these syndromes very similar to EEC, but their mutations are often the same as those found in EEC. LMS is similar to EEC but is also characterized by additional nipple and/or mammary gland hypoplasia, while ADULT is similar to LMS but lacks cleft lip/palate. Due to the wide range of phenotypic variability and overlapping mutations, it was proposed in 2011 to classify EEC, LMS, and ADULT syndromes into a single entity called ELA (EEC, LMS, and ADULT) syndrome [82] (Fig. 6.3).

6.5.2 *Non-syndromic Diseases Associated with* TP63 *Mutations*

Loss-of-function mutations dispersed throughout the *TP63* gene are associated with non-syndromic diseases, such as SHFM4 and OFC8 [83–86]. SHFM4 is a limb malformation characterized by the absence of central rays of the autopod, resulting in syndactyly and median clefts of the hands and/or feet. Mutations associated with this defect are often located in the C-terminal domain and involve sumoylation sites, impacting p63 protein stability [16, 35, 87]. Mutational overlap between EEC and SHFM4 has also been described. In particular, the R243Q mutation was found in both conditions [88].

Likewise, OFC8, a complex disorder characterized by unilateral or bilateral cleft lip or cleft lip/palate, is also associated with heterozygous mutations in the *TP63* gene, distributed across the entire p63 sequence [89, 90]. These mutations are usually associated with the introduction of a premature stop codon in the DBD resulting in loss-of-function mutations [91].

6.6 Molecular Diagnosis of p63-Associated Syndromes

Individuals with clinical signs of ED, hand/foot abnormalities, and/or facial clefting should be screened for *TP63* mutations. To this end, genomic DNA is isolated from peripheral blood and subjected to genetic testing by different technologies including Sanger sequencing or next generation sequencing (exome sequencing) to detect small deletions or insertions, non-sense and missense mutations, and mutations in splicing sites (see below). The proportion of individuals with a *TP63*-related disorder caused by a de novo *TP63* pathogenic variant is approximately 70%, whereas in the remaining 30% of the cases, the variant is inherited by a parent. The absence of clinical symptoms in the parents of the proband does not necessarily mean that they do not carry the mutation, as paucisymptomatic or non-symptomatic individuals giving rise to affected children have been observed. If a parent of the proband is affected and/or has the pathogenic variant identified in the proband, the risk to the sibs is 50% given the autosomal dominant nature of the TP63 disorders. Once the

TP63 pathogenic variant has been identified in an affected family member, prenatal and preimplantation genetic testing are possible by targeted mutation analysis.

In the presence of a proband with clinical symptoms typical of p63-associated syndromes, the molecular diagnosis can be based specifically on the analysis of the *TP63* gene (single-gene testing). The entire coding sequence, including intron-exon boundaries of the *TP63* gene, is amplified by Polymerase Chain Reaction (PCR) and subsequently sequenced by Sanger sequencing (for oligonucleotide sequences and detailed protocol, see [78]). Alternatively, if the condition is not clinically distinguishable from similar conditions, a panel of genes can be employed (multigene panel). The use of multigene panels that include *TP63* and other genes of interest is more likely to uncover the genetic etiology of the disorder while reducing the detection of variants of unknown importance. Multigene panels for p63-related syndromes are available in several diagnostic centers in Europe (https://www.orpha.net) and include between 12 and 253 genes. Genes mutated in ED classified in OMIM are 88 (https://www.omim.org), most of which are transcriptional targets of p63 itself and/or NF-KB, or IRF6 [92].

In addition to focused gene panels, genome-wide screening using exome sequencing or whole-genome sequencing (WGS) can be performed to identify novel causative genes, regulatory sequences, or modifier genes. Exome sequencing allows the recognition of the majority of current disease-causing variants, most of which fall in the coding regions. With currently available techniques, WGS is more rarely employed because it is less cost effective and more difficult to interpret. However, WGS has the potential to identify variants in transcription regulatory regions such as enhancers and promoters that may be relevant modifiers of the expressivity of the disorder.Thousands of genetic variants have been identified as the cause of monogenic disorders, mostly determined through small clinical studies, and thus, the penetrance and expressivity of these variants may be overestimated when compared to their effect on the general population. However, bioinformatic analyses of WGS and exome sequencing data available for thousands of individuals have revealed that none of the p63 causative mutations reported in patients is found in the general population (unpublished observation).

Other genetic screenings have recently been employed in a large study to identify deletions or loss-of-function mutations in the *TP63* gene associated with OFC [91]. This multiple approach has revealed for the first time that loss-of-function alleles in *TP63* can also contribute to the development of OFC. Single nucleotide polymorphism (SNP) microarrays and copy number variation (CNV) arrays have been used to identify deletions encompassing parts of the *TP63* gene. Using these methods, three large deletions at 3q28 encompassing *TP63* have been identified [91]. In the same study, targeted multiplex sequencing using molecular inversion probes (MIPs) has been used, which is a reliable and economical approach for target-specific capture and re-sequence candidate genes in thousands of patients [93, 94]. Among the identified variants, two were loss-of-function alleles, including one frameshift and one-stop variant in the DBD [91].

6.7 Potential Therapeutic Approaches to Treat Severe Manifestations of p63-Associated Syndromes

Given the complexity of p63-associated disorders, a multidisciplinary team of specialists in clinical genetics, dermatology, ophthalmology, otolaryngology, audiology, dentistry and prosthodontics, plastic surgery, nutrition/gastroenterology, nephrology, and psychology is recommended.

Skin erosions are treated with gentle wound care and periodic dilute bleach soaks or potassium permanganate baths/soaks and medical honey to prevent secondary infection [55]. Infants with severe skin erosions should be closely monitored and treated for dehydration, electrolyte imbalances, and malnutrition.

Studies of induced pluripotent stem cells (iPS) derived from individuals affected by EEC or AEC syndrome have shown that a p53-reactivating compound called APR-246 or PRIMA-1MET can rescue morphological features and gene expression during epidermal and corneal differentiation [95, 96]. Some features of epidermal differentiation were also rescued by PRIMA-1MET treatment in primary keratinocytes isolated from two AEC patients [97]. On this basis, these patients were treated topically with PRIMA-1MET, and significant improvement in chronic skin erosions was observed [97]. Further studies will be required to understand the molecular basis of PRIMA-1MET's action and to validate the encouraging results obtained on skin erosions. Other approaches are currently being tested by combining genetic and cellular correction or in vivo topical therapy, such as those that have been applied successfully for EB [98, 99].

Ocular manifestations are also critical to address; early correct diagnosis and appropriate therapy are needed to avoid excessive ocular surface insults and to maintain ocular surface integrity. As described above, reduced limbal stem cell performance in the cornea is associated with meibomian gland dysfunction, lacrimal duct obstruction, lacrimal duct deficiency, and ankyloblepharon. Given the various defects, corneal transplantation has not been successful, and other potential strategies have been extensively discussed elsewhere [100]. A potentially interesting approach is the use of mutant allele-specific small interfering RNAs [101], but such a strategy should be developed ad hoc for each single mutation, and the efficiency of small interfering RNA internalization in limbal stem cells should be tested *in vivo*.

Acknowledgements We thank Virgina Sybert, M.D. for providing photographs of individuals with AEC syndrome, and Lorenzo Manduca (manducalorenzo@gmail.com) for the illustrations. We acknowledge the support of the Telethon Foundation (Italy) (GGP20124 to C.M.) for research on AEC syndrome. We also wish to acknowledge the Italian Association for Cancer Research (AIRC) for its continuous support of p63-related research in cancer (IG2022).

References

1. Sethi I, Romano RA, Gluck C, Smalley K, Vojtesek B, Buck MJ, et al. A global analysis of the complex landscape of isoforms and regulatory networks of p63 in human cells and tissues. BMC Genomics. 2015;16:584. https://doi.org/10.1186/s12864-015-1793-9.
2. Marshall CB, Beeler JS, Lehmann BD, Gonzalez-Ericsson P, Sanchez V, Sanders ME, et al. Tissue-specific expression of p73 and p63 isoforms in human tissues. Cell Death Dis. 2021;12(8):745. https://doi.org/10.1038/s41419-021-04017-8.
3. Yang A, Kaghad M, Wang Y, Gillett E, Fleming MD, Dotsch V, et al. p63, a p53 homolog at 3q27-29, encodes multiple products with transactivating, death-inducing, and dominant-negative activities. Mol Cell. 1998;2(3):305–16. https://doi.org/10.1016/s1097-2765(00)80275-0.
4. Mangiulli M, Valletti A, Caratozzolo MF, Tullo A, Sbisa E, Pesole G, et al. Identification and functional characterization of two new transcriptional variants of the human p63 gene. Nucleic Acids Res. 2009;37(18):6092–104. https://doi.org/10.1093/nar/gkp674.
5. Suh EK, Yang A, Kettenbach A, Bamberger C, Michaelis AH, Zhu Z, et al. p63 protects the female germ line during meiotic arrest. Nature. 2006;444(7119):624–8. https://doi.org/10.1038/nature05337.
6. Lena AM, Rossi V, Osterburg S, Smirnov A, Osterburg C, Tuppi M, et al. The p63 C-terminus is essential for murine oocyte integrity. Nat Commun. 2021;12(1):383. https://doi.org/10.1038/s41467-020-20669-0.
7. Chen C, Gorlatova N, Kelman Z, Herzberg O. Structures of p63 DNA binding domain in complexes with half-site and with spacer-containing full response elements. Proc Natl Acad Sci USA. 2011;108(16):6456–61. https://doi.org/10.1073/pnas.1013657108.
8. Osterburg C, Dotsch V. Structural diversity of p63 and p73 isoforms. Cell Death Differ. 2022;29(5):921–37. https://doi.org/10.1038/s41418-022-00975-4.
9. Osterburg C, Osterburg S, Zhou H, Missero C, Dotsch V. Isoform-specific roles of mutant p63 in human diseases. Cancers (Basel). 2021;13(3):536. https://doi.org/10.3390/cancers13030536.
10. Thanos CD, Bowie JU. p53 family members p63 and p73 are SAM domain-containing proteins. Protein Sci. 1999;8(8):1708–10. https://doi.org/10.1110/ps.8.8.1708.
11. Sathyamurthy A, Freund SM, Johnson CM, Allen MD, Bycroft M. Structural basis of p63alpha SAM domain mutants involved in AEC syndrome. FEBS J. 2011;278(15):2680–8. https://doi.org/10.1111/j.1742-4658.2011.08194.x.
12. Wang N, Guo L, Rueda BR, Tilly JL. Cables1 protects p63 from proteasomal degradation to ensure deletion of cells after genotoxic stress. EMBO Rep. 2010;11(8):633–9. https://doi.org/10.1038/embor.2010.82.
13. Fomenkov A, Huang YP, Topaloglu O, Brechman A, Osada M, Fomenkova T, et al. P63 alpha mutations lead to aberrant splicing of keratinocyte growth factor receptor in the Hay-Wells syndrome. J Biol Chem. 2003;278(26):23906–14. https://doi.org/10.1074/jbc.M300746200.
14. Ou HD, Lohr F, Vogel V, Mantele W, Dotsch V. Structural evolution of C-terminal domains in the p53 family. EMBO J. 2007;26(14):3463–73. https://doi.org/10.1038/sj.emboj.7601764.
15. Straub WE, Weber TA, Schafer B, Candi E, Durst F, Ou HD, et al. The C-terminus of p63 contains multiple regulatory elements with different functions. Cell Death Dis. 2010;1(1):e5. https://doi.org/10.1038/cddis.2009.1.
16. Huang YP, Wu G, Guo Z, Osada M, Fomenkov T, Park HL, et al. Altered sumoylation of p63alpha contributes to the split-hand/foot malformation phenotype. Cell Cycle. 2004;3(12):1587–96. https://doi.org/10.4161/cc.3.12.1290.
17. Tadeu AM, Horsley V. Notch signaling represses p63 expression in the developing surface ectoderm. Development. 2013;140(18):3777–86. https://doi.org/10.1242/dev.093948.

18. Fan X, Wang D, Burgmaier JE, Teng Y, Romano RA, Sinha S, et al. Single cell and open chromatin analysis reveals molecular origin of epidermal cells of the skin. Dev Cell. 2018;47(1):21–37 e5. https://doi.org/10.1016/j.devcel.2018.08.010.
19. Koster MI, Kim S, Mills AA, DeMayo FJ, Roop DR. p63 is the molecular switch for initiation of an epithelial stratification program. Genes Dev. 2004;18(2):126–31. https://doi.org/10.1101/gad.1165104.
20. Richardson RJ, Hammond NL, Coulombe PA, Saloranta C, Nousiainen HO, Salonen R, et al. Periderm prevents pathological epithelial adhesions during embryogenesis. J Clin Invest. 2014;124(9):3891–900. https://doi.org/10.1172/JCI71946.
21. Senoo M, Pinto F, Crum CP, McKeon F. p63 is essential for the proliferative potential of stem cells in stratified epithelia. Cell. 2007;129(3):523–36. https://doi.org/10.1016/j.cell.2007.02.045.
22. Yang A, Schweitzer R, Sun D, Kaghad M, Walker N, Bronson RT, et al. p63 is essential for regenerative proliferation in limb, craniofacial and epithelial development. Nature. 1999;398(6729):714–8. https://doi.org/10.1038/19539.
23. Mills AA, Zheng B, Wang XJ, Vogel H, Roop DR, Bradley A. p63 is a p53 homologue required for limb and epidermal morphogenesis. Nature. 1999;398(6729):708–13. https://doi.org/10.1038/19531.
24. Thomason HA, Dixon MJ, Dixon J. Facial clefting in Tp63 deficient mice results from altered Bmp4, Fgf8 and Shh signaling. Dev Biol. 2008;321(1):273–82. https://doi.org/10.1016/j.ydbio.2008.06.030.
25. Lo Iacono N, Mantero S, Chiarelli A, Garcia E, Mills AA, Morasso MI, et al. Regulation of Dlx5 and Dlx6 gene expression by p63 is involved in EEC and SHFM congenital limb defects. Development. 2008;135(7):1377–88. https://doi.org/10.1242/dev.011759.
26. Romano RA, Smalley K, Magraw C, Serna VA, Kurita T, Raghavan S, et al. DeltaNp63 knockout mice reveal its indispensable role as a master regulator of epithelial development and differentiation. Development. 2012;139(4):772–82. https://doi.org/10.1242/dev.071191.
27. Aberdam E, Barak E, Rouleau M, de LaForest S, Berrih-Aknin S, Suter DM, et al. A pure population of ectodermal cells derived from human embryonic stem cells. Stem Cells. 2008;26(2):440–4. https://doi.org/10.1634/stemcells.2007-0588.
28. Shalom-Feuerstein R, Lena AM, Zhou H, De La Forest DS, Van Bokhoven H, Candi E, et al. DeltaNp63 is an ectodermal gatekeeper of epidermal morphogenesis. Cell Death Differ. 2011;18(5):887–96. https://doi.org/10.1038/cdd.2010.159.
29. Medawar A, Virolle T, Rostagno P, de la Forest-Divonne S, Gambaro K, Rouleau M, et al. DeltaNp63 is essential for epidermal commitment of embryonic stem cells. PLoS One. 2008;3(10):e3441. https://doi.org/10.1371/journal.pone.0003441.
30. Gambaro K, Aberdam E, Virolle T, Aberdam D, Rouleau M. BMP-4 induces a Smad-dependent apoptotic cell death of mouse embryonic stem cell-derived neural precursors. Cell Death Differ. 2006;13(7):1075–87. https://doi.org/10.1038/sj.cdd.4401799.
31. Li L, Wang Y, Torkelson JL, Shankar G, Pattison JM, Zhen HH, et al. TFAP2C- and p63-dependent networks sequentially rearrange chromatin landscapes to drive human epidermal lineage commitment. Cell Stem Cell. 2019;24(2):271–84 e8. https://doi.org/10.1016/j.stem.2018.12.012.
32. Antonini D, Sirico A, Aberdam E, Ambrosio R, Campanile C, Fagoonee S, et al. A composite enhancer regulates p63 gene expression in epidermal morphogenesis and in keratinocyte differentiation by multiple mechanisms. Nucleic Acids Res. 2015;43(2):862–74. https://doi.org/10.1093/nar/gku1396.
33. Antonini D, Rossi B, Han R, Minichiello A, Di Palma T, Corrado M, et al. An autoregulatory loop directs the tissue-specific expression of p63 through a long-range evolutionarily conserved enhancer. Mol Cell Biol. 2006;26(8):3308–18. https://doi.org/10.1128/MCB.26.8.3308-3318.2006.
34. Truong AB, Kretz M, Ridky TW, Kimmel R, Khavari PA. p63 regulates proliferation and differentiation of developmentally mature keratinocytes. Genes Dev. 2006;20(22):3185–97. https://doi.org/10.1101/gad.1463206.

35. Rinne T, Brunner HG, van Bokhoven H. p63-associated disorders. Cell Cycle. 2007;6(3):262–8. https://doi.org/10.4161/cc.6.3.3796.
36. Rinne T, Bolat E, Meijer R, Scheffer H, van Bokhoven H. Spectrum of p63 mutations in a selected patient cohort affected with ankyloblepharon-ectodermal defects-cleft lip/palate syndrome (AEC). Am J Med Genet A. 2009;149A(9):1948–51. https://doi.org/10.1002/ajmg.a.32793.
37. Russo C, Osterburg C, Sirico A, Antonini D, Ambrosio R, Wurz JM, et al. Protein aggregation of the p63 transcription factor underlies severe skin fragility in AEC syndrome. Proc Natl Acad Sci USA. 2018;115(5):E906–E15. https://doi.org/10.1073/pnas.1713773115.
38. Hay RJ, Wells RS. The syndrome of ankyloblepharon, ectodermal defects and cleft lip and palate: an autosomal dominant condition. Br J Dermatol. 1976;94(3):277–89.
39. Clements SE, Techanukul T, Holden ST, Mellerio JE, Dorkins H, Escande F, et al. Rapp-Hodgkin and Hay-Wells ectodermal dysplasia syndromes represent a variable spectrum of the same genetic disorder. Br J Dermatol. 2010;163(3):624–9. https://doi.org/10.1111/j.1365-2133.2010.09859.x.
40. Rinne T, Clements SE, Lamme E, Duijf PH, Bolat E, Meijer R, et al. A novel translation re-initiation mechanism for the p63 gene revealed by amino-terminal truncating mutations in Rapp-Hodgkin/Hay-Wells-like syndromes. Hum Mol Genet. 2008;17(13):1968–77. https://doi.org/10.1093/hmg/ddn094.
41. McGrath JA, Duijf PH, Doetsch V, Irvine AD, de Waal R, Vanmolkot KR, et al. Hay-Wells syndrome is caused by heterozygous missense mutations in the SAM domain of p63. Hum Mol Genet. 2001;10(3):221–9. https://doi.org/10.1093/hmg/10.3.221.
42. Bree AF. Clinical lessons learned from the international research symposium on ankyloblepharon-ectodermal defects-cleft lip/palate (AEC) syndrome. Am J Med Genet A. 2009;149A(9):1894–9. https://doi.org/10.1002/ajmg.a.32788.
43. Sutton VR, van Bokhoven H. TP63-related disorders. In: Adam MP, Feldman J, Mirzaa GM, Pagon RA, Wallace SE, Bean LJH, et al., editors. . Seattle, WA: GeneReviews((R)); 1993.
44. Siegfried E, Bree A, Fete M, Sybert VP. Skin erosions and wound healing in ankyloblepharon-ectodermal defect-cleft lip and/or palate. Arch Dermatol. 2005;141(12):1591–4. https://doi.org/10.1001/archderm.141.12.1591.
45. Cole P, Hatef DA, Kaufman Y, Magruder A, Bree A, Friedman E, et al. Facial clefting and oroauditory pathway manifestations in ankyloblepharon-ectodermal defects-cleft lip/palate (AEC) syndrome. Am J Med Genet A. 2009;149A(9):1910–5. https://doi.org/10.1002/ajmg.a.32836.
46. Farrington F, Lausten L. Oral findings in ankyloblepharon-ectodermal dysplasia-cleft lip/palate (AEC) syndrome. Am J Med Genet A. 2009;149A(9):1907–9. https://doi.org/10.1002/ajmg.a.32790.
47. Julapalli MR, Scher RK, Sybert VP, Siegfried EC, Bree AF. Dermatologic findings of ankyloblepharon-ectodermal defects-cleft lip/palate (AEC) syndrome. Am J Med Genet A. 2009;149A(9):1900–6. https://doi.org/10.1002/ajmg.a.32797.
48. Dishop MK, Bree AF, Hicks MJ. Pathologic changes of skin and hair in ankyloblepharon-ectodermal defects-cleft lip/palate (AEC) syndrome. Am J Med Genet A. 2009;149A(9):1935–41. https://doi.org/10.1002/ajmg.a.32826.
49. Payne AS, Yan AC, Ilyas E, Li W, Seykora JT, Young TL, et al. Two novel TP63 mutations associated with the ankyloblepharon, ectodermal defects, and cleft lip and palate syndrome: a skin fragility phenotype. Arch Dermatol. 2005;141(12):1567–73. https://doi.org/10.1001/archderm.141.12.1567.
50. Kantaputra PN, Hamada T, Kumchai T, McGrath JA. Heterozygous mutation in the SAM domain of p63 underlies Rapp-Hodgkin ectodermal dysplasia. J Dent Res. 2003;82(6):433–7. https://doi.org/10.1177/154405910308200606.
51. Zhang Z, Cheng R, Liang J, Lu Z, Wang Y, Li M, et al. Ankyloblepharon-ectodermal dysplasia-clefting syndrome misdiagnosed as epidermolysis bullosa and congenital ichthyosiform erythroderma: case report and review of published work. J Dermatol. 2019;46(5):422–5. https://doi.org/10.1111/1346-8138.14837.

52. Ferstl P, Wohlfart S, Schneider H. Sweating ability of patients with p63-associated syndromes. Eur J Pediatr. 2018;177(11):1727–31. https://doi.org/10.1007/s00431-018-3227-6.
53. Celik TH, Buyukcam A, Simsek-Kiper PO, Utine GE, Ersoy-Evans S, Korkmaz A, et al. A newborn with overlapping features of AEC and EEC syndromes. Am J Med Genet A. 2011;155A(12):3100–3. https://doi.org/10.1002/ajmg.a.34328.
54. Chiu YE, Drolet BA, Duffy KJ, Holland KE. A case of ankyloblepharon, ectodermal dysplasia, and cleft lip/palate syndrome with ectrodactyly: are the p63 syndromes distinct after all? Pediatr Dermatol. 2011;28(1):15–9. https://doi.org/10.1111/j.1525-1470.2009.00976.x.
55. Helenius K, Ojala L, Kainulainen L, Peltonen S, Hietala M, Pohjola P, et al. Overlap between EEC and AEC syndrome and immunodeficiency in a preterm infant with a TP63 variant. Eur J Med Genet. 2023;66(5):104735. https://doi.org/10.1016/j.ejmg.2023.104735.
56. Motil KJ, Fete TJ. Growth, nutritional, and gastrointestinal aspects of ankyloblepharon-ectodermal defect-cleft lip and/or palate (AEC) syndrome. Am J Med Genet A. 2009;149A(9):1922–5. https://doi.org/10.1002/ajmg.a.32789.
57. Sawardekar SS, Zaenglein AL. Ankyloblepharon-ectodermal dysplasia-clefting syndrome: a novel p63 mutation associated with generalized neonatal erosions. Pediatr Dermatol. 2011;28(3):313–7. https://doi.org/10.1111/j.1525-1470.2010.01207.x.
58. Fete M, vanBokhoven H, Clements SE, McKeon F, Roop DR, Koster MI, et al. International research symposium on ankyloblepharon-ectodermal defects-cleft lip/palate (AEC) syndrome. Am J Med Genet A. 2009;149A(9):1885–93. https://doi.org/10.1002/ajmg.a.32761.
59. Steele JA, Hansen H, Arn P, Kwong PC. Spectrum of phenotypic manifestations from a single point mutation of the p63 gene, including new cutaneous and immunologic findings. Pediatr Dermatol. 2005;22(5):415–9. https://doi.org/10.1111/j.1525-1470.2005.00105.x.
60. Stefanski HE, Xing Y, Nicholls J, Jonart L, Goren E, Taylor PA, et al. P63 targeted deletion under the FOXN1 promoter disrupts pre-and post-natal thymus development, function and maintenance as well as induces severe hair loss. PLoS One. 2022;17(1):e0261770. https://doi.org/10.1371/journal.pone.0261770.
61. Ferone G, Mollo MR, Thomason HA, Antonini D, Zhou H, Ambrosio R, et al. p63 control of desmosome gene expression and adhesion is compromised in AEC syndrome. Hum Mol Genet. 2013;22(3):531–43. https://doi.org/10.1093/hmg/dds464.
62. Beaudry VG, Pathak N, Koster MI, Attardi LD. Differential PERP regulation by TP63 mutants provides insight into AEC pathogenesis. Am J Med Genet Part A. 2009;149A(9):1952–7. https://doi.org/10.1002/ajmg.a.32760.
63. Mollo MR, Antonini D, Mitchell K, Fortugno P, Costanzo A, Dixon J, et al. p63-dependent and independent mechanisms of nectin-1 and nectin-4 regulation in the epidermis. Exp Dermatol. 2015;24(2):114–9. https://doi.org/10.1111/exd.12593.
64. Clements SE, Techanukul T, Lai-Cheong JE, Mee JB, South AP, Pourreyron C, et al. Mutations in AEC syndrome skin reveal a role for p63 in basement membrane adhesion, skin barrier integrity and hair follicle biology. Br J Dermatol. 2012;167(1):134–44. https://doi.org/10.1111/j.1365-2133.2012.10888.x.
65. De Moerlooze L, Spencer-Dene B, Revest JM, Hajihosseini M, Rosewell I, Dickson C. An important role for the IIIb isoform of fibroblast growth factor receptor 2 (FGFR2) in mesenchymal-epithelial signalling during mouse organogenesis. Development. 2000;127(3):483–92. https://doi.org/10.1242/dev.127.3.483.
66. Ferone G, Thomason HA, Antonini D, De Rosa L, Hu B, Gemei M, et al. Mutant p63 causes defective expansion of ectodermal progenitor cells and impaired FGF signalling in AEC syndrome. EMBO Mol Med. 2012;4(3):192–205. https://doi.org/10.1002/emmm.201100199.
67. Celli J, Duijf P, Hamel BC, Bamshad M, Kramer B, Smits AP, et al. Heterozygous germline mutations in the p53 homolog p63 are the cause of EEC syndrome. Cell. 1999;99(2):143–53. https://doi.org/10.1016/s0092-8674(00)81646-3.
68. Rinne T, Spadoni E, Kjaer KW, Danesino C, Larizza D, Kock M, et al. Delineation of the ADULT syndrome phenotype due to arginine 298 mutations of the p63 gene. Eur J Hum Genet. 2006;14(8):904–10. https://doi.org/10.1038/sj.ejhg.5201640.

69. Osterburg C, Ferniani M, Antonini D, Frombach AS, D'Auria L, Osterburg S, et al. Disease-related p63 DBD mutations impair DNA binding by distinct mechanisms and varying degree. Cell Death Dis. 2023;14(4):274. https://doi.org/10.1038/s41419-023-05796-y.
70. Browne G, Cipollone R, Lena AM, Serra V, Zhou H, van Bokhoven H, et al. Differential altered stability and transcriptional activity of DeltaNp63 mutants in distinct ectodermal dysplasias. J Cell Sci. 2011;124(Pt 13):2200–7. https://doi.org/10.1242/jcs.079327.
71. Rosenberg JB, Butrus S, Bazemore MG. Ectrodactyly-ectodermal dysplasia-clefting syndrome causing blindness in a child. J AAPOS. 2011;15(1):80–2. https://doi.org/10.1016/j.jaapos.2010.12.001.
72. Di Iorio E, Kaye SB, Ponzin D, Barbaro V, Ferrari S, Bohm E, et al. Limbal stem cell deficiency and ocular phenotype in ectrodactyly-ectodermal dysplasia-clefting syndrome caused by p63 mutations. Ophthalmology. 2012;119(1):74–83. https://doi.org/10.1016/j.ophtha.2011.06.044.
73. Kennedy DP, Chandler JW, McCulley JP. Ocular surface involvements in ectrodactyly-ectodermal dysplasia-cleft syndrome. Cont Lens Anterior Eye. 2015;38(3):228–31. https://doi.org/10.1016/j.clae.2015.02.002.
74. Akahoshi K, Sakazume S, Kosaki K, Ohashi H, Fukushima Y. EEC syndrome type 3 with a heterozygous germline mutation in the P63 gene and B cell lymphoma. Am J Med Genet A. 2003;120A(3):370–3. https://doi.org/10.1002/ajmg.a.20064.
75. Balci S, Engiz O, Okten G, Sipahier M, Gursu G, Kandemir B. A 19-year follow-up of a patient with type 3 ectrodactyly-ectodermal dysplasia-clefting syndrome who developed non-Hodgkin lymphoma. Oral Surg Oral Med Oral Pathol Oral Radiol Endod. 2009;108(3):e91–5. https://doi.org/10.1016/j.tripleo.2009.04.043.
76. Valenzise M, Arrigo T, De Luca F, Privitera A, Frigiola A, Carando A, et al. R298Q mutation of p63 gene in autosomal dominant ectodermal dysplasia associated with arrhythmogenic right ventricular cardiomyopathy. Eur J Med Genet. 2008;51(5):497–500. https://doi.org/10.1016/j.ejmg.2008.05.005.
77. Poloni G, Calore M, Rigato I, Marras E, Minervini G, Mazzotti E, et al. A targeted next-generation gene panel reveals a novel heterozygous nonsense variant in the TP63 gene in patients with arrhythmogenic cardiomyopathy. Heart Rhythm. 2019;16(5):773–80. https://doi.org/10.1016/j.hrthm.2018.11.015.
78. van Bokhoven H, Hamel BC, Bamshad M, Sangiorgi E, Gurrieri F, Duijf PH, et al. p63 gene mutations in eec syndrome, limb-mammary syndrome, and isolated split hand-split foot malformation suggest a genotype-phenotype correlation. Am J Hum Genet. 2001;69(3):481–92. https://doi.org/10.1086/323123.
79. Duijf PH, Vanmolkot KR, Propping P, Friedl W, Krieger E, McKeon F, et al. Gain-of- function mutation in ADULT syndrome reveals the presence of a second transactivation domain in p63. Hum Mol Genet. 2002;11(7):799–804. https://doi.org/10.1093/hmg/11.7.799.
80. Avitan-Hersh E, Indelman M, Bergman R, Sprecher E. ADULT syndrome caused by a mutation previously associated with EEC syndrome. Pediatr Dermatol. 2010;27(6):643–5. https://doi.org/10.1111/j.1525-1470.2010.01131.x.
81. Reisler TT, Patton MA, Meagher PP. Further phenotypic and genetic variation in ADULT syndrome. Am J Med Genet A. 2006;140(22):2495–500. https://doi.org/10.1002/ajmg.a.31482.
82. Prontera P, Garelli E, Isidori I, Mencarelli A, Carando A, Silengo MC, et al. Cleft palate and ADULT phenotype in a patient with a novel TP63 mutation suggests lumping of EEC/LM/ADULT syndromes into a unique entity: ELA syndrome. Am J Med Genet A. 2011;155A(11):2746–9. https://doi.org/10.1002/ajmg.a.34270.
83. Ianakiev P, van Baren MJ, Daly MJ, Toledo SP, Cavalcanti MG, Neto JC, et al. Acheiropodia is caused by a genomic deletion in C7orf2, the human orthologue of the Lmbr1 gene. Am J Hum Genet. 2001;68(1):38–45. https://doi.org/10.1086/316955.
84. Jin JY, Zeng L, Li K, He JQ, Pang X, Huang H, et al. A novel mutation (c.1010G>T; p.R337L) in TP63 as a cause of split-hand/foot malformation with hypodontia. J Gene Med. 2019;21(10):e3122. https://doi.org/10.1002/jgm.3122.

85. Otsuki Y, Ueda K, Satoh C, Maekawa R, Yoshiura KI, Iseki S. Intermediate phenotype between ADULT syndrome and EEC syndrome caused by R243Q mutation in TP63. Plast Reconstr Surg Glob Open. 2016;4(12):e1185. https://doi.org/10.1097/GOX.0000000000001185.
86. Ianakiev P, Kilpatrick MW, Toudjarska I, Basel D, Beighton P, Tsipouras P. Split-hand/split-foot malformation is caused by mutations in the p63 gene on 3q27. Am J Hum Genet. 2000;67(1):59–66. https://doi.org/10.1086/302972.
87. Kouwenhoven EN, van Heeringen SJ, Tena JJ, Oti M, Dutilh BE, Alonso ME, et al. Genome-wide profiling of p63 DNA-binding sites identifies an element that regulates gene expression during limb development in the 7q21 SHFM1 locus. PLoS Genet. 2010;6(8):e1001065. https://doi.org/10.1371/journal.pgen.1001065.
88. Yang X, Lin X, Zhu Y, Luo J, Lin G. Genetic analysis of a congenital split-hand/split-foot malformation 4 pedigree. Mol Med Rep. 2018;17(6):7553–8. https://doi.org/10.3892/mmr.2018.8838.
89. Basha M, Demeer B, Revencu N, Helaers R, Theys S, Bou Saba S, et al. Whole exome sequencing identifies mutations in 10% of patients with familial non-syndromic cleft lip and/or palate in genes mutated in well-known syndromes. J Med Genet. 2018;55(7):449–58. https://doi.org/10.1136/jmedgenet-2017-105110.
90. Leoyklang P, Siriwan P, Shotelersuk V. A mutation of the p63 gene in non-syndromic cleft lip. J Med Genet. 2006;43(6):e28. https://doi.org/10.1136/jmg.2005.036442.
91. Khandelwal KD, van den Boogaard MH, Mehrem SL, Gebel J, Fagerberg C, van Beusekom E, et al. Deletions and loss-of-function variants in TP63 associated with orofacial clefting. Eur J Hum Genet. 2019;27(7):1101–12. https://doi.org/10.1038/s41431-019-0370-0.
92. Wright JT, Fete M, Schneider H, Zinser M, Koster MI, Clarke AJ, et al. Ectodermal dysplasias: classification and organization by phenotype, genotype and molecular pathway. Am J Med Genet A. 2019;179(3):442–7. https://doi.org/10.1002/ajmg.a.61045.
93. Absalan F, Ronaghi M. Molecular inversion probe assay. Methods Mol Biol. 2007;396:315–30. https://doi.org/10.1007/978-1-59745-515-2_20.
94. O'Roak BJ, Vives L, Fu W, Egertson JD, Stanaway IB, Phelps IG, et al. Multiplex targeted sequencing identifies recurrently mutated genes in autism spectrum disorders. Science. 2012;338(6114):1619–22. https://doi.org/10.1126/science.1227764.
95. Shen J, van den Bogaard EH, Kouwenhoven EN, Bykov VJ, Rinne T, Zhang Q, et al. APR-246/PRIMA-1(MET) rescues epidermal differentiation in skin keratinocytes derived from EEC syndrome patients with p63 mutations. Proc Natl Acad Sci USA. 2013;110(6):2157–62. https://doi.org/10.1073/pnas.1201993110.
96. Shalom-Feuerstein R, Serror L, Aberdam E, Muller FJ, van Bokhoven H, Wiman KG, et al. Impaired epithelial differentiation of induced pluripotent stem cells from ectodermal dysplasia-related patients is rescued by the small compound APR-246/PRIMA-1MET. Proc Natl Acad Sci USA. 2013;110(6):2152–6. https://doi.org/10.1073/pnas.1201753109.
97. Aberdam E, Roux LN, Secretan PH, Boralevi F, Schlatter J, Morice-Picard F, et al. Improvement of epidermal covering on AEC patients with severe skin erosions by PRIMA-1(MET)/APR-246. Cell Death Dis. 2020;11(1):30. https://doi.org/10.1038/s41419-020-2223-8.
98. Gurevich I, Agarwal P, Zhang P, Dolorito JA, Oliver S, Liu H, et al. In vivo topical gene therapy for recessive dystrophic epidermolysis bullosa: a phase 1 and 2 trial. Nat Med. 2022;28(4):780–8. https://doi.org/10.1038/s41591-022-01737-y.
99. Hirsch T, Rothoeft T, Teig N, Bauer JW, Pellegrini G, De Rosa L, et al. Regeneration of the entire human epidermis using transgenic stem cells. Nature. 2017;551(7680):327–32. https://doi.org/10.1038/nature24487.
100. Barbaro V, Bonelli F, Ferrari S, La Vella G, Di Iorio E. Innovative therapeutic approaches for the treatment of the ocular morbidities in patients with EEC syndrome. Cells. 2023;12(3):495. https://doi.org/10.3390/cells12030495.
101. Barbaro V, Nasti AA, Del Vecchio C, Ferrari S, Migliorati A, Raffa P, et al. Correction of mutant p63 in EEC syndrome using siRNA mediated allele-specific silencing restores defective stem cell function. Stem Cells. 2016;34(6):1588–600. https://doi.org/10.1002/stem.2343.

Chapter 7
Focal Dermal Hypoplasia (FDH) and WNT10A-Related Ectodermal Dysplasia (ED)

Alessandra Gelmetti and Gianluca Tadini

Keywords Focal dermal hypoplasia · WNT pathway · Phenotypes

Also known as Goltz syndrome, focal dermal hypoplasia (FDH) is a rare congenital multisystemic genodermatosis affecting tissues of both ectodermal and mesodermal origin, leading to skin, central nervous system, ocular, skeletal, dental, and cardiac anomalies [1].

Skin features are those most commonly described in association with the syndrome, with diffuse linear areas of skin atrophy and pigmentation due to dermal hypoplasia as characteristic features, in association with skin fragility and appendage anomalies [1].

FDH is caused by pathogenic mutations such as nonsense, missense, frameshift and splicing variants, deletions, and insertions in the PORCN gene, located on the X-chromosome at the gene map locus Xp11.23. According to the most recent classification of ectodermal dysplasia (ED) [2, 3], being PORCN one of the genes involved in the Wingless Type MMTV Integration Site Family Member (WNT) signaling pathway showing a direct interrelationship with WNT, FDH can be included in the great chapter of ED, together with the WNT10A-related diseases.

PORCN encodes a 461 amino acid-sized (52 kDa) protein named porcupine, located in the endoplasmic reticulum and involved in the secretion and signaling of Wnt proteins, which play a central role in the interaction between ectodermal and mesodermal structures during embryogenesis. Recently, among the 257 PORCN variants registered online, 219 have been reported as pathogenetic while 19 as variants of uncertain significance (VUS) [3].

A. Gelmetti (✉)
Department of Experimental, Diagnostic and Specialty Medicine, Alma Mater Studiorum University of Bologna, Bologna, Italy

G. Tadini
Center for Inherited Cutaneous Diseases, University of Milan, Milan, Italy

G. Tadini et al. (eds.), *Multidisciplinary Approach to Ectodermal Dysplasia*,
https://doi.org/10.1007/978-3-031-75790-7_7

FDH is an X-linked dominantly inherited disease; thus, most of the patients described in the literature are females, showing heterozygosity of a pathogenic mutation in the PORCN gene. Postzygotic somatic mosaicism is also possible and explains the few reports of male patients [4, 5]. True mosaic female cases are reported with a phenotype very similar to classical FDH. Non-mosaic surviving male patients have been exceedingly rarely reported, thus suggesting the presence of less pathogenic mutations and the consequent need for further molecular genetics investigations [3].

To date, there is still no evidence of genotype-phenotype correlation, and it is debated whether the severity of the clinical picture is related to the level of X-chromosome inactivation or not [6, 7].

Lastly, since the number and diversity of clinical features described in patients affected by FDH, some authors speculate that epigenetic factors might play a role in modulating the phenotype of the disease [5].

7.1 Clinical Features

A constellation of cutaneous and extracutaneous signs have been reported in the literature, with skin and skeletal findings being present in most of the patients, in association with oral, ocular, neurologic, and visceral anomalies.

Since the prevalence of cutaneous and bone abnormalities in FDH patients, clinical diagnostic criteria have been proposed, including three or more skin manifestations and at least one characteristic limb malformation [8].

7.1.1 Skin, Mucosae, and Appendage Manifestations

As first described by Goltz, skin manifestations are one of the pivotal features of FDH. Typical lesions are evident at birth, with linear areas of atrophic skin following the Blaschko lines. At birth and in infancy, linear mosaic lesions may not be so obvious and easy to recognize; lines are fragmented (Fig. 7.1). In some patients, lesions are initially erythematous, and skin fragility can lead to erosions, blistering, and exudation, sometimes healing with stellate or hypertrophic scars [6]. Herniation of fat tissue in the form of yellowish papules (Fig. 7.2) and, with age, linear or reticular hyper or hypopigmentation can be observed [1] (Fig. 7.3).

Lesions can be bilateral, usually asymmetrical, and of different shapes and sizes [1, 5] and remain stable and persistent with age [6].

Histology of atrophic areas shows either significantly thinned or absent dermis, completely replaced by fat cells [9]. The presence of adipocytes in the upper dermis is thought to result from herniation of subcutaneous fat, facilitated by the absence of dermis, but some authors speculated that those cells represent a fat nevus resulting from dysplasia and not hypoplasia [10].

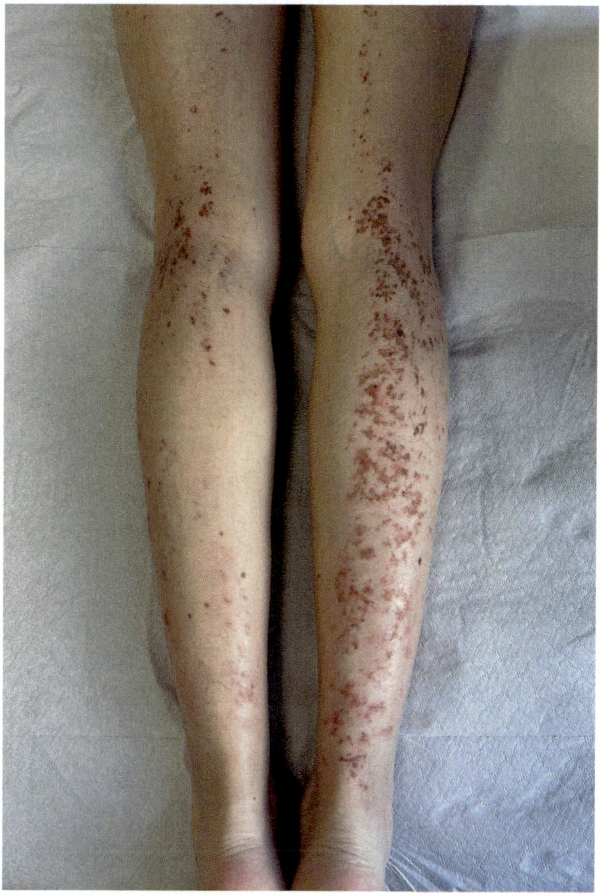

Fig. 7.1 Atrophic and pigmented lesions distributed in fragmented blaschkolinear fashion

Furthermore, in some cases described in the literature, dermal hypoplasia is not present. In the latter cases, the decrease and fragmentation of elastic fibers of the upper dermis might be a useful histologic feature to guide the diagnosis of FDH [4].

Another feature of the syndrome is the presence of cutaneous and mucosal papillomas. These are pink papular asymptomatic lesions which usually develop around the lips and nose, gums, oral, esophageal, gastrointestinal, and genital mucosae [5] (Fig. 7.4), with histological aspects of fibrovascular angiofibromas/papillomas [4]. Although usually small in size, multiple giant papillomas have been reported [11].

Regarding the oral cavity, the absence of a lingual frenulum has been reported, leading to the ability to touch the nose through tongue hyperextension [7], as visible in a subset of Ehlers-Danlos patients.

Hair anomalies are reported, clinically presenting as patchy alopecia and diffusely sparse scalp hair and eyelashes. On trichoscopy, hair shaft abnormalities have been described, such as atrophic hairs, pili torti, pili trianguli, and canaliculi [6].

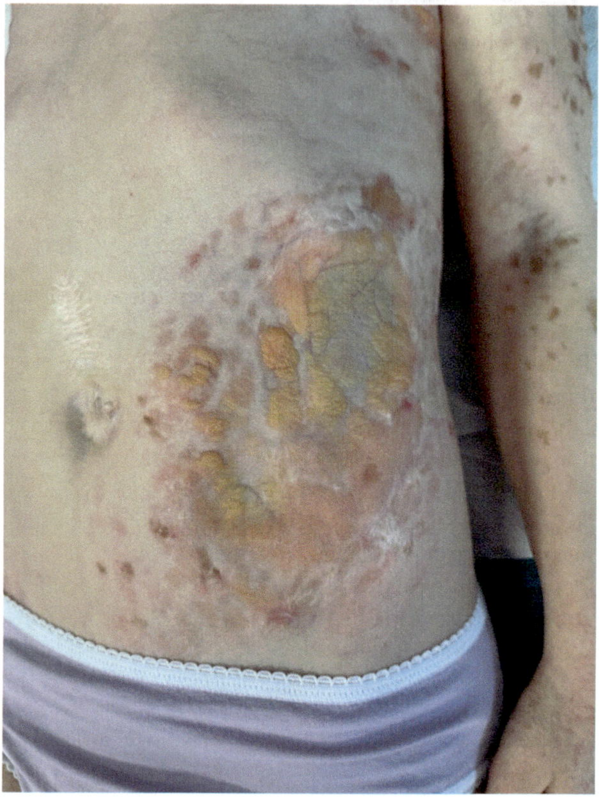

Fig. 7.2 Herniation of fatty tissue in the form of yellowish papules

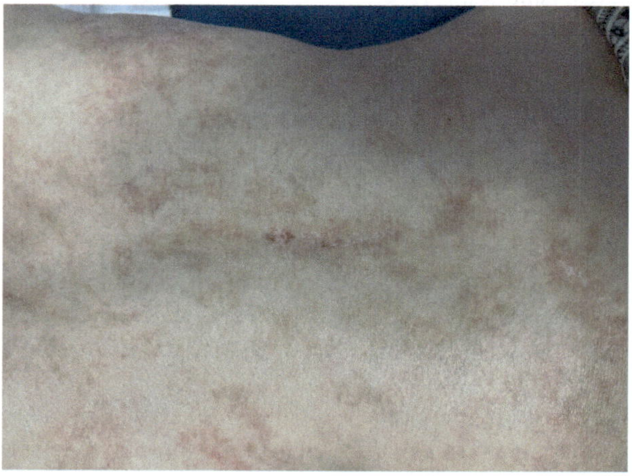

Fig. 7.3 Linear and reticular hypo-hyperpigmented lesions

Nails can be interested in FDH, and changes may vary in type and severity: longitudinal ridging of the nail plate, V-shaped splitting of the distal nail plate, micronychia, and, less frequently, anonychia [6]. Hypohidrosis, characteristically with mosaic distribution in a subset of patients.

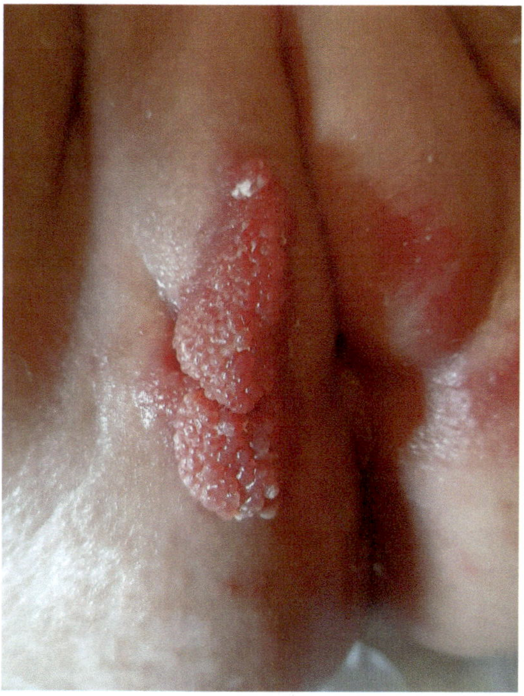

Fig. 7.4 Pink "grape-like" papillomatous lesions on genital mucosae

7.1.2 Skeletal Malformations

Skeletal anomalies are the second most common findings in FDH regarding skull, vertebrae, and limbs, with hypoplastic digits, syndactyly, ectrodactyly ("lobster-claw" hand defect), oligodactyly, transverse limb, and long bone reduction defects being commonly described so as to be included in the above-mentioned proposed clinical diagnostic criteria [3, 8, 12] (Figs. 7.5, 7.6, and 7.7). Short stature and scoliosis might also be observed [7]. At routine RX examination, "osteopathia striata" is visible and is the osseous counterpart of mosaic defects, a kind of bones' Blaschko lines.

As concerns the skull, defective ossification of the cranial bones leads to microcephaly and bossing in different cranial areas, while vertebral anomalies consist in the fusion of vertebral bodies and spina bifida [5, 13]. Osteolytic lesions described as benign giant cell tumor-like lesions of bones have been reported, possibly leading to pathologic fractures [14].

Odontodysplasia, oligodontia, and enamel hypoplasia are the most observed anomalies of the teeth; cleft lip and palate are visible in a minority of cases [5, 7].

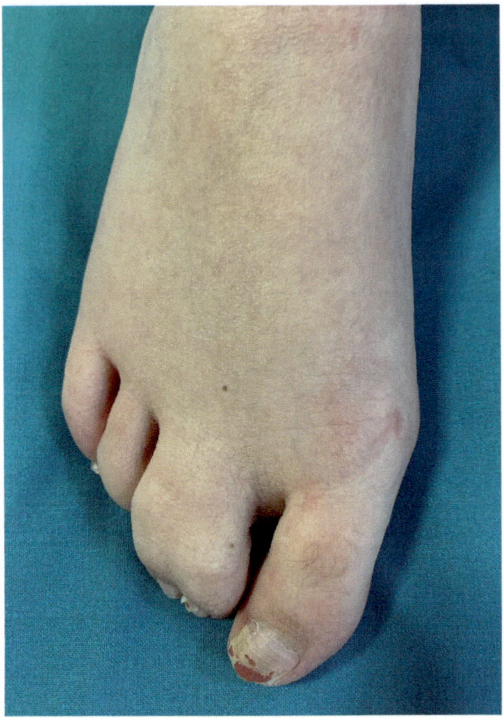

Fig. 7.5 Syndactily of the II and III toe

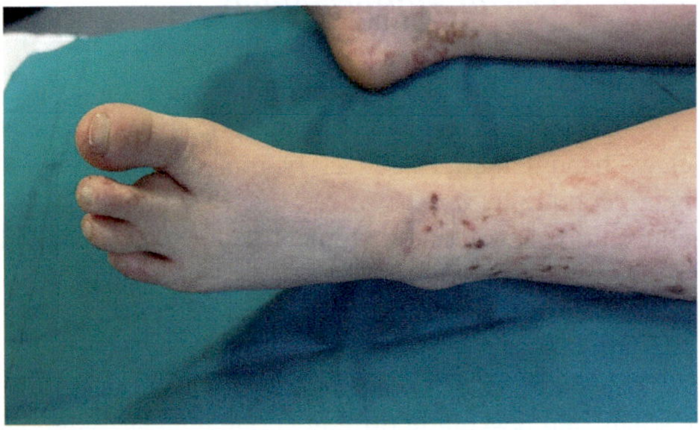

Fig. 7.6 Defective bones in adult patient foot

7.1.3 Ocular Involvement

A variety of ocular anomalies have been reported in FDH, of both ectodermal and mesenchymal origin, such as cataracts, anophthalmia, microphthalmia, colobomas, lacrimal duct anomalies, strabismus, nystagmus, optic atrophy, and patchy retinal hypo/hyperpigmentation. Photophobia and visual impairment are the most reported resulting symptoms [13, 15].

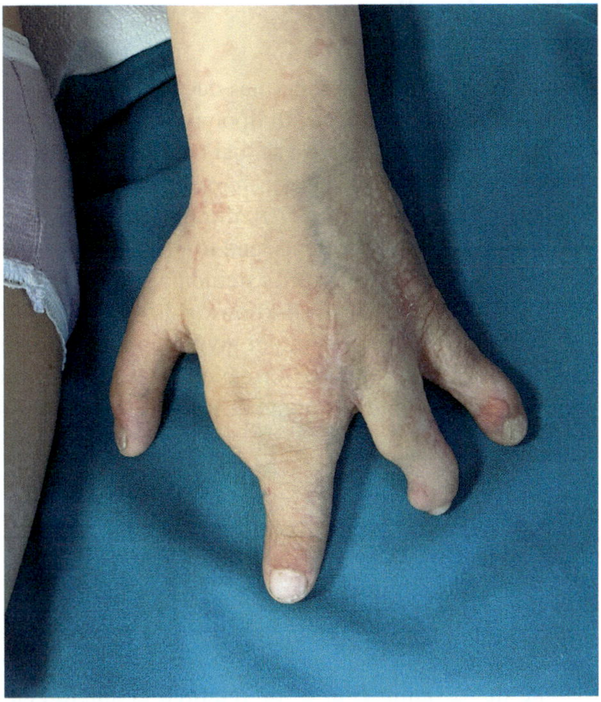

Fig. 7.7 Ectrodactyly with evident post-orthopedic surgery procedures

7.1.4 Neurologic Anomalies

In vivo mice models, studies showed that heterozygous mutations in the PORCN gene were lethal in males while leading to defects in neural tubes in females, and these results have been postulated to be similar to what happens in humans in the uterus, thus explaining both the rarity of nervous system reported anomalies and prevalence in female patients [16].

Despite the scarcity of cases of central nervous system (CNS) anomalies reported in association with FDH, even in the first description of the syndrome, "central nervous system and optical defects" were mentioned among the main clinical features of Goltz syndrome [1].

Microcrania, mental retardation, epileptiform seizures, spina bifida occulta, neurosensory hearing loss, hydrocephalus, myelomeningocele, Arnold-Chiari malformation, agenesis of the corpus callosum, cerebral atrophy, and cerebellar dysplasia have been reported [16, 17].

Although rare, CNS anomalies must always be excluded in FDH syndrome suspected individuals, thus suggesting the importance of a neurologic evaluation of these patients.

7.1.5 Miscellaneous

Omphalocele and visceral hernias due to abdominal wall defects might be observed soon after birth, together with lipomas and osteochondromas [7, 18].

Amenorrhea and delayed sexual development are frequent.

Visceral anomalies include horseshoe kidney [19], intestinal malrotation and mediastinal dextroposition [20], intrathoracic herniation of abdominal viscera, cardiac ventricular septal defects, and truncus arteriosus, unilateral renal agenesis [21].

A case of papillary thyroid carcinoma in adolescent patients affected by FDH has been reported, and the well-known role of the Wnt/β-catenin pathway in cancer initiation and progression might give rise to the possible role of PORCN mutations in susceptibility to tumor formation. Cancer proneness with a well-established increased risk of internal organ cancers leads to multidisciplinary diagnostic protocol [22, 23]..

7.2 Diagnosis

Clinical findings of the above-described cutaneous and extracutaneous features must lead to the suspicion of FDH, which has to be confirmed by genetic testing.

The first examination to be required is single-gene testing of PORCN from a peripheral blood sample, and, in case no pathogenic variants are found, chromosomal microarray analysis should be performed.

Second testing is performed in case of negativity of the above-mentioned first assays or in case somatic mosaicism is suspected: a sequence analysis or deletion/duplication analysis is performed on saliva or affected tissues.

If both first and second tests do not detect any pathogenic variant, in the presence of a highly suggestive phenotype, further investigations might be considered such as either a multigene panel including PORCN and other genes determined by the clinicians, or a comprehensive genomic testing with an exome or, less frequently, genome sequencing [24].

Once the diagnosis of FDH, a multidisciplinary approach is mandatory for the systemic management of patients. Specialist consultations, skin biopsies, and imaging studies according to the specific observed anomalies have to be performed.

7.3 Novel Variants

In recent years, novel PORCN variants have been described, both as a result of a deeper knowledge of the disease and the support of increasingly precise diagnostic techniques.

A novel de novo heterozygous frameshift c.375delG p.(Ala126HisfsTer3) protein-truncating PORCN mutation was identified in an Egyptian female patient presenting the typical FDH clinical features in association with partial fusion of labia majora, ventral hernia, and bladder extrophy [25].

Through whole exome sequencing (WES), it is now possible to identify even intronic variants, as found in a mother and a daughter in whom a new intronic PORCN variant creating an alternative splice acceptor site explained the FDH phenotype [26].

A novel hemizygous missense PORCN variant p.Asp283His (hg19:chrX:48372914; c.847G>C, p.Asp283His) was found using WES in a male patient presenting mainly CNS anomalies in the absence of cutaneous involvement. The same variant was identified in the asymptomatic mother, and since skewed X-chromosome inactivation was excluded, it was speculated that other factors such as epigenetics, modifiers expression, or other associated mutations might influence the phenotypic expression of this variant [3].

A novel large deletion with an 181.374 kb region of copy number loss from peripheral blood leukocytes and both lesional and non-lesional skin was identified in an adult female patient [27].

Precocious puberty, not previously reported in association with FDH, was found in a female patient with a novel missense PORCN variant in association with mild intellectual disability and left-side diaphragm eventration [28].

7.3.1 WNT10A-Related ED

Mutations in the WNT10A gene (WNT-beta catenin pathway) cause autosomal dominant and recessive hypohidrotic ED. Epidemiologically, in our cohort of more than 300 ED cases, WNT10A accounts for at least 15–20% of patients. Moreover, WNT10A gene mutations account per se for more than 50% of isolated non-syndromic oligodontia.

The associated phenotype is highly variable, even in the same family, but mainly consists of oligo-hypodontia that may be associated with minor defects in the body, scalp hair, and nails. Hyperhidrosis may be present but is less severe than in Ectodysplasin A (EDA)-pathway-affected patients and rarely leads to heat intolerance episodes. Moreover, WNT10-affected ED patients do not show the facial dysmorphism of EDA patients and can be easily recognized and differentiated with advanced facial recognition imaging systems (Figs. 7.8, 7.9, 7.10, and 7.11).

Furthermore, mutations in the WNT10 gene have been related to other two recessively inherited phenotypes known as, respectively, Odonto-Onycho-Dermal dysplasia and Schopf-Schultz-Passarge syndrome. Recent findings clearly demonstrate that these two entities are only a continuum of signs and not two different diseases, sharing different degrees of hypodontia, nail dystrophy, hair abnormalities with pili

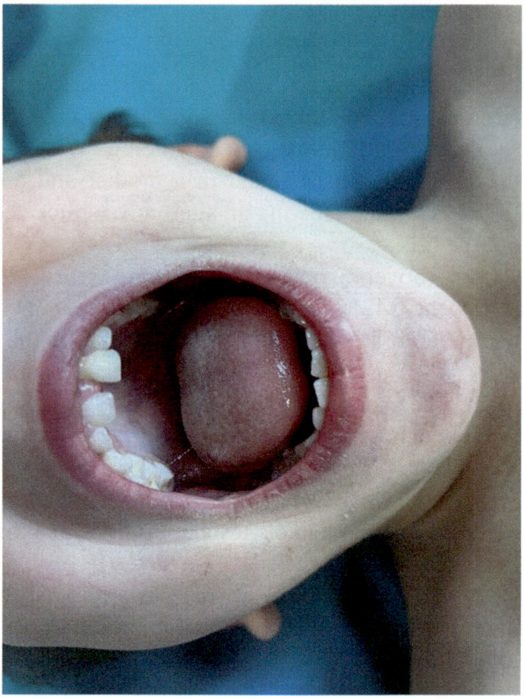

Fig. 7.8 Dental anomalies in WNT10-mutated patient

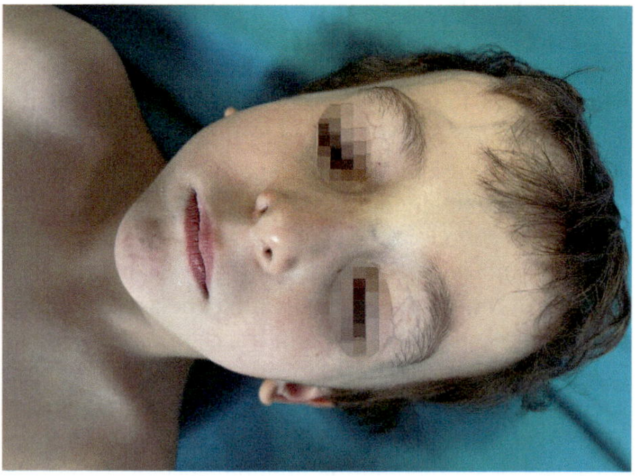

Fig. 7.9 Facies with frontal bossing and hypotrichosis in WNT 10 mutated

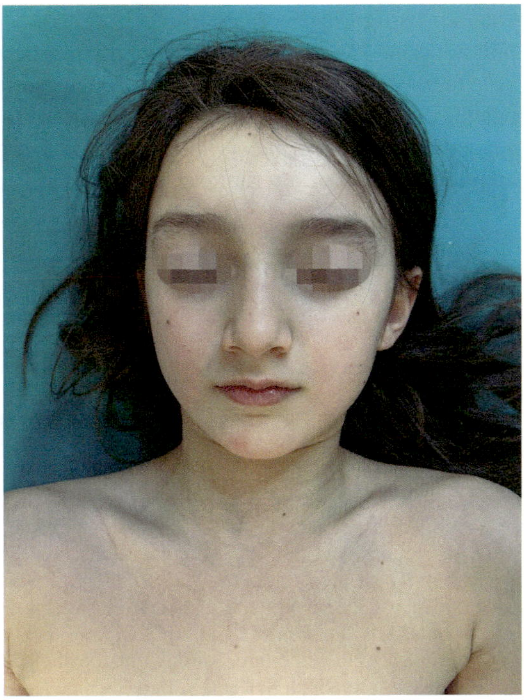

Fig. 7.10 Frontal view of facies in WNT10 mutated young female

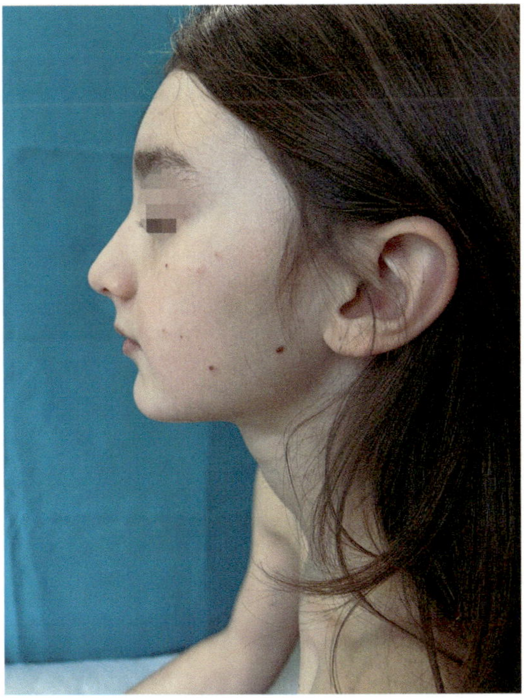

Fig. 7.11 Profile of the same patient in Fig. 7.9 with evidence of low-set ears

annulati pattern, palmoplantar hyperkeratosis, or pitting. Peculiar signs are palpebral apocrine hydrocystomas, whitish papules in periorbital and malar areas, multiple facial milia, and, in a subset of patients, a rosacea-like appearance with papules pustules and erythema in midfacial areas. As expected, the tendency to develop skin cancers, namely, eccrine syringoadenomas and poromas, is described together with an increased risk of internal organ cancers in these patients.

References

1. Goltz RW, Peterson WC, Gorlin RJ, Ravits HG. Focal dermal hypoplasia. Arch Dermatol. 1962;86:708–17.
2. Peschel N, Wright JT, Clarke AJ, Tadini G, Fete M, Hadj-Rabia S, Sybert VP, Norderyd J, Maier-Wolfhart S, Fete JT, Pagnan N, Visinoni AF, Schneider H. Molecular pathway-based classification of ectodermal dysplasias: first five-yearly update. Genes (Basel). 2022;13(12):2327.
3. Arlt A, Kohlschmidt N, Hentschel A, Bartels E, Groß C, Töpf A, Edem P, Szabo N, Sickmann A, Meyer N, Schara-Schmidt U, Lau J, Lochmüller H, Horvath R, Oktay Y, Roos A, Hiz S. Novel insights into PORCN mutations, associated phenotypes and pathophysiological aspects. Orphanet J Rare Dis. 2022;17(1):29.
4. Rohdenburg C, Liersch J, Kutsche K, Schaller J. Fragmented elastic fibers in focal dermal hypoplasia (Goltz-Gorlin syndrome) without focal dermal hypoplasia: report of a male case and review of the literature. Am J Dermatopathol. 2020;42(9):653–61.
5. Al Kaissi A, Ryabykh S, Kenis V, Ben Chehida F, Al Kaissi H, Kircher SG, Grill F. Cutaneous, cranial, and skeletal defects in children and adults with focal dermal hypoplasia. Children (Basel). 2023;10(10):1715.
6. Bree AF, Grange DK, Hicks MJ, Goltz RW. Dermatologic findings of focal dermal hypoplasia (Goltz syndrome). Am J Med Genet C Semin Med Genet. 2016;172C(1):44–51.
7. Murakami C, de Oliveira Lira Ortega A, Guimarães AS, Gonçalves-Bittar D, Bönecker M, Ciamponi AL. Focal dermal hypoplasia: a case report and literature review. Oral Surg Oral Med Oral Pathol Oral Radiol Endod. 2011;112(2):e11–8.
8. Bostwick B, Fang P, Patel A, Sutton VR. Phenotypic and molecular characterization of focal dermal hypoplasia in 18 individuals. Am J Med Genet C Semin Med Genet. 2016;172C(1):9–20.
9. Bolognia JL, Schaffer JV, Cerroni L, editors. Dermatology. 4th ed. China: Elsevier; 2018. ISBN 978–0-7020–6275–9
10. Howell JB, Freeman RG. Cutaneous defects of focal dermal hypoplasia: an ectomesodermal dysplasia syndrome. J Cutan Pathol. 1989;16(5):237–58.
11. Kore-Eda S, Yoneda K, Ohtani T, Tachibana T, Furukawa F, Imamura S. Focal dermal hypoplasia (Goltz syndrome) associated with multiple giant papillomas. Br J Dermatol. 1995;133(6):997–9.
12. Cox NH, Paterson WD. Osteochondroma of humerus in focal dermal hypoplasia (Goltz) syndrome. Clin Exp Dermatol. 1991;16(4):283–4.
13. Thomas JV, Yoshizumi MO, Beyer CK, Craft JL, Albert DM. Ocular manifestations of focal dermal hypoplasia syndrome. Arch Ophthalmol. 1977;95(11):1997–2001.
14. D'Alise MD, Timmons CF, Swift DM. Focal dermal hypoplasia (Goltz syndrome) with vertebral solid aneurysmal bone cyst variant. A case report. Pediatr Neurosurg. 1996;24(3):151–4.
15. Nobre ÁVV, Taba M, Silva AR, de Souza SLS, Motta ACF. Focal dermal hypoplasia (Goltz syndrome): a case report showing a wide variety of systemic and oral manifestations. Ann Dermatol. 2022;34(4):291–6.

16. Peters T, Perrier R, Haber RM. Focal dermal hypoplasia: report of a case with myelomeningocele, Arnold-Chiari malformation and hydrocephalus with a review of neurologic manifestations of Goltz syndrome. Pediatr Dermatol. 2014;31(2):220–4.
17. Goltz RW, Henderson RR, Hitch JM, Ott JE. Focal dermal hypoplasia syndrome. A review of the literature and report of two cases. Arch Dermatol. 1970;101(1):1–11.
18. Bhatia AM, Clericuzio CL, Musemeche CA. Congenital ventral hernia in association with focal dermal hypoplasia. Pediatr Dermatol. 1995;12(4):336–9.
19. Suskan E, Kürkçüoğlu N, Uluoğlu O. Focal dermal hypoplasia (Goltz syndrome) with horseshoe kidney abnormality. Pediatr Dermatol. 1990;7(4):283–6.
20. Irvine AD, Stewart FJ, Bingham EA, Nevin NC, Boston VE. Focal dermal hypoplasia (Goltz syndrome) associated with intestinal malrotation and mediastinal dextroposition. Am J Med Genet. 1996;62(3):213–5.
21. Han XY, Wu SS, Conway DH, Pawel BR, Punnett HH, Martin RA, de Chadarevian JP. Truncus arteriosus and other lethal internal anomalies in Goltz syndrome. Am J Med Genet. 2000;90(1):45–8.
22. Costanza F, Papi G, Corrado S, Pontecorvi A. Case report: papillary thyroid carcinoma in Goltz-Gorlin syndrome. Front Endocrinol (Lausanne). 2023;14:1243540.
23. Reya T, Clevers H. Wnt signalling in stem cells and cancer. Nature. 2005;434(7035):843–50.
24. Sutton VR. PORCN-related developmental disorders. 2008 May 15 [updated 2023 Jun 15]. In: Adam MP, Feldman J, Mirzaa GM, Pagon RA, Wallace SE, LJH B, Gripp KW, Amemiya A, editors. GeneReviews® [Internet]. Seattle, WA: University of Washington, Seattle; 1993–2024.
25. Elhossini RM, Abdel-Hamid MS, Ashaat E, Otaify GA, Dawoud H, Elshimy K, El Ruby M, Aglan M. Two new patients with focal dermal hypoplasia: a novel PORCN variant and insights on the diagnostic considerations. Congenit Anom (Kyoto). 2022;62(2):68–77.
26. Yamoto K, Okada S, Kato F, Fujisawa Y, Fukami M, Saitsu H, Ogata T. A novel intronic PORCN variant creating an alternative splice acceptor site in a mother and her daughter with focal dermal hypoplasia. Am J Med Genet A. 2022;188(5):1612–7.
27. Wu R, Zhong W, Chen J, Dou X. A novel large deletion mutation involving the PORCN gene in a Chinese patient with focal dermal hypoplasia and literature review. Int J Dermatol. 2023;62(9):1164–7.
28. Akalin A, Grzeschik KH, Utine E, Boduroğlu K, Simsek-Kiper PÖ. A long-term follow-up of a patient with a novel *PORCN* variant and additional clinical features. Mol Syndromol. 2024;15:217–24. https://doi.org/10.1159/000535681.

Chapter 8
Nectinopathies: Ectodermal Dysplasia Syndromes Caused by Mutations in *PVRL1/4* Genes Encoding Cell Adhesion Molecules Nectins-1/4

Paola Fortugno and Francesco Brancati

Keywords Nectins · Syndactily · Molecular diagnosis

8.1 History and Terminology: Toward a Molecularly Driven Dyadic Approach

Among more than 200 clinically recognized ectodermal dysplasias (EDs), a rather distinctive association is represented by cutaneous syndactyly and ectodermal defects (mainly abnormalities of the hair shaft and alopecia), with or without: cleft lip/palate, palmoplantar hyperkeratosis, mild cognitive impairment.

Several clinical reports in the medical literature have described such a combination of features over the past 40 years under the umbrella term "ectodermal dysplasia syndactyly syndrome (EDSS)." Since the 2000s, when the genetic bases of these conditions began to be deciphered, light was finally shed on the molecular mechanisms, prompting an etiological classification of these (and other) EDs. This is a fascinating example of how, in the age of molecular medicine, the initial recognition of distinct clinical pictures led us to catalog genetically distinct disorders later reunified by shared pathways or molecular function.

P. Fortugno
Università Telematica San Raffaele, Rome, Italy

IRCCS San Raffaele Roma, Rome, Italy

F. Brancati (✉)
IRCCS San Raffaele Roma, Rome, Italy

Human Genetics, Department of Life, Health and Environmental Sciences, University of L'Aquila, L'Aquila, Italy
e-mail: francesco.brancati@univaq.it

G. Tadini et al. (eds.), *Multidisciplinary Approach to Ectodermal Dysplasia*,
https://doi.org/10.1007/978-3-031-75790-7_8

In this book chapter, we will refer to ED syndromes caused by a deficiency in nectin molecules as "nectinopathies" [1]. Following the indication by Biesecker et al. [2], according to which the name of the disease may follow a dyad that includes the molecular etiology and the phenotype name, we will refer to the two currently known nectinopathies as nectin-1 ED and nectin-4 ED, caused by mutations in *PVRL1* and *PVRL4* genes, respectively.

Initially, Zlotogora et al. [3] and Ogür and Yuksel [4] independently reported children with a syndrome including cleft lip and palate, syndactyly, ED, and psychomotor retardation. The significant overlap between these clinical entities has led to the definition of Zlotogora-Ogür syndrome. Later, Bustos et al. [5] reported several families from Margarita Island the Caribbean Sea (Venezuela) with a similar phenotype and termed this novel entity *Margarita Island ectodermal dysplasia*. The large number of affected individuals related to a single founder in Margarita Island allowed, by linkage disequilibrium analysis, the mapping of the disease to the 11q23 region [6] and, subsequently, the identification of *PVRL1*, which encodes the cell adhesion molecule (CAM) nectin-1, as the disease-causative gene [7]. Different homozygous mutations were characterized in the *PVRL1* gene in the patients from Margarita Island and in the two families with the Zlotogora Ogür syndrome previously described, confirming that indeed they represent different presentations of the same cleft lip/palate ectodermal dysplasia syndrome (CLPED) (OMIM #225060).

Next, Brancati et al. [8] demonstrated genetic heterogeneity of nectin-related ED by identification of mutations in the *PVRL4* gene in two families presenting a syndromic phenotype with ED and syndactyly strongly overlapping with CLPED. *PVRL4*, located at 1q23 locus, encodes nectin-4, an adhesion molecule belonging to the nectin family and specifically interacting with nectin-1 at cell-cell junction in epithelial cells of skin and placenta [8]. In that study, the authors reported homozygous missense variants in four affected sibs previously reported by Boudghene-Stambouli and Merad-Boudia [9] and described a second Italian family with two affected sibs sharing compound heterozygous variants in *PVRL4*, outlining the existence of a newly defined entity termed EDSS1 (OMIM #613573).

8.2 Nectin-1 ED

The summary of the clinical features was done on 26 patients from 10 different families affected by CLPED1 syndrome described in the literature so far, for which reports of the clinical features and corresponding mutations in the *PVRL1* gene are available (Table 8.1). In addition to the 7 families from Margarita Island [5] and the 2 families from Israel [3] and Brazil [10], in which Suzuki et al. [7] identified homozygous prematurely truncating mutations in *PVRL1*, a 7-year-old Japanese boy with homozygous nonsense mutations has been reported by Yoshida et al. [37].

The appearance of affected individuals is very similar due to the shape of the face, the abnormal and sparse hair, and the scanty or absent lateral eyebrows. The majority of the patients present cleft lip and/or palate, or rarely an abnormal

Table 8.1 Known patients with nectinopathies and detailed genotypes at *PVRL1* and *PVRL4* loci

Gene	Genotype	State	No. of patients (families)	Reference
PVRL1	c.554G>A (p.Trp185Ter)	Homo	20 + 7 (7)	Bustos et al. [5] Suzuki et al. [7]
	c.554delG (p.Glu186LysfsTer4)	Homo	2 (1)	Zlotogora et al. [3, 36] Suzuki et al. [7]
	c.969dupT (p.Thr324TyrfsTer65)	Homo	3 + 2 (1)	Rodini and Richieri-Costa [10] Suzuki et al. [7]
	c.400C>T (p.Arg134Ter)	Homo	1 (1)	Yoshida et al. [37]
PVRL4	c.851G>A (p.Arg284Gln)	Homo	4 (1)	Boudghene-Stambouli and Merad-Boudia [9] Brancati et al. [8]
	c.554C>T + c.906delT (p.Thr185Met + p.Pro304HisfsTer2)	Comp het	2 (1)	Brancati et al. [8]
	c.635C>G (p.Pro212Arg)	Homo	10 (1)	Jelani et al. [11]
	c.724G4A (p.Val242Met)	Homo	3 (1)	Fortugno et al. [12]
	Exon 2 in frame deletion	Homo	1 (1)	Svendsen et al. [38]
	c.181C>T (p.AspGln61Ter)	Homo	3 (1)	Raza et al. [13]
	c.247C>T (p.His83Tyr)	Homo	1 (1)	Dardour et al. [14]
	c.242T>C (p.Leu81Pro)	Homo	4 (1)	Ahmad et al. [39]
	c.229C>T (p.Gln77Ter)	Homo	1 (1)	Florian et al. [15]
	c.1150delC (p.Gln384ArgfsTer7)	Homo	1 (1)	Rotunno et al. [16]
	c.1117C>T (p.Arg373Ter)	Homo	1 (1)	Carroppo et al. [17]
	c.163C>T (p.Arg55Ter)	Homo	3 + 12 (1)	Hajra et al. [40]

philtrum. Only 7 out of the 26 do not have lip or palate defects; all of them belong to the Margarita Island families.

In addition, partial cutaneous syndactyly is almost always present at fingers 2–3 and/or 3–4, and toes 2–3; syndactyly 1–2 or 4–5 has never been reported in these patients. In seven of the Margarita Island affected individuals, no syndactyly was detected.

The skin is dry and thick on the palms and soles. Palmar and plantar hyperkeratosis worsen with age. The nails are mostly normal, but onychodysplasia is occasionally reported.

Anomalies of the teeth are prominent with microdontia, hypodontia, delayed eruption, and anodontia reported in adults.

While mental retardation was thought to be a mandatory feature when the syndrome was first delineated, it is now clear that cognitive involvement differs from family to family. In the Israeli, Brazilian, and Japanese families, all affected children presented cognitive impairment [3, 10], not recorded in the Margarita Island patients [5]. Such many individuals deriving from a founder effect offers a unique opportunity to unravel the full spectrum of the disease, although one cannot exclude concurrent, yet independent, phenotypes unrelated to the underlying gene defect (and unlinked to nectin-1 deficiency). Among *PVRL1* reported individuals, the most severely affected patients were mentally retarded and presented with all the features of the syndrome. On the other hand of the clinical spectrum, in two affected individuals from Margarita Island with the typical faces, scanty eyebrows, sparse, short and brittle hairs, anodontia and hyperkeratosis of palms and soles were not retarded without either cleft lip/palate or cutaneous syndactyly.

Affected individuals appear to have a normal life span, and affected adults have been reported; however, several patients died in infancy with no apparent cause. In the Israeli family, one of the two affected siblings died suddenly at the age of 8 months, and in the Brazilian family, two boys out of 5 affected died, one at the age of 10 days and the other neonatally. None of the affected patients from Margarita Island died neonatally or in infancy. It seems therefore that there may be two different forms of the syndrome: a severe form with mental retardation and risk for infantile death and a milder form with normal mental development and life span.

Four different homozygous mutations have been identified in the *PVRL1* gene, all encoding a prematurely truncated nectin-1 protein that lacks the transmembrane and intracellular domains. Two of them, identified by Suzuki et al. [7] in the Israeli and Margarita Island families, affect the same codon (c.554delG p.Glu186Lysfs*4, and c.554G>A p.Trp185*). These findings are summarized in Table 8.1. Possible nonsense-mediated mRNA decay has not been investigated; however, loss of the intracellular domain might disrupt the cell-cell adhesion function of the protein.

8.3 Nectin 4-ED

Brancati et al. [8] identified biallelic mutations in the *PVRL4* gene, encoding CAM nectin-4, as the underlying cause of this syndrome. One of the families was previously reported by Boudghene-Stambouli and Merad-Boudia in 1991 [9]. Later, additional reports have described single patients broadening the allelic spectrum of this entity, although the clinical features are quite homogeneous. The summary of the clinical features was performed by reviewing 46 individuals from 12 families affected by this syndrome and harboring biallelic (homozygous or, more rarely, compound heterozygous) variants in the *PVRL4* gene (Table 8.1).

Syndactyly and defects of hair and teeth are pathognomonic of the disease. In particular, cutaneous syndactyly of toes 2–3 is a consistent finding, and sometimes toes 4–5 too. Cutaneous syndactyly of fingers 2–3–4 has been observed in different combinations and absent in two affected individuals. Syndactyly of fingers 1–2 or 4–5 and toes 1–2 has never been reported.

Hypotrichosis with progressive alopecia is present in all patients, and a family with congenital alopecia has also been described. Hair, eyelashes, and eyebrows are dry, sparse, and fragile. Hair abnormalities suggestive of pili torti have been observed by trichoscopic evaluation performed in several cases.

Teeth are mainly small, peg shaped, and widely spaced; enamel defects and other dental anomalies, such as delayed eruption, microdontia, hypodontia, and anodontia in adults, have also been found in several patients.

Most of the patients present dry skin and palmoplantar keratosis that progressively worsens with age. Nails can be hyperkeratotic and discolored; hypoplastic nails were reported by Jelani et al. [11].

None of the patients presented with either cleft lip/palate or mental retardation, and the life span of the affected individuals appears to be in the normal range.

Finally, additional findings were described in a few patients, such as deformed pinnae, abnormal nipples, and heat intolerance. A complete absence of sweat gland units was observed in the palm biopsy of one of the patients [13].

8.4 Possible existence of genetic heterogeneity

Further genetic heterogeneity may be suspected. Indeed, in a single family reported by Tariq et al. [18], including 4 affected patients, the responsible gene was linked to a haplotype of 7p21.1-p14.3.

The patient is the first child of healthy parents of Turkish descent. The parents are related; first cousins once removed. Family history is negative with regard to congenital malformations or similar disorders as seen in the child.

The child presents hypotrichosis and slow-growing hair on the scalp, but pili torti was not observed. The teeth were conical and cylindrical shaped with ill-defined surface morphology. Mild epidermolytic hyperkeratosis and mild to severe dystrophic palmoplantar keratoderma were observed in the patients. Due to the strong similarity to the EDSS1 phenotype, the disease was named EDSS2. This second EDSS was never confirmed in the literature so far; rather distinct partially overlapping phenotypes may mimic nectin-4 ED (see differential diagnosis).

8.5 Differential Diagnosis Among Families with Ectodermal Dysplasia and Syndactyly

The resemblance between patients that have been classified as affected with an EDSS1 or EDSS2 and those with CLPED1 is striking. Similar features include the hair changes often described as pili torti, dental abnormalities, progressive palmar and plantar hyperkeratosis, and cutaneous syndactyly of fingers and toes in various combinations sparing the first and last fingers and toes. The major differences are the potential presence of cleft lip/palate, mental retardation, and early mortality in CLPED1. Cleft lip/palate was present in at least one member of CLPED1-affected families, while it has never been described in EDSS-affected families. Interfamilial variability is significant in CLPED1. For example, infantile mortality and mental retardation described in two families are absent in all the members of the Margarita Island families. These manifestations are absent also in the EDSS families, and they may represent distinctive CLPED1 features or simply they will be identified when other EDSS families are described. While clinically the syndromes appear to be distinct, the existing overlap between individual patients does not allow classifying with certainty on a clinical basis patients with syndactyly and ED.

In 1994, according to the clinical features, six families were included in the delineation of what was known as the Zlotogora Ogür syndrome [42]. As described above, in three families, a mutation in the *PVRL1* gene was characterized, and two of the other families are probably affected by the syndrome. These families are the one reported by Ogür and Yuksel that probably represents another example of the severe form of CLPED1 syndrome and the family reported by Richieri-Costa et al. with the mild form of the syndrome. The report of Richieri-Costa included the description of a single affected individual with normal neuropsychological development, bilateral cleft lip and palate, and typical facial features of CLPED1.

The family reported by Wiedemann in 1978 that was thought to represent the first description of the Zlotogora Ogür syndrome included three children with pili torti, sparse eyebrows and eyelashes, abnormal teeth with hyperkeratosis of the palmoplantar region, as well as a distal third of the trunk and lower limbs. Syndactyly of fingers and toes were present at diverse degrees. The intelligence was normal, and there was no cleft lip/palate. Accordingly, they were probably affected by one of the ED syndactyly syndromes [3].

In one Italian family with two sibs exhibiting features overlapping nectin 4-ED, Fortugno et al. [41] identified biallelic variants in the *RIPK4* gene, previously involved in Bartsocas-Papas syndrome (BPS) (OMIM 263650), a more severe disorder with overlapping features and a mild form termed curly hair-ankyloblepharon-nail dysplasia (CHAND) syndrome, characterized by ankyloblepharon, sparse, curly, and woolly hair, nail dysplasia, and oral frenula [19]. The authors provided convincing evidence on the functional link between RIPK4 and nectin-mediated cell adhesion which may mirror phenotypic overlap. Interestingly, they provided evidence that other ED syndromes such as TP63-pathies (Hay-Wells, OMIM#106260 and ectrodactyly, ectodermal dysplasia, and cleft lip/palate syndrome, EEC, OMIM#604292) and IRF6-pathies (Popliteal pterygium syndrome, OMIM#119500 and van der Woude syndrome, OMIM#119300) display both functional and clinical convergences. These overlapping manifestations demonstrate how apparently unrelated molecules may act with different functions in converging pathways to cause distinct, yet overlapping, ED syndromes [41].

Several other examples in the medical literature exist, potentially representing examples of patients with nectinopathies. This observation is based on the association of distinct hair defects (often referred to as pili torti et canaliculi), cutaneous syndactyly, and variable developmental delay/cognitive defects. Examples of such clinical reports include Ackerman et al. [20] and Argenziano et al. [21], but the authors were not able to recall such patients for genetic analysis of *PVRL1/4* genes.

8.6 Molecular Pathology of Nectinopathies

The nectin family is composed of four members, nectin-1 to -4, all sharing the same domain organization. They contain an extracellular region with three immunoglobulin-like loops, a single membrane-spanning region, and a cytoplasmic tail, through which they directly bind afadin, an F-actin-binding protein [22, 23]. Nectins are known to promote cell-cell adhesion through homophilic or heterophilic interaction mediated by their Ig-like ectodomains both in *cis* and *trans*. In particular, nectins first form *cis*-homodimers, which then undergo lateral cluster formation on the cell surface [24]. Homogeneous clusters interact in *trans*, either homophilically or heterophilically, with those present on the opposing cell surface. Heterophilic interactions (such as nectin-1 and -4) are typically stronger than homophilic ones [23]. During adherens junctions (AJ) formation, nectin-enriched clusters assemble earlier at cell-cell contact sites and, through Rho GTPase activation, contribute to the recruitment of cadherin-enriched clusters, to which they are connected by junction-associated actin filament bundles [25, 26].

AJs significantly contribute to cell adhesion in the epidermis and in the hair follicle, both during organogenesis and in skin homeostasis [27]. During tissue development, physiological renewal, and repair, cells migrate to particular places through directional and/or random cell movement and then adhere to neighboring cells, through cell-cell adhesion junctions, to form tissues with well-defined structure and function. A finely driven cell migration and positioning is indispensable for correct development and, in this context, CAMs, such as nectins, play a crucial role [22].

In particular, *trans*-heterodimer formation is the molecular basis for a unique function of nectins in modulating specific cell-cell interactions and arranging cells in precise patterns [23]. Indeed, in the context of ectodermal development and skin homeostasis, nectin-1 and -4 operate in synergy as also demonstrated not only by the broad phenotypic overlap observed in EDSS1 and CLPED1 ([1, 3, 8]), but also by the specific and by some means complementary pattern of expression in skin, hair follicles, developing tooth, and palate [8, 12, 28]. It has been shown, both in patient skin biopsies and in vitro cultured keratinocytes, that nectin-4-altered expression perturbs nectin-1 clustering at cell-cell contact sites and delays, but does not impede, cadherin recruitment at AJs and cell aggregation [12]. Moreover, *trans*-interaction between specific nectins expressed in the different epithelial compartments of the developing tooth is involved in the formation of cell-cell junctions between ameloblasts and cells of the neighboring stratum intermedium (nectin-1 and -2 expressed in ameloblasts interact with nectin-3 and -4 present on the surface of stratum intermedium cells) [23].

Besides nectins 1/4, other CAMs (i.e., P-cadherin and plakophilins (PKP)) or their regulators (i.e., the transcription factors p63 and IRF6) and the protein kinase RIPK4 have been implicated in the pathogenesis of ED syndromes, validating the importance of investigating this class of molecules in other as yet uncharacterized EDs [41].

8.7 Role of Nectins as Viral Receptors

The high frequency of CLPED1 reported on Margarita Island might be a consequence of another peculiar function of nectins. Indeed, members of nectins have also been reported as viral receptors. In particular, nectin-1 (and -2) was shown to be the principal receptor used by α-herpesviruses to mediate entry into human cells [29]; PVRL1 mutation, therefore, might protect carriers from infection by α-herpesviruses, including HSV1 and HSV2 [7]. As well, nectin-4 has been demonstrated to be a receptor for the measles virus (a paramyxovirus) and to sustain measles virus entry and noncytopathic spread in differentiated human epithelial airway sheets [30, 31].

8.8 Role of Nectins in Cancer

In the adult organism, dysfunction of cell-cell adhesion plays a crucial role in the development and progression of cancers. Altered expression of both nectin-1 and -4 has been reported in various cancer types. However, while loss of nectin-1 expression has been associated with reduced cell-cell adhesion and increased invasiveness and metastasis (*reviewed in* [32, 33]), nectin-4 is specifically overexpressed in various cancer types, including breast cancer, ovarian cancer, and pancreatic cancer, and is closely related to tumor oncogenesis and the poor prognosis of affected patients [34]. The biological role of Nectin-4 in promoting proliferation, migration, and triggering metastasis in carcinogenesis is under intensive research focus. Despite the fact that the expression level or the positive rate of Nectin-4 is different among selected types of tumor specimens, most studies have confirmed Nectin-4 as a prognostic and diagnostic biomarker with strong evidence to use it as a target for cancer therapy [34].

Acknowledgments The authors wish to thank first all families and patients participating in their studies on nectin-related EDs as well as their mentors Professor Bruno Dallapiccola and Giovanna Zambruno, pioneers in the field of medical genetics and genodermatoses.

References

1. Brancati F, Agolini E, Fortugno P. Nectinopathies: an emerging group of ectodermal dysplasia syndromes. G Ital Dermatol Venereol. 2013;148:59–64.
2. Biesecker LG, Adam MP, Alkuraya FS, Amemiya AR, Bamshad MJ, Beck AE, Bennett JT, Bird LM, Carey JC, Chung B, Clark RD, Cox TC, Curry C, Dinulos MBP, Dobyns WB, Giampietro PF, Girisha KM, Glass IA, Graham JM Jr, Gripp KW, Haldeman-Englert CR, Hall BD, Innes AM, Kalish JM, Keppler-Noreuil KM, Kosaki K, Kozel BA, Mirzaa GM, Mulvihill JJ, Nowaczyk MJM, Pagon RA, Retterer K, Rope AF, Sanchez-Lara PA, Seaver LH, Shieh JT, Slavotinek AM, Sobering AK, Stevens CA, Stevenson DA, Tan TY, Tan WH, Tsai AC, Weaver

DD, Williams MS, Zackai E, Zarate YA. A dyadic approach to the delineation of diagnostic entities in clinical genomics. Am J Hum Genet. 2021;108(1):8–15.

3. Zlotogora J, Zilberman Y, Tenenbaum A, Wexler MR. Cleft lip and palate, pili torti, malformed ears, partial syndactyly of fingers and toes, and mental retardation: a new syndrome? J Med Genet. 1987;24:291–3.
4. Oğur G, Yüksel M. Association of syndactyly, ectodermal dysplasia, and cleft lip and palate: report of two sibs from Turkey. J Med Genet. 1988;25:37–40.
5. Bustos T, Simosa V, Pinto-Cisternas J, Abramovits W, Jolay L, Rodriguez L, Fernandez L, Ramela M. Autosomal recessive ectodermal dysplasia: I. An undescribed dysplasia/malformation syndrome. Am J Med Genet. 1991;41:398–404.
6. Suzuki K, Bustos T, Spritz RA. Linkage disequilibrium mapping of the gene for Margarita Island ectodermal dysplasia (ED4) to 11q23. Am J Hum Genet. 1998;63:1102–7.
7. Suzuki K, Hu D, Bustos T, Zlotogora J, Richieri-Costa A, Helms JA, Spritz RA. Mutations of PVRL1, encoding a cell-cell adhesion molecule/herpesvirus receptor, in cleft lip/palate-ectodermal dysplasia. Nat Genet. 2000;25:427–30.
8. Brancati F, Fortugno P, Bottillo I, Lopez M, Josselin E, Boudghene-Stambouli O, Agolini E, Bernardini L, Bellacchio E, Iannicelli M, Rossi A, Dib-Lachachi A, Stuppia L, Palka G, Mundlos S, Stricker S, Kornak U, Zambruno G, Dallapiccola B. Mutations in PVRL4, encoding cell adhesion molecule nectin-4, cause ectodermal dysplasia-syndactyly syndrome. Am J Hum Genet. 2010;87:265–73.
9. Boudghene-Stambouli O, Merad-Boudia A. Association of ectodermal dysplasia and syndactylia. Ann Dermatol Venereol. 1991;118:107–10.
10. Rodini ES, Richieri-Costa A. Autosomal recessive ectodermal dysplasia, cleft lip/palate, mental retardation, and syndactyly: the Zlotogora-Ogur syndrome. Am J Med Genet. 1990;36:473–6.
11. Jelani M, Chishti MS, Ahmad W. Mutation in PVRL4 gene encoding nectin-4 underlies ectodermal-dysplasia-syndactyly syndrome (EDSS1). J Hum Genet. 2011;56:352–7.
12. Fortugno P, Josselin E, Tsiakas K, Agolini E, Cestra G, Teson M, Santer R, Castiglia D, Novelli G, Dallapiccola B, Kurth I, Lopez M, Zambruno G, Brancati F. Nectin-4 mutations causing ectodermal dysplasia with syndactyly perturb the Rac1 pathway and the kinetics of adherens junction formation. J Invest Dermatol. 2014;134(8):2146–53.
13. Raza SI, Nasser Dar R, Shah AA, Ahmad W. A novel homozygous nonsense mutation in the PVRL4 gene and expansion of clinical spectrum of EDSS1. Ann. Hum. Genet. 2015;79:92–8.
14. Dardour L, Cosyns K, Devriendt K. A novel missense variant in the *PVRL4* gene underlying ectodermal dysplasia-syndactyly syndrome in a Turkish child. Mol Syndromol. 2017;9(1):22–4.
15. Florian R, Gruber R, Volc-Platzer B. A novel homozygous mutation in PVRL4 causes ectodermal dysplasia-syndactyly syndrome 1. Int J Dermatol. 2018;57(2):223–6.
16. Rotunno R, Diociaiuti A, Dentici ML, Rinelli M, Callea M, Retrosi C, Zambruno G, Bellacchio E, El Hachem M. Ectodermal dysplasia-syndactyly syndrome with toe-only minimal syndactyly due to a novel mutation in NECTIN4: a case report and literature review. Genes (Basel). 2021;12(5):748.
17. Caroppo F, Fagotto L, Fortina AB. A novel pathogenic variant of NECTIN4 gene in a child with ectodermal dysplasia-syndactyly syndrome. Indian Dermatol Online J. 2023;14:110–1.
18. Tariq M, Khan MN, Ahmad W. Ectodermal dysplasia-cutaneous syndactyly syndrome maps to chromosome 7p21.1-p14.3. Hum. Genet. 2009;125:421–9.
19. Busa T, Jeraiby M, Clemenson A, Manouvrier S, Granados V, Philip N, Touraine R. Confirmation that RIPK4 mutations cause not only bartsocas-papas syndrome but also CHAND syndrome. Am J Med Genet. 2017;173A:3114–7.
20. Abramovits-Ackerman W, Bustos T, Simosa-Leon V, Fernandez L, Ramella M. Cutaneous findings in a new syndrome of autosomal recessive ectodermal dysplasia with corkscrew hairs. J Am Acad Dermatol. 1992;27(6 Pt 1):917–21.
21. Argenziano G, Monsurrò MR, Pazienza R, Delfino M. A case of probable autosomal recessive ectodermal dysplasia with corkscrew hairs and mental retardation in a family with tuberous sclerosis. J Am Acad Dermatol. 1998;38(2 Pt 2):344–8.

22. Mandai K, Rikitake Y, Mori M, Takai Y. Nectins and nectin-like molecules in development and disease. Curr Top Dev Biol. 2015;112:197–231.
23. Rikitake Y, Mandai K, Takai Y. The role of nectins in different types of cell-cell adhesion. J Cell Sci. 2012;125(Pt 16):3713–22.
24. Irie K, Shimizu K, Sakisaka T, Ikeda W, Takai Y. Roles and modes of action of nectins in cell-cell adhesion. Semin Cell Dev Biol. 2004;15(6):643–56.
25. Honda T, Shimizu K, Kawakatsu T, Yasumi M, Shingai T, Fukuhara A, Ozaki-Kuroda K, Irie K, Nakanishi H, Takai Y. Antagonistic and agonistic effects of an extracellular fragment of nectin on formation of E-cadherin-based cell-cell adhesion. Genes Cells. 2003;8(1):51–63.
26. Indra I, Hong S, Troyanovsky R, Kormos B, Troyanovsky S. The adherens junction: a mosaic of cadherin and nectin clusters bundled by actin filaments. J Invest Dermatol. 2013;133(11):2546–54.
27. Jamora C, Fuchs E. Intercellular adhesion, signalling and the cytoskeleton. Nat Cell Biol. 2002;4(4):E101–8.
28. Mollo MR, Antonini D, Mitchell K, Fortugno P, Costanzo A, Dixon J, Brancati F, Missero C. p63-dependent and independent mechanisms of nectin-1 and nectin-4 regulation in the epidermis. Exp Dermatol. 2015;24(2):114–9.
29. Geraghty RJ, Krummenacher C, Cohen GH, Eisenberg RJ, Spear PG. Entry of alphaherpesviruses mediated by poliovirus receptor-related protein 1 and poliovirus receptor. Science. 1998;280:1618–20.
30. Laksono BM, Fortugno P, Nijmeijer BM, de Vries RD, Cordisco S, Kuiken T, Geijtenbeek TBH, Duprex WP, Brancati F, de Swart RL. Measles skin rash: Infection of lymphoid and myeloid cells in the dermis precedes viral dissemination to the epidermis. PLoS Pathog. 2020;16(10):e1008253.
31. Mühlebach MD, Mateo M, Sinn PL, Prüfer S, Uhlig KM, Leonard VH, Navaratnarajah CK, Frenzke M, Wong XX, Sawatsky B, Ramachandran S, McCray PB Jr, Cichutek K, von Messling V, Lopez M, Cattaneo R. Adherens junction protein nectin-4 is the epithelial receptor for measles virus. Nature. 2011;480(7378):530–3.
32. Barcelo J, Sanz-Moreno V. NECTIN1 is a melanoma metastasis suppressor gene. Nat Genet. 2022;54(12):1776–7.
33. Duraivelan K, Samanta D. Emerging roles of the nectin family of cell adhesion molecules in tumour-associated pathways. Biochim Biophys Acta Rev Cancer. 2021;1876(2):188589.
34. Liu Y, Han X, Li L, Zhang Y, Huang X, Li G, Xu C, Yin M, Zhou P. Role of nectin-4 protein in cancer. Int J Oncol. 2021;59:1–14.
35. Richieri-Costa A, Guion-Almeida ML, Freire-Maia N, Pinheiro M. Autosomal recessive cleft lip/palate, ectodermal dysplasia, and minor acral anomalies: report of a Brazilian family. Am J Med Genet. 1992;44:158–62.
36. Zlotogora J, Ogur G. Syndactyly, ectodermal dysplasia, and cleft lip and palate. J Med Genet. 1988;25:503.
37. Yoshida K, Hayashi R, Fujita H, Kubota M, Kondo M, Shimomura Y, Niizeki H. Novel homozygous mutation, c.400C>T (p.Arg134*), in the PVRL1 gene underlies cleft lip/palate-ectodermal dysplasia syndrome in an Asian patient. J Dermatol. 2015;42(7):715–9. doi: 10.1111/1346-8138.12882. Epub 2015 Apr 24. PMID: 25913853.
38. Svendsen T, Henningsen E, Hertz JM, Vestergaard Grejsen D, Bygum A. A retrospective study of clinical and mutational findings in 45 Danish families with ectodermal dysplasia. Acta Derm Venereol. 2014;94(5):531–3.
39. Ahmad F, Nasir A, Thiele H, Umair M, Borck G, Ahmad W. A novel homozygous missense variant in NECTIN4 (PVRL4) causing ectodermal dysplasia cutaneous syndactyly syndrome. Ann Hum Genet. 2018;82(4):232–8.
40. Hajra B, Abdullah, Bibi N, Syed F, Ullah A, Ahmad W, Umm-E-Kalsoom. A novel homozygous nonsense mutation in NECTIN4 gene in a Pakistani family with ectodermal dysplasia syndactyly syndrome 1. An Bras Dermatol. 2023;98(5):580–6.

41. Fortugno P, Monetta R, Belli M, Botti E, Angelucci F, Palmerini MG, Nottola SA, De Luca C, Ceccarini M, Salvatore M, Bianchi L, Macioce P, Teson M, Ricci F; Italian Undiagnosed Diseases Network; Macchiarelli G, Didona B, Costanzo A, Castiglia D, Brancati F. RIPK4 regulates cell-cell adhesion in epidermal development and homeostasis. Hum Mol Genet. 2022;31(15):2535–47.
42. Zlotogora J. Syndactyly, ectodermal dysplasia, and cleft lip/palate. J Med Genet. 1994;31(12):957–9.

Chapter 9
Other Syndromes with Prominent Ectodermal Dysplasia Signs

Gianluca Tadini, Beatrice Carcano, and Michela Brena

Keywords WNT · P63 · Eda pathways

9.1 KREMEN-1-Related ED

"Kringle containing transmembrane protein 1" acts in the WNT/beta-catenin pathway via low-density lipoprotein receptor-related protein 6 (LRP6; positive modulation)- and via DKK1-mediated WNT inhibition. Autosomal recessive mutations in few families are reported, primarily with hypodontia of both dentitions. Some family members show abnormal hair distribution, brittle and oily scalp hair, and facial dysmorphism (hypertelorism and downslanting palpebral fissures, broad nose and protruding lips, and soft facial skin). Sweat glands and nails are usually unaffected (Fig. 9.1) [1, 2].

9.2 LEF1-Related ED

Lymphoid enhancer-binding factor 1 (LEF1) is a downstream effector of the WNT pathway together with beta-catenin. 4q25 deletions encompassing LEF1 and haploinsufficiency lead to the ectodermal dysplasia (ED) phenotype.

WNT-stabilized beta-catenin translocates to the nucleus and requires LEF1 for activation of gene expression, especially EDA pathway gene expression. In mouse

G. Tadini · B. Carcano
Center for Inherited Cutaneous Diseases, University of Milan, Milan, Italy
e-mail: gtadinicmce@unimi.it

M. Brena (✉)
Center for Inherited Cutaneous Diseases, University of Milan, Milan, Italy

Pediatric Dermatology Unit, Department of Clinical Sciences and Community Health, Fondazione IRCCS Ca' Granda Ospedale Maggiore Policlinico, Milan, Italy
e-mail: michela.brena@policlinico.mi.it

G. Tadini et al. (eds.), *Multidisciplinary Approach to Ectodermal Dysplasia*,
https://doi.org/10.1007/978-3-031-75790-7_9

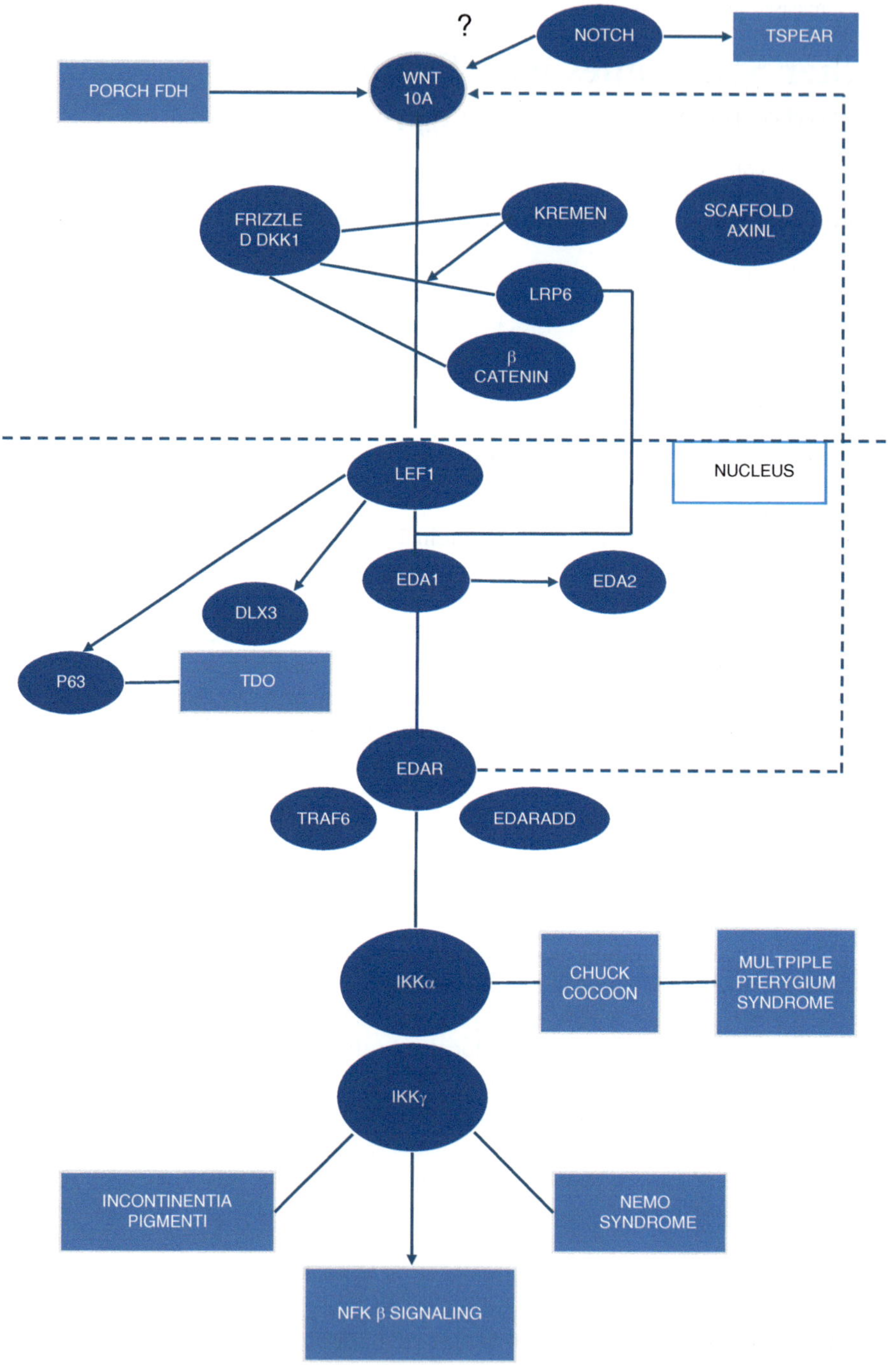

Fig. 9.1 WNT-EDA pathway and related phenotypes

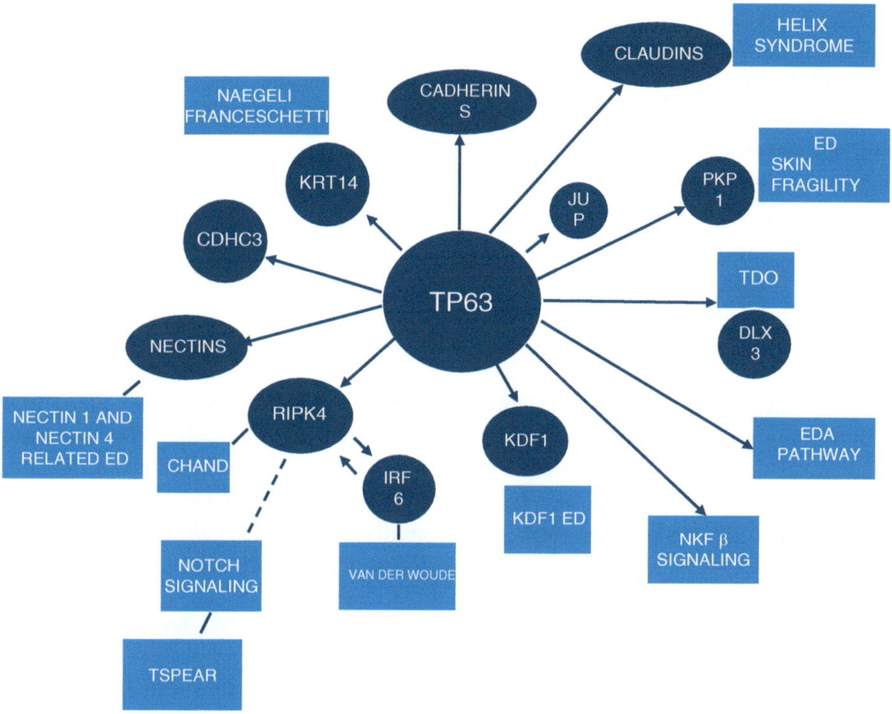

Fig. 9.2 P63 pathway and related phenotypes

models, LEF1 is essential for mesenchymal interactions and in tooth and hair development, exerting a crucial role in embryogenesis. Knockout mice may have also limb defects and split hand and foot malformations, similar to those observed in p63-related ED (Fig. 9.2).

Usually, affected patients present with oligodontia of various degrees, taurodontism, and alveolar bone defects. Sparse fine hair, dry skin, and hypohidrosis are reported in some patients. Nipples and mammary malformations may be associated [3].

9.3 AXIN2-Related ED

Axis inhibition protein 2 (AXIN2) is a scaffolding component of the beta-catenin degradation protein complex. AXIN2 autosomal dominant mutations disrupt the WNT signaling pathway (negative regulation).

Affected patients present with "facies": hypognathia, malar hypoplasia, broad nasal bridge, and upslanting palpebral fissures. Oligodontia and cleft lip/palate may be associated.

Skin signs are fine scalp hair and eyebrows with normal body hair. Sweat glands and nails appear unaffected.

AXIN2 mutations are primarily involved in early-onset colorectal cancers (CRC) and adenomatous polyposis coli (APC) and increased the risk of occurrence of other internal organ cancers (mammary).

Teeth, skin, and CRC/APC may be present in the same subject or may be present separately [4].

9.4 LRP6

Low-density lipoprotein receptor-related protein 6 (LRP6)-encoding gene acts in the formation of a complex with WNTs and Frizzled to activate the WNT signaling pathway, translocating beta-catenin into the nucleus and interacting with LEF1 that facilitates the transcription of WNT target genes, that is, EDA pathway genes. Mutations in the LRP6 gene have been recently associated with autosomal dominant tooth agenesis, cleft lip/palate, and anatomical defects of fingers and external ears.

LRP6 is also associated with neurological disturbances (Alzheimer's disease), osteoporosis, and coronary artery disease.

In some patients, triangular facies together with sparse hair and hypohidrosis may be present. Incomplete intrafamilial penetrance is possible [5].

9.5 KDF1-Related ED

Keratinocyte differentiation factor 1 (KDF1) is a promoter of the proliferation and differentiation of progenitor epidermal cells. Mutations in exon 2 demonstrate that haploinsufficiency is enough to cause the related phenotype.

Affected patients may have ED signs, like nonsyndromic tooth agenesis or a syndromic ED characterized by severe oligodontia, cleft lift/palate, punctal agenesis, hypo-athelia and skin defects with sparse hair, rudimentary eyebrows and eyelashes, and xerotic skin with a facies very similar to the EDA1 facial phenotype. Nails are brittle, hypoplastic, and convex with pitting and keratosis of the nail bed.

Hypospadias and urethral stenosis are reported together with an increased risk of infections.

9.6 HELIX Syndrome

An autosomal recessive syndrome due to mutations in Claudin-10 causes HELIX syndrome. Claudins, in number of 27, are protein involved in the formations of tight junctions, structures located in the upper part of the lateral epithelial cell membranes that selectively control the passage of water and small ions, maintain cell polarity, and modulate signal transduction acting as a regulator of paracellular selectivity and pore permeability to electrolytes.

That is, CLDN19 mutations are responsible for hypoMg and hyperK syndrome, mutations of CLDN1 are responsible for ichthyosis and sclerosing cholangitis syndrome, and CLDN14 mutations are involved in a subset of nonsyndromic deafness.

HELIX syndrome-affected patients show xerostomia, whole-body hypohidrosis, mild diffuse ichthyosis, palmoplantar keratoderma with hyperlinearity, hypoalacrimia, enamel defects, hypokalemia, and muscle cramps. Hair and nails are unaffected. Skin biopsies reveal an increased number of dilated eccrine glands with acantholytic appearance of sweat gland epithelia.

Signs and symptoms are explained by total loss of Na transport across the tight junctions [6].

9.7 TSPEAR-Related ED

Autosomal recessive mutations lead to the ED phenotype.

ThromboSpondin-type laminin G domain and Epilepsy Associated Repeats (TSPEAR) is related to the NOTCH signaling pathway. Even if the function of this structure is largely unknown, it may interact with the NF-kbeta pathway and the WNT pathway. TSPEAR shows an analogy with the Drosophila counterpart "CLOSCA" that is an extracellular matrix-dependent regulator. TSPEAR and WNT knockout zebrafish show epithelial stem cell disturbances of self-renewal and decreased capacity of damage repair and fin anomalies.

In our cohort, TSPEAR accounts for the majority of recessive ED syndromes, even though the published cases account for only 30 patients.

Skin signs are abnormality of hair texture and fine sparse hair in 50–60% of cases; nail anomalies in up to 40%; and xerosis in one-third of patients (Figs. 9.3, 9.4, 9.5, 9.6, and 9.7). Hypohidrosis of different severity is reported in 20% of cases but, on the contrary, is the hallmark in our six TSPEAR mutated patients from 3 different families.

Hypodontia and oligodontia are reported in almost all patients with conical teeth requiring odontostomatological survey and treatment.

No internal organ involvement is reported [7].

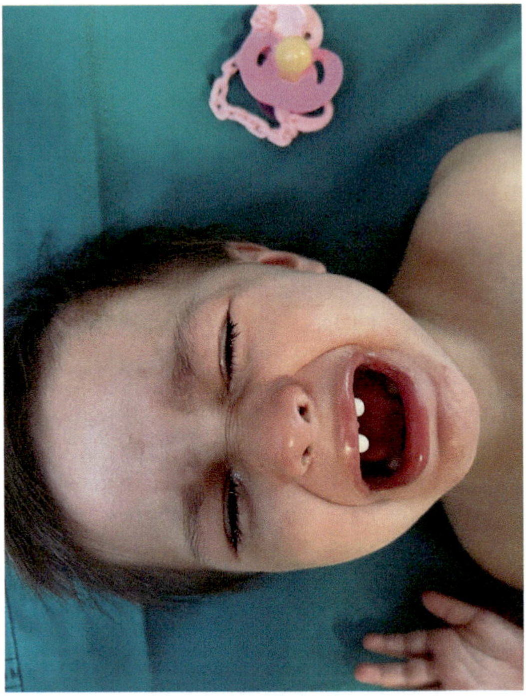

Fig. 9.3 Dental anomalies in a 5-year-old boy with TSPEAR mutation

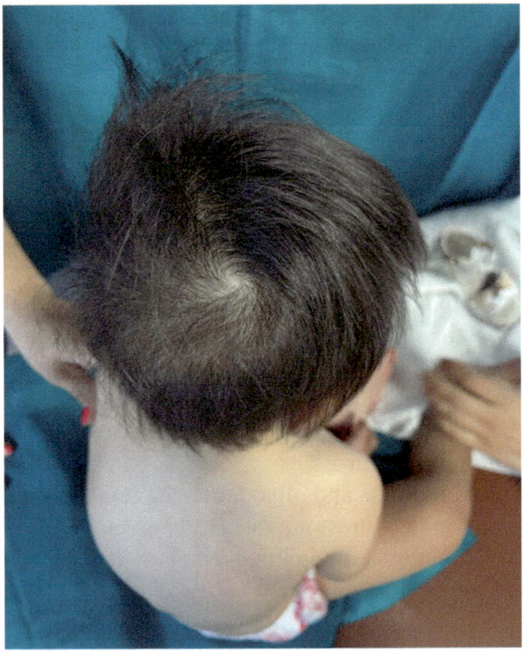

Fig. 9.4 Hair defects in a 2-year-old boy with TSPEAR mutation

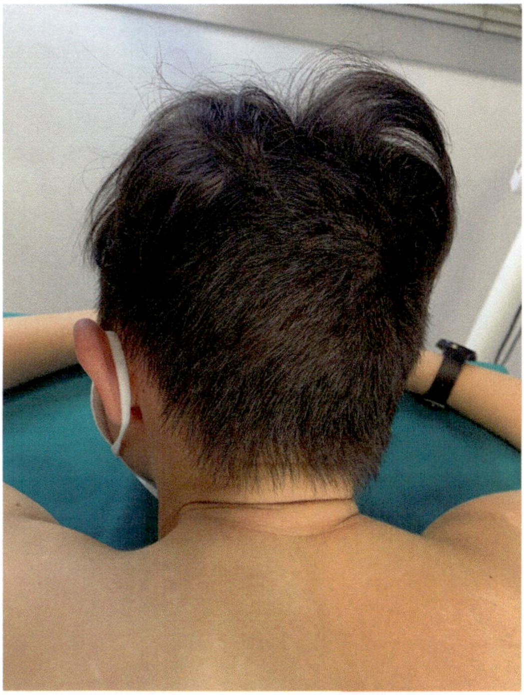

Fig. 9.5 Peculiar hair distribution in a 7-year-old boy with TSPEAR mutation

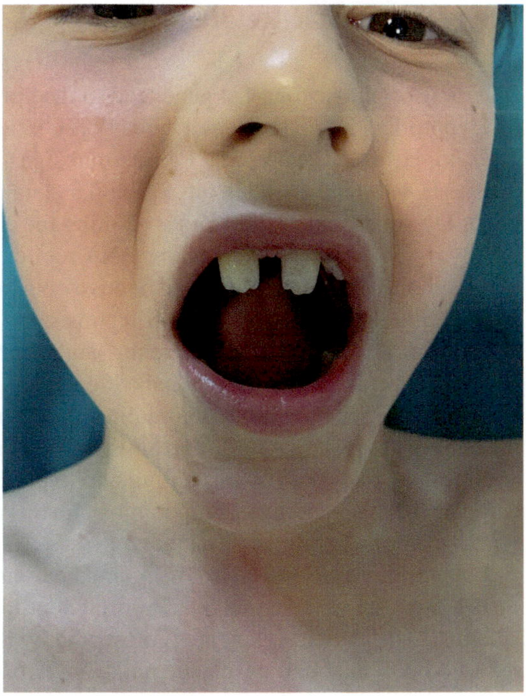

Fig. 9.6 TSPEAR-4

Fig. 9.7 TSPEAR-5

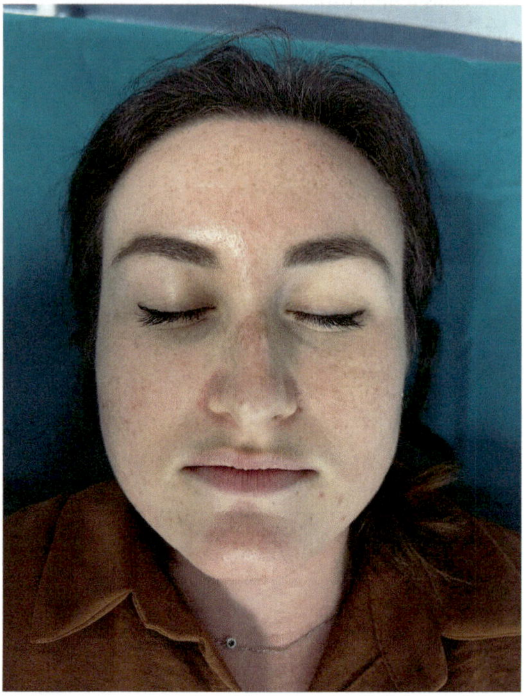

9.8 HIST1H1E-Related ED

Mutations in the histone 1-4 gene lead to the autosomal dominant syndrome.

Hypotonia, Intellectual and behavioral issues, Skeletal, undescended Testes, Thyroid, Heart anomalies and Ectodermal signs (HIST1H1E).

The H 1-4 gene encodes for a globular domain-containing factor that binds the linker DNA between nucleosomes forming the chromatin fibers. This structure intimately modulates gene expression, DNA replication, recombination, and repair. As expected, these patients show a distinctive epigenetic signature with increased DNA methylation that is very useful for diagnosis.

First recognized in schizophrenia- and neurodevelopmental-affected patients, now a syndromic pattern is recognizable in the about 50 described pedigrees, characterized by: generalized hypotonia in infancy, mild-to-severe intellectual disability, behavioral issues (ADHD and autism spectrum), and facies with frontal bossing, and deep-set eyes with downslanting and hypertelorism. Skeletal anomalies are the hallmark of this syndrome with craniosynostosis, kyphoscoliosis, limb asymmetry, brachy-camptodactyly, and fractures.

Cryptorchidism, hypothyroidism, and heart anomalies are reported.

ED signs are represented by abnormal dentitions with enamel dysplasia and caries. In 30% of patients, they are represented by thin brittle slow-growing scalp hair, reduced body hair, and dysplastic nails. No hypohidrosis is reported [8].

9.9 MAP3K20-Related ED

Rare biallelic pathogenic variants in Mitogen-Activated Protein 3-Kinase 20 (MAP3K20) cause split hand and foot malformation, hearing loss, and nail abnormalities.

Heterozygous de novo mutations show craniosynostosis, camptodactyly, and limb anomalies similar to p63-related cases and sensorineural hearing loss.

Facies with hypertelorism, telecanthus, palpebral fibromas of inner canthus, micrognathia, small nose, and anteverted ears are reported.

Skin signs are blaschkoid streaks of dystrophic lichenoid hypoplastic dry skin visible also at palmoplantar level, psoriasiform plaques, keratosis pilaris, and xerotic skin. Nails may be brittle, small, and dysplastic. Sparse hair and eyebrows with trichorrhexis nodosa are reported. Overheating episodes and hypohidrosis are reported, together with skin fragility [9].

9.10 CHAND Syndrome

Curly and sparse Hair, Ankyloblepharon, Nail dysplasia, and Dry skin (CHAND) syndrome is a very rare autosomal recessive disorder due to the mutation in the RIPK4 gene (receptor-interacting serine/threonine kinase protein 4). The function of RIPK4 is largely unknown. It is involved in the canonical NF-kbeta pathway together with CHUK (IKKgamma protein).

Associated signs may be visible as, for example, oral frenula and commissural labial pits.

RIPK4 mutations also cause Bartsocas-Papas phenotype, a severe form of multiple pterygia syndrome. Intermediate severity cases have been reported [10].

9.11 CHUK-Related ED

CHUK is a component of the inhibitor of nuclear factor kappa B kinase complex, known also the IKKalpha subunit of modulation of the NF-kbeta signaling pathway.

IKKalpha is a direct downstream target of p63 and is critical for epidermal morphogenesis and for developing spine, limb buds, cranial structures, and apoptosis of interdigital tissue during embryogenesis.

Homozygous CHUK mutations have been reported in the so-called cocoon syndrome in two fetuses with severe malformations similar to the Bartsocas-Papas phenotype of multiple pterygia syndrome. Heterozygous missense mutations, both inherited and "de novo," may cause a less severe phenotype with intrauterine growth retardation and reduced fetal movements. At birth, cleft lip and palate with buccal synechiae are visible and associated with ankyloblepharon, sparse hair eyebrows and eyelashes, hypohidrosis, abnormal palmar creases, dysplastic nails, and tooth anomalies. V finger clinodactyly and different complex bone abnormalities of hands and feet may coexist. Moreover, these patients may suffer from severe gastrointestinal reflux, hypogammaglobulinemia, and frequent lower respiratory infections [11].

9.12 Basan Syndrome

It is characterized by congenital multiple milia and partial or total adermatoglyphia, acral erosions and skin fragility, fine sparse hair, dystrophic nails, and brachydactyly of the V finger. Mutations in the SMARCAD1 gene are responsible for this phenotype that may present in some pedigrees with only minor palmar hyperhidrosis and partial adermatoglyphia.

SMARCAD1 (matrix-associated actin-dependent regulator of chromatin) short isoform is mainly expressed in skin fibroblast and acts in the regulation of DNA methylation [12].

9.13 ARF1-Related ED

The ADP-ribosylation factor is relevant for neuronal motility and migration, vesicle formation, lipid transport, and cytoskeleton regulation. Mutations in the ARF1 gene cause periventricular nodular heterotopia, intellectual impairment, seizures, and ED signs such as thin brittle hair, sparse eyebrows, dark palpebral wrinkles, dystrophic fingernails, and hypohidrosis [13].

9.14 SEN (Scalp-Ear-Nipple) Syndrome

SEN syndrome is due to mutations in the KCTD1 gene (potassium channel tetramerization domain), causing ad autosomal dominant disorder characterized by aplasia cutis congenita, malformation of breast, and minor anomalies of external ears, digits, and nails). KCTD1 acts in modulating of AP-2alpha transcription factor and as a putative suppressor of the WNT/beta-catenin pathway [14].

9.15 NEMO Syndrome

Hypomorphic mutations of IKBKG account for about 200 patients. This clinical picture is also known as “Hypo-anhidrotic ED with immunodeficiency.” The phenotype is characterized by immune deficiency, recurrent infections, and inflammatory bowel disease. ED signs with sparse hair and hypohidrosis are associated with oral, acral, and perianal ulcers, poor wound healing, diffuse ichthyosis-like presentation, eczematous atopic-like dermatitis, palmoplantar keratoderma, and hypopigmented papules [15].

9.16 Sensenbrenner Syndrome

Also known as cranioectodermal syndrome is a "ciliopathy" due to many genes (intraflagellar transport genes and WDR genes), encoding components of ciliary transport machinery.

Patients show a peculiar craniofacial pattern with sagittal craniosynostosis, dolichocephaly, frontal bossing, long narrow face, epicanthal folds, telecanthus, broad nasal bridge, full cheeks, and low-set ears. Bone defects lead to brachysyndactyly, narrow thorax, and pectus excavatum. Less frequently, joint and skin laxity and inguinal hernias are present. Renal insufficiency and liver dysfunctions are present in >50% of patients with a relatively high mortality rate.

Sparse hair with hypotrichosis and alopecia, nail abnormalities, and small and widely spaced teeth complete the phenotype. Of note, large intra- and inter-familial phenotypic variability is reported.

The ORAI1 gene, coding for a component of calcium channel and the formation of the pore subunit of calcium channels, plays a role in the T-cell receptor signaling, showing a hypohidrotic ED with myopathy.

In the same way as perturbation of small ion (Ca++) penetration in the cytoplasm, STIM1 gene mutations are responsible for a complex of symptoms with hepatomegaly, lymphadenopathy, autoimmune diseases, myopathy, and dental dysplasia.

The following syndromes are historically inserted in the chapter of ED syndromes [14].

9.17 Tricho-Dento-Osseous Syndrome

Inherited as an autosomal dominant trait due to mutations of the DLX3 gene, a transcription expressed preferentially during tooth and hair follicle development, giving rise to a perturbed epithelial-mesenchymal interaction. DLX3 interacts with other proteins such as MSX and with Cbfa1, an osteoblast differentiation factor, explaining the increased bone density that is the hallmark of this syndrome.

The disease accounts for at least 100 reports in the literature and is characterized by increased bone density of the bones and can have dolichocephaly and frontal bossing (without CNS involvement), tall stature, "taurodontism" with enamel defects and discoloration, and decreased sinuses' pneumatization.

ED signs are represented by kinky and curly, uncombable hair, brittle nails with peeling and transverse bands, dystrophic eyebrows and eyelashes, and diffuse xerosis.

9.18 Tricho-Rhino-Phalangeal Syndrome

This autosomal dominant syndrome is due to mutations in the TRPS1 gene that acts as a localization signal nuclear protein.

Peculiar facies with pear-shaped nose, tented alae, long philtrum, thin upper lip, full cheeks, and micrognathia are associated with fine sparse slow-growing scalp hair and rudimentary eyebrows.

Brachyphalangia with deviation of the fingers and toes, shortened phalanges, and metacarpals is reported. Multiple cartilaginous exostosis, microcephaly, short stature, cone-shaped epiphyses, and ankylosing spondylitis may be visible in a subset of patients.

9.19 "Pure Hair-Nail" ED

It leads to a rare autosomal dominant or recessively inherited phenotype due to mutations in KRTH85 and HOXC13 genes.

KRTH85 deficiency probably affects intermediate filament assembly in hair follicle development, whereas HOXC13 is an evolutionarily conserved gene that acts as a transcription factor regulating the activity of various hair keratins.

Patients show "beak-like" nose, curly dark hair with areas of folliculitis decalvans, and alopecia in frontal and nuchal regions together with severe onycodystrophy.

Sweat glands and teeth are unaffected. Normal neurological functions are reported.

9.20 ED with Skin Fragility

This rare autosomal recessive syndrome is due to mutations in the PKP1 gene, coding for plakophilin 1 protein, a major component of desmosomal structures, leading to defective cell-cell adhesion and interactions, as well as abnormal architecture of the keratin network.

Patients present with diffuse blisters at birth followed during time by bulla formation even after minor trauma and in friction/pressure points, together with sparse hair, thickened and dystrophic nails, and palmoplantar hyperkeratosis, leading to the formation of thick large plaques with impaired walking. Hypohidrosis is reported in a subset of patients.

Electron microscopy of skin biopsies reveals poorly formed rudimentary desmosomes, disrupted keratin filament networks, and cytolysis.

Mosaic presentations are reported to be both classical and revertant.

9.21 Naegeli-Franceschetti Syndrome

The disease is inherited as an autosomal dominant trait. More than 100 patients are described.

Mutations in the KRT14 gene are responsible for that peculiar clinical picture with primarily reticulate, brownish, hyperpigmented macules of small dimensions on periocular and perioral areas, progressively extending to the neck and trunk. Furthermore, patients show classical ED signs, namely, dysplastic hyperkeratotic nails with malalignment, punctate palmoplantar keratoderma with possible hypoplasia/absence of dermatoglyphics and transient blistering, partial noncicatricial alopecia of scalp and eyebrows, and finally decreased sweating and heat intolerance.

9.22 Witkop Syndrome

Also called "tooth and nail" syndrome is a low incidence autosomal dominant disease due to mutations in the MSX1 gene that is crucial for the formation of dental buds and nail matrix.

The phenotype shows an almost normal primary dentition that is followed by permanent dentition abnormalities, either partial or total, and retention of primary teeth. Orthopantomography easily demonstrates permanent dentition anomalies.

Koilonychia and thin laminae and anonychia are reported. Toenails are more severely affected than fingernails. Malalignment of the first toe is frequent. Hair anomalies are rarely reported.

Ellis-van Creveld (EVC)-Weyers Acrofacial Dysostosis (WAD) complex.

These disorders are allelic: Ellis-van Creveld (EVC) is inherited recessively (homozygous loss-of-function mutations). WAD is the dominantly inherited, usually less severe, counterpart.

EVC1 and EVC2 genes are expressed in the developing bones, heart (septa), kidney, and lung.

Disproportionate dwarfism with short distal extremities and less severe proximal defects, short ribs and narrow thorax, hypoplastic iliac bones, abnormalities of hand rays, and possible post-axial polydactyly is reported. Congenital heart defects in about 50% of patients, cryptorchidism and hypospadias, and mental retardation of various degrees are reported.

ED signs are neonatal teeth, hypo-oligodontia, delayed eruption for both dentitions, and obliterations of upper and lower buccal vestibule with “pterigia” and frenulum anomalies. Fine and sparse hair in some patients may be associated with nail dysplasia with hypoplastic laminae and koilonychia [16].

9.23 Connexins-Related Syndromes

Connexin proteins are components of gap junctions, which are aqueous pores that allow intercellular exchange of ions and small molecules, causing influence on epidermal proliferation and differentiation. Connexins are integral membrane proteins that allow the diffusional exchange of ions and small metabolites between cells in multicellular tissues. These proteins are thought to play a role in maintaining epidermal integrity and homeostasis.

There are many dermatologic diseases caused by diverse connexin mutations, and confusingly, the diseases share many similarities.

9.23.1 Clouston Syndrome

It is a rare autosomal dominant disease with early onset due to mutations of Connexin 30 and Connexin 26 (cell-cell signal transduction).

Skin changes are represented by the following:

Diffuse xerotic skin, with accentuated thickening and discoloration at friction areas.

Hypohidrosis (never severe).

Severe palmoplantar keratoderma (that rarely in some subjects may be absent or mild).

Hypotrichosis: sparse-to-mild brittle hair with pili canaliculi and pili torti to almost complete hair loss. Same defects for all body hair comprising eyelashes and eyebrows that may be hypotrophic or absent.

Nail abnormalities of different degrees.

Less frequently, oral plaques.

From the point of view of other organs, there are some reports of intellectual disability and also of ophthalmological anomalies such as decreased lacrimation and conjunctival scars.

The course of the disease is progressive; there are some reports in the literature of cancer in palmoplantar areas.

Differential diagnosis is versus KID syndrome, pachyonychia congenita, and other diseases with alopecias like Ichthyosis Follicularis, Atrichia, and Photophobia (IFAP syndrome) or Alopecia Areata Universalis.

We recommend follow-up for neurological disorders and treatment of eventual neoplasms.

Skin may be treated with emollients and keratolytic agents. Nail change assessment is mandatory [17–21].

9.23.2 Oculo-Dento-Digital Dysplasia (ODDD)

Less than 30 cases are described in the literature for this syndrome due to mutations of Connexin 43, a product of the GJA1 gene also responsible for Hallermann-Streiff syndrome and for a subset of Bart-Pumphrey phenotypes.

Peculiar facies with microphthalmia and microcornea and with iris abnormalities are reported.

Anomalies of IV and V fingers with camptodactyly and syndactyly are reported.

Dystrophic ribs and clavicles and other long bones that are hyperostotic for abnormal trabecula formation are reported.

Reduced paranasal sinuses due to hypertrophy of osseous tissue are reported.

Hypomyelination and compression due to hyperostosis may lead to neurological symptoms.

Conductive deafness and glaucoma are reported.

Ectodermal issues are represented by enamel defects, hypotrichosis of different degrees of hair body hair, eyebrows, and eyelashes but with nonaffected sweating and nails.

Differential diagnosis with MIDAS syndrome and with other ED with syndactyly is reported.

We recommend surgical treatment for syndactyly and follow-up for hearing loss and glaucoma [22–24].

9.23.3 KID Syndrome

KID syndrome, also known as Keratitis-ichthyosis-deafness syndrome, is a rare disease. About 100 cases are described in the literature, with an age of onset at birth or shortly thereafter.

Some of the cutaneous findings in this disease are diffuse, and progressive erythematous-hyperkeratotic plaques with a surface are described as grainy or leathery, spiny hyperkeratosis (head and extremities, palmoplantar hyperkeratosis, angular cheilitis, chronically fissured lips, and gingival hyperemia). Additionally, patients have absent or sparse hair, onychodystrophy, hypohidrosis, and higher occurrence of squamous cell carcinomas (on mucosae). Rarely, linear hyperkeratotic lesions are superimposed, explained by allelic loss.

Some of the extracutaneous findings may be neurosensorial deafness of variable degrees, corneal ulcerations, and opacities. Moreover, vascularizing keratitis, keratoconjunctivitis, blepharitis, and photophobia are present in more than 75% of patients. Neurological manifestations, such as cerebellar hypoplasia and Dandy-Walker malformations, are reported. Usually there's no cognitive impairment.

Severe hearing loss may lead to impaired speech and psychomotor development. Ocular involvement is progressive during life, leading rarely to blindness. There is an increased risk of severe infection with pyogenic bacteria and fungi.

The disease is autosomal dominant with mainly de novo cases, even if some rare cases of recessive inheritance have been described as KIDAR (caused by loss-of-function mutations in the *AP1B1* gene, which codes for the 1B subunit of the heterotetrameric adaptor protein complex 1 that mediates endomembrane polarization, sorting, and transport).

The GJB2 gene, which encodes Connexin 26, is the gene involved in pathogenesis of the disease. Together with other connexin-related human skin diseases, patients have palmoplantar keratoderma and deafness. The V37E mutant of Connexin 30 (loss of function), previously linked distinctly to Clouston syndrome, has now also been found in KID patients. Connexin 26 and 30 mutations are involved in a broad spectrum of diseases, ranging from isolated central sensorineural deafness, Vohwinkel disease and Bart-Pumphrey variant, Clouston, KID, to PEODDN (Porokeratotic Eccrine and Ostial Dermal Duct Nevus).

Differential diagnosis includes epidermolytic hyperkeratosis, IFAP syndrome, and Clouston syndrome. The so-called hystrix-like ichthyosis and deafness (HID) syndrome is merely a different presentation of KID syndrome and not a separate entity.

Follow-up and therapy are based on a survey for squamous cell carcinomas in skin and mucosae, antibiotics, and antifungal therapy for infections, keratolytics, and emollients to relieve pruritus and xerosis. Ophthalmological management is needed for keratitis, whereas otorhinolaryngologist is mandatory in order to detect and stage neurosensory hearing loss. Oral retinoids give controversial results [25–27].

References

1. Lee Y, Zhang H, Seymen F, et al. Novel homozygous KREMEN1 mutation causes ectodermal dysplasia. Oral Dis. 2022;28(3):843–5. https://doi.org/10.1111/odi.13921.
2. Issa YA, Kamal L, Rayyan AA, et al. Mutation of KREMEN1, a modulator of Wnt signaling, is responsible for ectodermal dysplasia including oligodontia in Palestinian families. Eur J Hum Genet. 2016;24(10):1430–5. https://doi.org/10.1038/ejhg.2016.29.
3. Lévy J, Capri Y, Rachid M, et al. LEF1 haploinsufficiency causes ectodermal dysplasia. Clin Genet. 2020;97(4):595–600. https://doi.org/10.1111/cge.13714.
4. Marvin ML, Mazzoni SM, Herron CM, Edwards S, Gruber SB, Petty EM. AXIN2-associated autosomal dominant ectodermal dysplasia and neoplastic syndrome. Am J Med Genet A. 2011;155A(4):898–902. https://doi.org/10.1002/ajmg.a.33927.

5. Yu M, Fan Z, Wong SW, et al. Lrp6 dynamic expression in tooth development and mutations in oligodontia. J Dent Res. 2021;100(4):415–22. https://doi.org/10.1177/0022034520970459.
6. Hadj-Rabia S, Brideau G, Al-Sarraj Y, et al. Multiplex epithelium dysfunction due to CLDN10 mutation: the HELIX syndrome. Genet Med. 2018;20(2):190–201. https://doi.org/10.1038/gim.2017.71.
7. Jackson A, Lin SJ, Jones EA, et al. Clinical, genetic, epidemiologic, evolutionary, and functional delineation of TSPEAR-related autosomal recessive ectodermal dysplasia 14. HGG Adv. 2023;4(2):100186. https://doi.org/10.1016/j.xhgg.2023.100186.
8. Zhao W, Zhang Y, Lv T, He J, Zhu B. A case report of a novel HIST1H1E mutation and a review of the bibliography to evaluate the genotype-phenotype correlations. Mol Genet Genomic Med. 2023;11(12):e2273. https://doi.org/10.1002/mgg3.2273.
9. Brooks D, Burke E, Lee S, et al. Heterozygous MAP3K20 variants cause ectodermal dysplasia, craniosynostosis, sensorineural hearing loss, and limb anomalies. Hum Genet. 2024;143(3):279–91. https://doi.org/10.1007/s00439-024-02657-2.
10. Busa T, Jeraiby M, Clémenson A, et al. Confirmation that RIPK4 mutations cause not only Bartsocas-Papas syndrome but also CHAND syndrome. Am J Med Genet A. 2017;173(11):3114–7. https://doi.org/10.1002/ajmg.a.38475.
11. Khandelwal KD, Ockeloen CW, Venselaar H, et al. Identification of a de novo variant in CHUK in a patient with an EEC/AEC syndrome-like phenotype and hypogammaglobulinemia. Am J Med Genet A. 2017;173(7):1813–20. https://doi.org/10.1002/ajmg.a.38274.
12. Nieto-Benito LM, Molina-López I, Feito-Rodríguez M, Martínez-González V, Suárez-Fernández R, Campos-Dominguez M. Ectodermal dysplasia with congenital adermatoglyphia (Basan syndrome): report of two cases presenting with extensive congenital milia. Pediatr Dermatol. 2021;38(2):530–2. https://doi.org/10.1111/pde.14512.
13. de Sainte Agathe JM, Pode-Shakked B, Naudion S, et al. ARF1-related disorder: phenotypic and molecular spectrum. J Med Genet. 2023;60(10):999–1005. https://doi.org/10.1136/jmg-2022-108803.
14. Tadini G, Brena M, Besagni F, Pezzani L. Atlas of genodermatoses. Boca Raton: CRC Press; 2024. isbn-10:0367643960.
15. Kohn LL, Braun M, Cordoro KM, et al. Skin and mucosal manifestations in NEMO syndrome: a case series and literature review. Pediatr Dermatol. 2022;39(1):84–90. https://doi.org/10.1111/pde.14905.
16. Peschel N, Wright JT, Koster MI, et al. Molecular pathway-based classification of ectodermal dysplasias: first five-yearly update. Genes (Basel). 2022;13(12):2327. https://doi.org/10.3390/genes13122327.
17. Ahmed C, Trope BM, Amorim G, Ribeiro M, Ramos-E-Silva M. Clouston syndrome. Skinmed. 2021;19(1):54.
18. Cammarata-Scalisi F, Rinelli M, et al. Novel clinical features associated with Clouston syndrome. Int J Dermatol. 2019;58(8):e143–6.
19. Kantaputra P, Intachai W, Kawasaki K, et al. Clouston syndrome with pili canaliculi, pili torti, overgrown hyponychium, onycholysis, taurodontism and absence of palmoplantar keratoderma. J Dermatol. 2020;47(6):e230–2.
20. Kelly JJ, Abitbol JM, Hulme S, Press ER, Laird DW, Allman BL. The connexin 30 A88V mutant reduces cochlear gap junction expression and confers long-term protection against hearing loss. J Cell Sci. 2019;132(2):jcs224097.
21. Lilly E, Sellitto C, Milstone LM, White TW. Connexin channels in congenital skin disorders. Semin Cell Dev Biol. 2016;50:4–12.
22. Michell-Robinson MA, Perrier S, Lucia C, et al. Oculodentodigital dysplasia: a cause of hypomyelinating leukodystrophy in adults. Neurology. 2022;98(16):675–7.
23. Sargiannidou I, Christophidou-Anastasiadou V, Hadjisavvas A, Tanteles GA, Kleopa KA. Novel GJA1/Cx43 variant associated with oculo-dento-digital dysplasia syndrome: clinical phenotype and cellular mechanisms. Front Genet. 2021;11:604806.

24. Wang Z, Sun L, Wang P, Chen C, Zhang A, Wang W, Ding X. Novel ocular findings in oculodentodigital dysplasia (ODDD): a case report and literature review. Ophthalmic Genet. 2019;40(1):54–9.
25. Asgari T, Naji M, Mansouri P, et al. Keratitis-ichthyosis-deafness syndrome: phenotypic heterogeneity and treatment perspective of patients with p.Asp50Asn GJB2 mutation. Dermatol Ther. 2020;33(6):e14493.
26. Cammarata-Scalisi F, Willoughby CE, Cárdenas Tadich A, Labrador N, Herrera A, Callea M. Clinical, etiopathogenic, and therapeutic aspects of KID syndrome. Dermatol Ther. 2020;33(4):e13507.
27. Godillot C, Severino-Freire M, Michaud V, Boralevi F, Labrèze C, Guigonis V, Onnis G, Morice-Picard F, Mazereeuw-Hautier J. Keratitis-ichthyosis-deafness syndrome: early death caused by the GJB2 mutation p.Gly12Arg. Acta Derm Venereol. 2019;99(10):921–2.

Chapter 10
Ectodermal Dysplasias: Orofacial Manifestations and Management

B. Meyer and John Timothy Wright

Keywords Facies · Embriology · Dentitions

10.1 Introduction

Ectodermal dysplasias (EDs) are a genetically and clinically diverse group of hereditary conditions that affect the development of ectodermal tissue derivatives including those of the face and oral cavity. Numerous genetic mutations are known to cause the EDs, and many of these genes are associated with the WNT, NFkB, and TP63 molecular pathways that are critical for the development of ectodermal tissues [1]. Multiple molecular mechanisms are involved in these different pathways altering signaling cascades and progenitor cell proliferation resulting in the spectrum of ED phenotypes observed clinically [2–8]. ED conditions are also caused by genes that are not associated with the WNT, NFkB, or TP63 pathways adding to the diversity of molecular mechanisms causing abnormal development and/or homeostasis of ectodermal tissues [1].

The most recent classification of EDs lists approximately 100 different hereditary conditions involving abnormal development of at least two tissues of ectodermal derivation [1]. The resulting clinical phenotypes vary substantially with tissues of ectodermal derivation, such as hair, sweat glands, fingernails, salivary glands, and teeth being commonly affected [9, 10]. In this chapter, we review the most prevalent oral and facial manifestations seen in association with the EDs and some

B. Meyer
Department of Pediatric Dentistry, School of Dentistry, The Ohio State University, Columbus, OH, USA

J. T. Wright (✉)
Division of Pediatric and Public Health, Adams School of Dentistry, University of North Carolina, Chapel Hill, NC, USA
e-mail: tim_wright@unc.edu

G. Tadini et al. (eds.), *Multidisciplinary Approach to Ectodermal Dysplasia*,
https://doi.org/10.1007/978-3-031-75790-7_10

of the therapeutic approaches for managing these manifestations. Specific clinical conditions are identified using the Online Mendelian Inheritance in Man (OMIM) nomenclature and numbering system [11].

10.2 Soft Tissues

The soft tissue manifestations associated with EDs are diverse, vary between the different conditions and genetic mutations, and are variably expressed. The facial features can be quite distinctive for some EDs such as X-linked hypohidrotic ED (XLHED) (OMIM# 305100) caused by mutations in the *EDA* gene. Facial features seen in XLHED, including prominent lips, changes in hair distribution, and pigmentation typically result in a distinctive facial phenotype [12]. Cleft lip/palate is frequently associated with EDs caused by *TP63* mutations but is not common in the EDs associated with the *EDA* or other molecular pathways. Reliable prevalence estimates do not exist for most of the oral soft tissue abnormalities seen in conditions under the ED umbrella as these conditions are rare and the phenotypes are variable. Here, we review the soft tissue phenotypes associated with the different forms of ED. We provide representative examples of some of the soft tissue phenotypes seen in different EDs, their causative genes, and, if known, the molecular pathways (Table 10.1).

Table 10.1 Ectodermal dysplasia soft tissue phenotypes

	Disorder	Gene	Inheritance	Soft tissue features
EDA pathway	Hypohidrotic ED (XHED)	*EDA*	XLR	Prominent lips, hypoplastic/absent mucous glands
	Incontinentia pigmenti	*IKBKG*	XLD	Mucocutaneous ulcers
	Ectodermal dysplasia (ED) and immunodeficiency 2	*NFKBIA*	AD	Oral candidiasis
WNT pathway	Focal dermal hypoplasia	PORCN	XLD	Gingival papilloma, gingival hyperplasia, cleft lip/palate
	Odonto-onycho-dermal dysplasia	*WNT10A*	AR	Smooth tongue, reduced fungiform, and filiform papillae
	Ablepharon-macrostomia syndrome	*TWIST2*	AD	Macrostomia, possible discontinuity of orbicularis oris muscle, long uvula
TP63 pathway	Ectrodactyly, ectodermal dysplasia and cleft lip/palate (EEC3)	*TP63*	AD	Cleft lip/palate, xerostomia
	Ankyloblepharon-ectodermal defects-cleft lip/palate (AEC)	*TP63*	AD	Hypodontia, conical teeth, cleft palate
	Rapp-Hodgkin	TP63	AD	Small mouth, cleft lip/palate/uvula, velopharyngeal incompetence

10.2.1 Cleft Lip/Palate

Facial clefting including cleft lip/palate is a clinical manifestation that occurs with increased frequency in some EDs including several of the *TP63* pathway-associated EDs. The allelic TP63 conditions have overlapping and variable phenotypes that can include cleft lip with or without cleft palate (Fig. 10.1). Clefting can include unilateral or bilateral cleft lip with or without cleft palate, cleft palate alone, or submucous cleft [13]. The prevalence and severity of clefting varies between the different *TP63*-associated EDs. For example, all individuals with AEC (OMIM# 106260) have clefts [14], whereas about 60–75% of individuals with ectrodactyly ED and cleft lip/palate syndrome (EEC3; OMIM# 604292) have clefting, half of which are bilateral [15]. The occurrence of cleft palate, hypodontia, and bifid uvula is less common in the *TP63-associated* condition limb-mammary syndrome (OMIM# 603543) compared with AEC and EEC3, and cleft lip/palate is not a feature of acro-dermato-ungual-lacrimal-tooth (ADULT) syndrome (OMIM# 103285) or split hand and foot malformation (OMIM# 605289). The influence of cleft lip/palate on the facial soft tissues, facial growth, and facial appearance depends on numerous factors such as the underlying causative gene effects, type of cleft, severity of the cleft, and treatment outcomes. Hard tissue elements of the cleft lip/palate phenotype are discussed in a subsequent section.

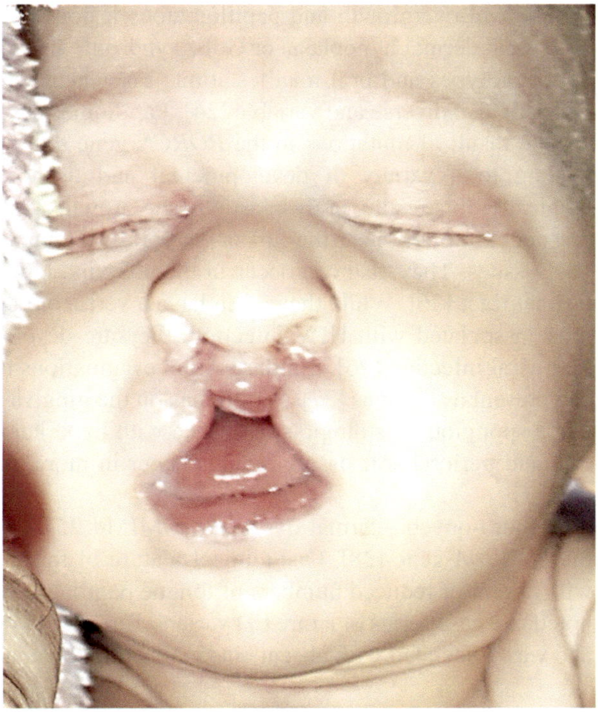

Fig. 10.1 Infant with ankyloblepharon-ectodermal defects-cleft lip/palate syndrome (AEC; OMIM# 106260) with bilateral cleft lip and cleft palate. Note the short and narrow philtrum of the upper lip

10.2.2 Oral Mucosa and Gingiva

Alteration of the soft tissues in people with ED is the result of changes in the pigmentation, architecture, and/or growth of the tissues. For example, individuals with incontinentia pigmenti (OMIM# 308300) that is caused by mutations in the *IKBKG* gene are reported to have an increased risk of oral and gastrointestinal ulceration [16]. The etiology of these ulcerative tissue changes is not fully understood, but the role of *IKGKG* and the NFkB pathway is known to be involved in inflammation and autoimmunity [17]. EED and Immunodeficiency 1 and 2 (OMIM# 300291 & 612132) due to mutations in the *IKBGK* and *NFKBIA* genes can have oral candidiasis as one of a variety of recurrent infections [18, 19].

Gingival changes can include alterations in pigmentation as occur in some cases of dermatopathia pigmentosa reticularis (OMIM# 125595) and Naegeli syndrome (OMIM# 161000). These are autosomal dominant disorders caused by allelic mutations in the *KRT14* gene. Some affected individuals have pigmentation of the oral mucosa that has a reticular or net-like appearance [20]. Chondroectodermal dysplasia or Ellis-van Creveld syndrome (EVC) (OMIM 225500) is a rare autosomal recessive condition caused by mutations in the *EVC* and *EVC2* genes. The oral soft tissue involvement is variable with supernumerary frenula being one of the more common features (46%) [21, 22]. Other soft tissue features include a flat philtrum, absent mucobuccal fold, abnormal tongue shape, cleft lip, and tongue depapillation [22].

Gingival overgrowth and papillomatous lesions can be observed in individuals with focal dermal hypoplasia or Goltz syndrome (OMIM# 305600) [23]. The clinical phenotypes and oral manifestations associated with mutations in the *PORCN* gene are also diverse and variable [24]. Papillomas associated with Goltz syndrome are the result of mutations in the *PORCN* gene that alters critical WNT signaling leading to a variety of developmental and tissue growth abnormalities [25]. Clinically, this results in dysplastic tissue growths, such as papillomas, which can present extraorally near the lips or intraorally on buccal mucosa, gingiva, and lingual tissues. They also can occur in the pharynx, larynx, esophagus, and gastrointestinal tract [26]. While they often have a verrucoid clinical appearance similar to those associated with HPV infection, they are developmental and not associated with viral infection [26]. Similarly, lipid evaginations through the connective tissue can present as lipomas [27]. Papillomas on the gingiva show epithelial proliferation and a spongiotic histologic appearance with hyperkeratosis [23]. Combined, these oral and perioral soft tissue findings occur in more than 50% of affected individuals [7].

Odonto-onycho-dermal dysplasia (OMIM# 257980) is caused by mutations in the *WNT10A* gene [28]. One clinical feature of this condition is a smooth tongue with absent or reduced numbers of tongue papillae [29]. Gingival fibromatosis was noted in a case series of a rare ED variant, Barber-Say syndrome (OMIM# 209885), and was associated with absent elastic fibers in the connective tissue [30].

10.2.3 Salivary Glands

The parotid, submandibular, and minor salivary glands all are of ectodermal origin and begin forming during early human embryonic development [31]. Saliva has multiple important roles in oral health and digestion. In addition to buffering pH and diluting oral substances, saliva serves as an ion reservoir for calcium, phosphate, and fluoride to promote enamel remineralization and the formation of apatite, which is more resistant to demineralization or breakdown due to dental caries [32]. Saliva also plays a critical role in digestion from chewing to initiating digestion to swallowing [33]. Hypoplastic development and salivary gland dysfunction accompanied by hyposalivation, and varying degrees of xerostomia are common ED manifestations. Between 60 and 80% of individuals with hypohidrotic ED have xerostomia, which also occurs in other forms of ED as well [34–36]. Histopathologic, imaging, and salivary function studies confirm altered salivary gland anatomy and reduced flow rates in individuals with ED. [37] Studies of salivary gland development and function show the salivary glands can have both a diminished size and abnormal function leading to a reduction in salivary flow and changes in salivary composition and properties [4, 37]. Clinical studies indicate that the submandibular gland is more commonly affected than the parotid gland, and that individuals with ED have saliva that is more concentrated with inorganic ions and proteins [37, 38].

10.2.4 Managing the Soft Tissues

Management for cleft lip/palate is often tailored to the severity and functional impact of the affected individual experience. Depending on the type of cleft, there can be a host of feeding, hearing, language, dental, and surgical issues that need to be addressed. Most, if not all, major children's hospitals maintain craniofacial teams to provide coordinated and multidisciplinary care for individuals with craniofacial anomalies, an umbrella term that sometimes includes EDs. Each center operates slightly differently, but the team often includes representatives from plastic surgery, otolaryngology, speech pathology, audiology, oral and maxillofacial surgery, orthodontics, pediatric dentistry, social work, and/or psychology [39]. Depending on the size of the hospital and team, disciplines like neurosurgery, ophthalmology, and genetics might also be included [39]. Teams operate a diagnostics clinic where patients and their families can be seen with regularity to be evaluated by the entire team for monitoring and/or planning coordinated treatment. Ideally, the team members meet after the patient evaluation to discuss and develop an individualized and coordinated plan of care. Team-based care offers clinical and psychosocial advantages over discipline-specific care [31, 39–41].

Confirmatory excisional biopsy can aid diagnosis of mucosal and gingival lesions such as those seen with Goltz syndrome. Excisional biopsy is often effective in management of these lesions. For individuals with supernumerary frenum attachments, frenum release can be completed if needed for improved oral function with nursing or oral prosthetic placement. Recurrence of excised lesions in patients with any of the ED variants is difficult to ascertain due to their overall limited and variable prevalence.

A variety of approaches can be used to assess salivary flow and function [42]. While diagnostic testing for salivary function may be helpful for some patients, obtaining a detailed history and physical assessment likely is sufficient for determining preliminary management. Managing hyposalivation typically entails the use of artificial saliva substitutes, saliva stimulants like chewing gums, and fluoride exposures to prevent secondary complications from dental caries. On the horizon, researchers are developing artificial salivary glands and novel therapeutic approaches to increase salivary production [43, 44].

10.3 Hard Tissues

As illustrated in the previous section on soft tissue involvement of EDs, the hard tissue manifestations are also diverse and variable. Many of the genes causing EDs are involved in formation of both the hard and soft tissues of the face and oral cavity (e.g., *EDA, TP63, PORCN, TBX3*). Consequently, there are phenotypic features that involve the craniofacial bones and their relationships to each other, bony alveolar development, palate formation, and the dentition [45]. The hard tissue manifestations, genes, and pathways of some EDs are summarized in Table 10.2 and reviewed in the following sections.

10.3.1 Face and Occlusion

The presence of cleft lip/palate is often associated with numerous changes in facial growth and facial morphology. The degree of midfacial involvement is highly variable for individuals with ED and cleft lip with or without cleft palate. The severity of the change is a function of both the genetic mutation involved in the development of the facial bones and the type and extent of surgeries and healing involved to repair the soft and hard tissues of the lip and palate. Even in the absence of cleft lip with or without cleft palate, individuals with ED often have their maxilla positioned posteriorly, or more retrusively, in relation to the other craniofacial structures compared to individuals unaffected by ED (OMIM# 305100, OMIM# 190320). Individuals with EEC and AEC syndrome typically have varying degrees of midface retrusion, and this can be coupled with a diminution in the upper and/or lower face height [46]. Midface retrusions in individuals with ED lead to an appearance of prognathism (Fig. 10.2) [47, 48]. However, cephalometric studies of jaw size and relationships show the mandible is typically of normal size and shape [48].

Table 10.2 Ectodermal dysplasias hard tissue phenotypes

	Disorder	Gene	Inheritance	Hard tissue features
EDA pathway	Hypohidrotic ED (XHED)	*EDA*	XLR	Hypodontia, anodontia, conical teeth, taurodontism, hypoplastic maxilla, reduced facial height
	Incontinentia pigmenti	*IKBKG*	XLD	Hypodontia, abnormal cusps and tooth morphology, delayed tooth eruption
WNT pathway	Focal dermal hypoplasia syndrome	*PORCN*	XLD	Hypodontia, enamel hypoplasia, delayed eruption, notched incisors, cleft lip/palate
	Odonto-onycho-dermal dysplasia	*WNT10A*	AR	Hypodontia
	Hypohidrotic ectodermal dysplasia (ED)	LEF1	AD	Hypodontia, taurodontism, alveolar defect
	Ablepharon-macrostomia syndrome	*TWIST2*	AD	Conical teeth
TP63 pathway	Ectrodactyly, ectodermal dysplasia and cleft lip/palate (EEC3)	*TP63*	AD	Hypodontia, microdontia, caries, cleft lip/palate
	Ankyloblepharon-ectodermal defects-cleft lip/palate (AEC)	*TP63*	AD	Hypodontia, conical teeth, cleft lip/palate
	Rapp-Hodgkin syndrome	*TP63*		Hypodontia, conical teeth, cleft lip/palate
	ADULT syndrome	*TP63*		Hypodontia, small and dysplastic teeth
	Tricho-dento-osseous syndrome	*DLX3*	AD	Small teeth, hypoplastic enamel, taurodontism, dense craniofacial bones

Defects in the articulation of the dentition and the dental occlusion are frequent in EDs. Dental articulation problems can stem from both the abnormal position of the jaws and the abnormal number, shape, size, and position of the dentition. These abnormalities often translate into individuals with ED having a reduced vertical facial dimension because of missing posterior teeth and in some cases having teeth that fail to articulate (e.g., posterior open bite) (Fig. 10.3). When the posterior teeth are not present, there may be no articulation of teeth to establish a normal vertical dimension and the mandible over-rotates on closure leading to a reduced vertical dimension in the lower face between the chin and the nose. This overclosure and lack of lip support from the dentition can result in a collapsed facial appearance and eversion and protrusion of the lower lip (Fig. 10.4). The combination of these features gives an appearance of mandibular prognathism, but the mandible is rarely prognathic in comparison with the cranial base [49].

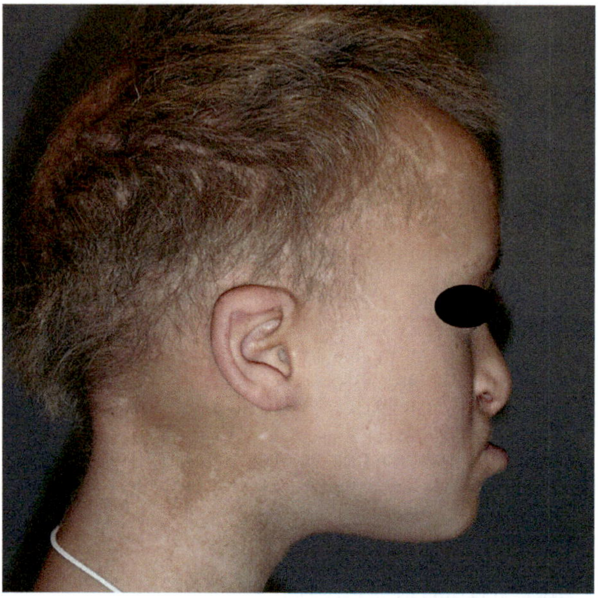

Fig. 10.2 This child with AEC shows the midface retrusion and prognathic appearance that is common in individuals with this *TP63*-associated condition

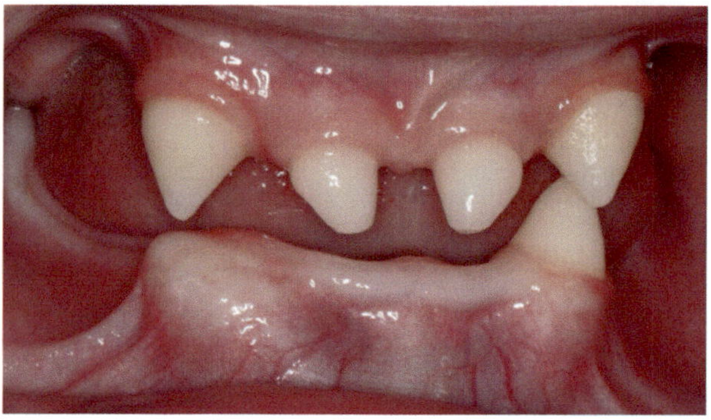

Fig. 10.3 This child affected with X-linked hypohidrotic ED (XLHED) due to a mutation in the *EDA* gene has no posterior teeth to articulate in either the maxillary or mandibular dental arch

10.3.2 Dentition

Abnormal development of the dentition is one of the most prevalent hard tissue signs of ED [50]. The teeth can be missing altogether, be diminished in number, and/or have an altered morphology and size [51]. Hypodontia refers to reduced numbers of teeth, and microdontia refers to reduced size (and may or may not be associated with changes in shape) of teeth. Many individuals with ED have missing and/or small cone-shaped teeth. Individuals with mild systemic manifestations of ED may not be diagnosed until the presence of missing primary and/or abnormally shaped teeth is noted (Fig. 10.3).

The developmental biology of tooth formation has been studied extensively for decades, and given the highly conserved and molecularly regulated formation of teeth, it is not surprising that tooth development is so frequently altered with EDs

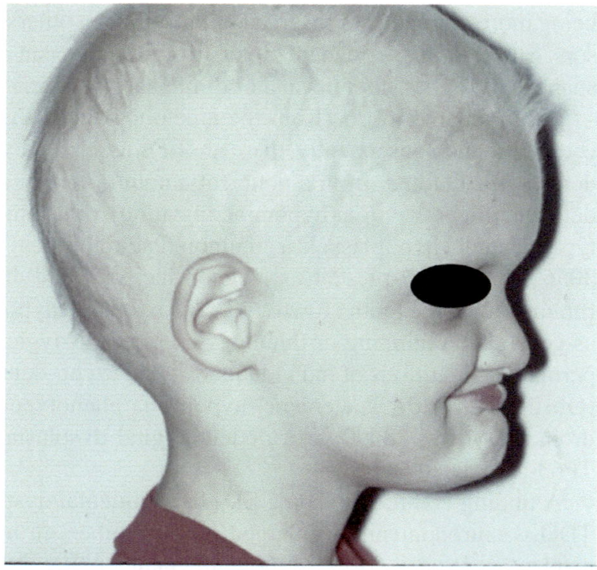

Fig. 10.4 This male child with XLHED has a reduced lower face height (distance from chin to nose) due to overclosure resulting from having only four primary teeth in the upper jaw and none in the lower jaw. Retrusion of the midface is also present

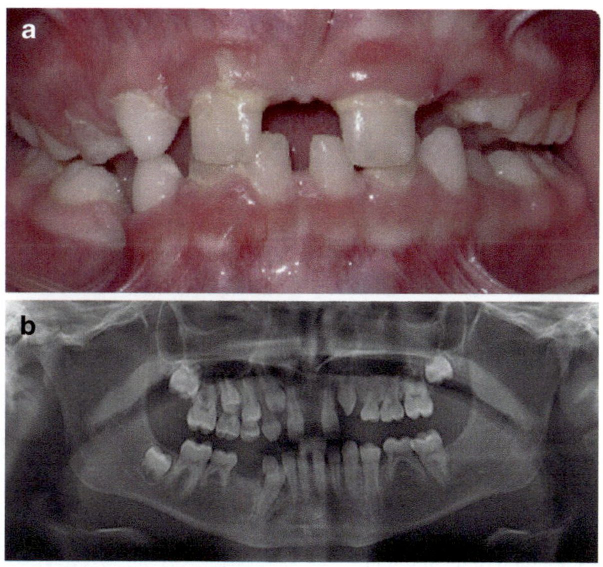

Fig. 10.5 This female child with incontinentia pigmenti is missing nine permanent teeth excluding her third molars. The maxillary lateral incisors and second premolars are commonly missing teeth in the general population and in people with EDs

[52]. Investigators have identified multiple genetic pathways that involve genes that are critical for early events in the initiation of tooth formation including *EDA* (OMIM# 305100) [53–58], *MSX1* (OMIM# 189500) [59, 60], and *WNT10A* (OMIM# 257980) [8, 58, 61–64]. These and many other genes play a role in normal tooth development, and their alteration in ED affects the developmental cascades and tissue interactions that occur at the dental placode or bud stage of tooth development [65]. However, the pattern of missing teeth across ED conditions varies widely (Fig. 10.5) [51]. The number of missing teeth is highly variable with certain teeth

being more commonly conserved or present than others (e.g., maxillary central incisors, canines, first permanent molars) [66]. Shapes can range from conical to normal shape and can be either normal or diminished in size.

Dental enamel forms from the ameloblast cells that are derived from the oral ectoderm, and consequently, there are EDs associated with enamel defects. Enamel defects in ED range from a deficient amount of enamel substructure (hypoplasia), deficient mineralization (hypomineralization), or a combination of these two phenotypes. Enamel hypoplasia is a common feature of focal dermal hypoplasia (OMIM# 305600) and may present as notched incisors, and enamel with vertical grooves running down the tooth crown (Fig. 10.6). Enamel hypoplasia that can either present as generalized thinning or thinning and pitting is typically seen in the primary and permanent dentitions of individuals with the tricho-dento-osseous (TDO) syndrome (OMIM# 190320). The enamel hypoplasia phenotype also is seen in Witkop syndrome (OMIM# 185900), oculodentodigital dysplasia (OMIM# 164200), and the TP63-associated EDs [67].

A finding common in some EDs like otodental dysplasia (OMIM# 166750) and TDO is taurodontism or enlarged pulp chambers in molar teeth due to the apical displacement of the floor of the pulp chamber (Fig. 10.7) [68–70]. TDO is caused by mutations in the transcription factor *DLX3* that is involved in the development of

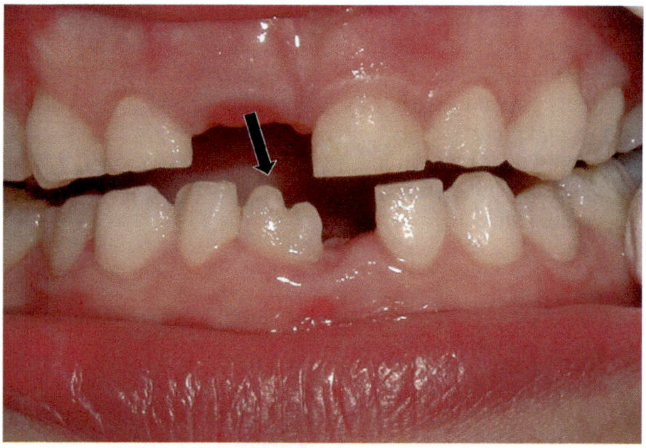

Fig. 10.6 This female child with focal dermal hypoplasia has a newly erupting mandibular incisor with a notched incisal edge

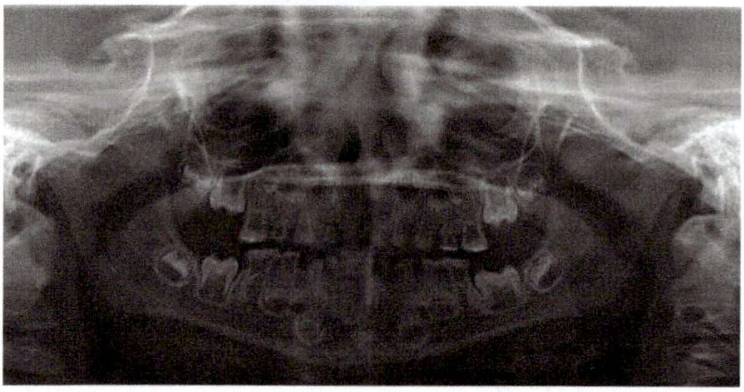

Fig. 10.7 This panoramic radiograph of a child with tricho-dento-osseous (TDO) syndrome illustrates the markedly enlarged pulp chambers in the erupted primary teeth and the developing permanent teeth

hair, teeth, and bone [71–73]. Individuals with TDO typically have taurodontism, which can help delineate this ED type from conditions with a similar enamel hypoplasia phenotype [74]. The kinky curly hair that is often present at birth is another diagnostic indicator. Taurodontism occurs more commonly in ED because the root morphology is defined by an epithelial cell lineage of Hertwig's epithelial root sheath [74, 75].

10.3.3 Other Hard Tissue Findings

Individuals with ED sometimes have delayed tooth eruption (OMIM# 189500, 129490, 209885). Natal and neonatal teeth are more prevalent in some types of ED compared with the general population including EVC syndrome (OMIM# 225500) and hypohidrotic ED type 12 (OMIM# 617337). Individuals also have thin or absent dentoalveolar bone in the areas where teeth are missing. The dentoalveolar bone exists to support the teeth, and without the teeth, the dental alveolus is hypoplastic and lacks normal development. In the maxilla, this can sometimes lead to a flat palate without depth or broad but short alveolar ridges. In patients with complete anodontia of the mandible, there is essentially no alveolus giving a mandible no alveolus to support a dental prosthesis.

10.3.4 Managing the Hard Tissues

Managing the hard tissue manifestations and defects for people with ED is predicated on the manifestations, severity of involvement, patient age, patient and family desires, financial and treatment support available, and a host of other factors. As each individual moves through the life course, their oral health care is likely to require teams of oral health care providers to address the myriad issues and developmental defects of the orofacial hard tissues. Treatment often involves the general dentist or pediatric dentist, orthodontist, prosthodontist, periodontist, oral surgeon, and others. Clinical management of facial clefting associated with ED is touched upon in the section on soft tissues and will only be briefly mentioned here. Treatment can involve bone grafting at various ages to close alveolar and palatal clefts [76]. At one time, bone grafts were used to help build a sufficient bony base for dental prostheses; however, this is less common with the advent of dental implant therapies and approaches. Orthognathic surgery is used in some cases of severe midface retrusion and dental malocclusion to help produce a more favorable facial form, jaw alignment, and dental occlusion [77].

Managing the dentition requires treatment over the affected individual's life course with multiple phases of therapy being required. Treatment may begin in early childhood to manage misshapen and missing teeth with treatment continuing through the transition to permanent dentition and into adulthood depending on the

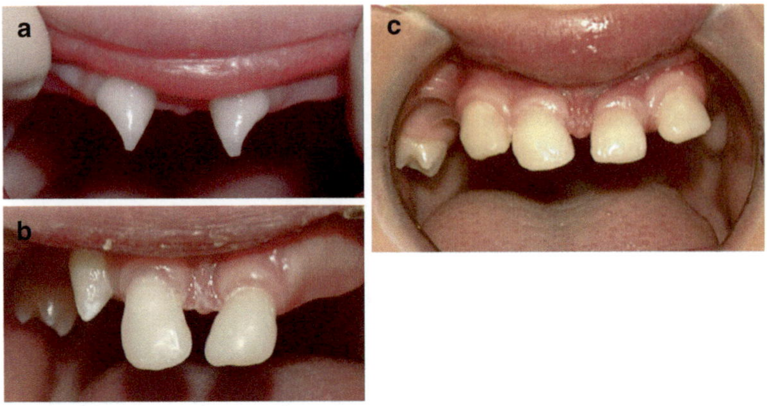

Fig. 10.8 This young male with XLHED had four maxillary anterior teeth with the central incisors erupting with a marked conical shape. The canines also erupted with a smaller and more conical shape than normal. The four primary anterior teeth were bonded for improved esthetics and to reduce the child's tendency to puncture his tongue and lips with these sharp pointed teeth

dental phenotype (Fig. 10.8). The goal for oral health management of the hard tissues is to preserve the dental tissues with appropriate preventive care, conservative treatments, and if necessary to create a dentition to improve function and enhance esthetics [78].

Managing small and misshapen teeth in the primary dentition and early permanent dentition is often accomplished using direct restorative techniques or crown forms with bonding and composite resin [79, 80]. Advances in digital dentistry offer new approaches for placing computer-designed and fabricated crowns and/or veneers for managing small and misshapen teeth. Usually, minimal, if any, tooth preparation or local anesthesia is necessary. Restorations can be placed freehand, with the use of lingual matrices, prefabricated celluloid crown forms, or digitally fabricated crown forms or restorations depending on provider preferences [81]. Preformed zirconia crowns for primary teeth offer a durable and esthetic treatment for microdont and conical-shaped teeth [82–84]. The following sequence offers a framework for clinicians:

1. Diagnostic visit
   (a) Obtain detailed histories and conduct clinical exam
   (b) Obtain diagnostic casts (intraoral scans or traditional alginate impressions)
   (c) Obtain necessary radiographs and clinical photographs
2. Between visits (if a lingual matrix is going to be used)
   (a) Traditional techniques
      - Make diagnostic wax-up on the casts to restore the size and shape of the teeth to "normal"
      - Make a polyvinyl siloxane mold of the lingual surface to serve as the restorative guide and trim to fit

   (b) Digital techniques [78, 85, 86]

      - Make a digital diagnostic wax-up on the intraoral scan
      - 3D print the model and make a vacuum formed retainer

         - Trim excess from the retainer to give access for direct restoration

3. Restorative visit

   (a) Follow well-established techniques for direct composite restorations [78, 81, 85, 86]

      - Isolation
      - Acid etch
      - Dental adhesive
      - Composite resin

   (b) Obtain clinical photographs

In the transitional and permanent dentitions, more treatment options are available depending on the extent of the microdontia and other dental comorbidities like hypodontia or periodontal disease. The same composite resin techniques described above can be applied to the adolescent or adult patient. In the transitional and permanent dentition, orthodontic treatment may be necessary to manage the space around the microdont teeth or to improve tooth positioning to improve the functional and esthetic outcome [78, 87]. Restoratively, indirect restoration techniques can be applied to offer improved esthetics. Veneers [88], onlays [89], and full coverage restorations could all be reasonable options depending on the type of tooth that is being restored. These techniques use different tooth materials, such as porcelain or zirconia, and likely require tooth preparation to achieve proper resistance form and parallelism to support the indirect restoration.

While microdontia can be treated any time a child and/or parent desires, managing hypodontia is much more dependent on growth and development and the ability of the child to cooperate with the required multiphasic treatment. Establishing which teeth are missing and those present but unerupted is critical before proceeding with prosthetic treatment of the dentition. Treatment approaches will vary across different time points as the individual progresses from the primary to the permanent dentition [90]. In all stages of dental development, as with microdontia, the goal for treating congenitally missing teeth is to maintain as much tissue as possible for as long as possible to improve function and enhance esthetics.

In the primary dentition, treatment depends on (a) how many teeth are missing, (b) where those missing teeth are located and the tooth and bony structures available to support a prosthesis, and (c) the child's motivation to replace the missing teeth. The combinations of these variables should dictate treatment planning. Goals for tooth replacement should consider the child's psychosocial impact of hypodontia, esthetics, function, and retaining all functional teeth whenever possible. For children missing one or two teeth, no replacement may be necessary in the primary dentition. If multiple teeth are missing in multiple quadrants, a removable partial or complete denture may be indicated (Fig. 10.9). Overdentures are sometimes a good option, depending on the location of the abutment teeth [91–96]. For example, when present and in an upright position, canines tend to serve as good abutment teeth for both removable partial dentures and overdentures, particularly in the mandible where denture success is generally poorer due to tongue movements during speech, chewing, and swallowing (Table 10.3) [101, 102].

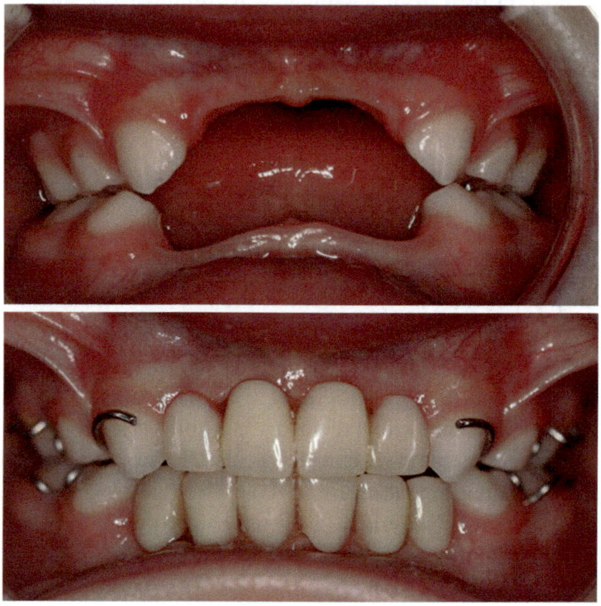

Fig. 10.9 This young child with a *WNT10A* mutation was missing her four maxillary incisors and all six of her mandibular anterior teeth. Upper and lower partial dentures were placed at the age of 3 years

Table 10.3 Dental prosthesis fabrication workflow [97–100]

Traditional visit number	Traditional workflow	Digital workflow	Digital visit number
1	Preliminary alginate impressions	Intraoral scans and bite registration to set vertical dimension	1
Between first and second visits	Make a custom tray	Digitally set teeth and print/mill esthetic try-in in monochromatic acrylic	Between first and second visits
2	Final impression using polyvinyl siloxane	Deliver printed try-in and trial wear for a few weeks	2
3	Wax rims to set vertical dimension and begin setting anterior teeth	Reprint/re-mill final prosthetic in multichromatic acrylic	Between second and third visits
4	Full try-in	Deliver final prosthesis	3
Between fourth and fifth visits	Final processing using traditional acrylic methods		
5	Deliver final prosthesis		

A major consideration for making dentures for the patients in the primary dentition is whether they want to wear them. Children not interested in wearing a denture will likely not wear one. Children should be counseled as to their interest and commitment to this type of treatment before proceeding, thus helping ensure a successful outcome. Otherwise, the experience may be negative and the time and cost of going through the extensive process to fabricate, maintain, and repair the denture may be greater than the perceived benefit. Longevity of dentures in a growing child will vary depending on dental and skeletal development and their ability to care for the appliance. Dentures in the primary dentition are typically serviceable for 2–3 years before needing to be relined or remade, though some can last longer depending on the child [103, 104]. Fixed appliances using lingual arches or bonded bridges are sometimes used for children in the primary, mixed, or even early permanent dentitions. More traditional fixed appliances such as dental bridges become an appropriate option in the permanent dentition.

Dental implants have markedly changed the approaches to managing missing teeth and have been shown to be useful in patients with ED. Implants are occasionally used in children when they have severe hypodontia or even anodontia and are not able to wear a tissue-supported removable appliance [105–110]. Dental implants being placed in proximity of natural teeth should be delayed until craniofacial growth is complete in early adulthood (late teens or early 20s) as teeth continue to erupt and jaw growth, though minor, continues throughout the life. In some cases where maxillary dentoalveolar bone levels are insufficient, zygomatic dental implants could be considered [111]. The number of dental implants and the type of restorative prosthesis will depend on the number of missing teeth, the span between implants, and the clinician's preferences.

No treatment for taurodontism is directly indicated; however, if restorative treatment is indicated on the taurodont, dentists should be aware of its presence. If pulp treatment is indicated, long-shanked dental burs may be needed to completely remove the chamber tissue and filling the chamber with a restorative material may make the tooth more prone to coronal fractures.

10.4 Summary

Since the discovery of the first ED-associated gene (*EDA*) in 1996, a great deal has been learned regarding the genotypes, phenotypes, and molecular pathways of these genetically and clinically diverse conditions [54]. Treatments have evolved with this understanding, and novel therapies such as protein replacement and gene therapy are being investigated [112, 113]. While these new therapeutic approaches show tremendous promise, it is unknown how the oral and craniofacial manifestations of the different EDs will be affected. The craniofacial manifestations of ED have a profound effect on affected individuals with current treatment approaches being costly and requiring expertise from team of health care providers [114–116]. Early identification of individuals with ED allows optimization of preventive and habilitative services that can help ensure that good oral health is realized throughout the individual's life course.

References

1. Peschel N, Wright JT, Koster MI, et al. Molecular pathway-based classification of ectodermal dysplasias: first five-yearly update. Genes (Basel). 2022;13(12):2327.
2. Häärä O, Fujimori S, Schmidt-Ullrich R, et al. Ectodysplasin and Wnt pathways are required for salivary gland branching morphogenesis. Development. 2011;138(13):2681–91.
3. Chibly AM, Aure MH, Patel VN, Hoffman MP. Salivary gland function, development, and regeneration. Physiol Rev. 2022;102(3):1495–552.
4. Mukaibo T, Munemasa T, Masaki C, Cui CY, Melvin JE. Defective NaCl reabsorption in salivary glands of Eda-null X-LHED mice. J Dent Res. 2018;97(11):1244–51.
5. Kowalczyk-Quintas C, Schneider P. Ectodysplasin A (EDA)—EDA receptor signalling and its pharmacological modulation. Cytokine Growth Factor Rev. 2014;25(2):195–203.
6. Arlt A, Kohlschmidt N, Hentschel A, et al. Novel insights into PORCN mutations, associated phenotypes and pathophysiological aspects. Orphanet J Rare Dis. 2022;17(1):29.
7. Wright JT, Puranik CP, Farrington F. Oral phenotype and variation in focal dermal hypoplasia. Am J Med Genet C Semin Med Genet. 2016;172C(1):52–8.
8. Xu M, Horrell J, Snitow M, et al. WNT10A mutation causes ectodermal dysplasia by impairing progenitor cell proliferation and KLF4-mediated differentiation. Nat Commun. 2017;8:15397.
9. Wright JT, Fete M, Schneider H, et al. Ectodermal dysplasias: classification and organization by phenotype, genotype and molecular pathway. Am J Med Genet A. 2019;179(3):442–7.
10. Itin PH. Etiology and pathogenesis of ectodermal dysplasias. Am J Med Genet A. 2014;164A(10):2472–7.
11. OMIM. Online Mendelian inheritance in man. Baltimore: Center for Medical Genetics, Johns Hopkins University and National Center for Biotechnology Information, National Library of Medicine; 2023. https://www.ncbi.nlm.gov/omim/ed.
12. Goodwin AF, Larson JR, Jones KB, et al. Craniofacial morphometric analysis of individuals with X-linked hypohidrotic ectodermal dysplasia. Mol Genet Genomic Med. 2014;2(5):422–9.
13. Sutton VR, van Bokhoven H. TP63-related disorders. In: Adam MP, Mirzaa GM, Pagon RA, Wallace SE, Bean LJH, Gripp KW, et al., editors. GeneReviews®. Seattle; 1993.
14. Cole P, Hatef DA, Kaufman Y, et al. Facial clefting and oroauditory pathway manifestations in ankyloblepharon-ectodermal defects-cleft lip/palate (AEC) syndrome. Am J Med Genet A. 2009;149A(9):1910–5.
15. Buss PW, Hughes HE, Clarke A. Twenty-four cases of the EEC syndrome: clinical presentation and management. J Med Genet. 1995;32(9):716–23.
16. Kohn LL, Braun M, Cordoro KM, et al. Skin and mucosal manifestations in NEMO syndrome: a case series and literature review. Pediatr Dermatol. 2022;39(1):84–90.
17. Perazzio SF, Allenspach EJ, Eklund KK, et al. Behcet disease (BD) and BD-like clinical phenotypes: NF-kappaB pathway in mucosal ulcerating diseases. Scand J Immunol. 2020;92(5):e12973.
18. Schimke LF, Rieber N, Rylaarsdam S, et al. A novel gain-of-function IKBA mutation underlies ectodermal dysplasia with immunodeficiency and polyendocrinopathy. J Clin Immunol. 2013;33(6):1088–99.
19. Bret Puvilland C, Boisson B, Fusaro M, et al. EDA-ID: a severe clinical presentation associated with a new IKBKG mutation. J Clin Immunol. 2021;41(5):1099–102.

20. Brar BK, Mehta V, Kubba A. Dermatopathia pigmentosa reticularis. Pediatr Dermatol. 2007;24(5):566–70.
21. Hegde K, Puthran RM, Nair G, Nair PP. Ellis van Creveld syndrome—a report of two siblings. BMJ Case Rep. 2011;2011:bcr0920114774.
22. Lauritano D, Attuati S, Besana M, et al. Oral and craniofacial manifestations of Ellis-van Creveld syndrome: a systematic review. Eur J Paediatr Dent. 2019;20(4):306–10.
23. Nobre AVV, Taba M, Silva AR, de Souza SLS, Motta ACF. Focal dermal hypoplasia (Goltz syndrome): a case report showing a wide variety of systemic and oral manifestations. Ann Dermatol. 2022;34(4):291–6.
24. Bostwick B, Van den Veyver IB, Sutton VR. Focal dermal hypoplasia. In: Adam MP, Mirzaa GM, Pagon RA, Wallace SE, Bean LJH, Gripp KW, et al., editors. GeneReviews®. Seattle; 1993.
25. Yu J, Liao PJ, Xu W, et al. Structural model of human PORCN illuminates disease-associated variants and drug-binding sites. J Cell Sci. 2021;134(24):jcs259383.
26. Gordjani N, Herdeg S, Ross UH, et al. Focal dermal hypoplasia (Goltz-Gorlin syndrome) associated with obstructive papillomatosis of the larynx and hypopharynx. Eur J Dermatol. 1999;9(8):618–20.
27. Ishii N, Baba N, Kanaizuka I, et al. Histopathological study of focal dermal hypoplasia (Goltz syndrome). Clin Exp Dermatol. 1992;17(1):24–6.
28. Adaimy L, Chouery E, Megarbane H, et al. Mutation in WNT10A is associated with an autosomal recessive ectodermal dysplasia: the odonto-onycho-dermal dysplasia. Am J Hum Genet. 2007;81(4):821–8.
29. Kantaputra P, Kaewgahya M, Jotikasthira D, Kantaputra W. Tricho-odonto-onycho-dermal dysplasia and WNT10A mutations. Am J Med Genet A. 2014;164A(4):1041–8.
30. Martins F, Ortega KL, Hiraoka C, Ricardo P, Magalhães M. Oral and dental abnormalities in Barber-Say syndrome. Am J Med Genet A. 2010;152A(10):2569–73.
31. Quiros-Terron L, Arraez-Aybar LA, Murillo-Gonzalez J, et al. Initial stages of development of the submandibular gland (human embryos at 5.5-8 weeks of development). J Anat. 2019;234(5):700–8.
32. Garcia-Godoy F, Hicks MJ. Maintaining the integrity of the enamel surface: the role of dental biofilm, saliva and preventive agents in enamel demineralization and remineralization. J Am Dent Assoc. 2008;139 Suppl:25S–34S.
33. Dawes C, Pedersen AM, Villa A, et al. The functions of human saliva: a review sponsored by the world workshop on oral medicine VI. Arch Oral Biol. 2015;60(6):863–74.
34. Yildirim M, Yorgancilar E, Gun R, Topcu I. Ectodermal dysplasia: otolaryngologic evaluation of 23 cases. Ear Nose Throat J. 2012;91(2):E28–33.
35. Semmler M, Kniesburges S, Pelka F, et al. Influence of reduced saliva production on phonation in patients with ectodermal dysplasia. J Voice. 2023;37(6):913–23.
36. Mohanan A, Varma BR, Kumar S, Kumaran P, Xavier AM. Assessment of salivary flow rate and antioxidant levels in ectodermal dysplasia patients: an in vivo study. Contemp Clin Dent. 2019;10(1):74–80.
37. Nordgarden H, Storhaug K, Lyngstadaas SP, Jensen JL. Salivary gland function in persons with ectodermal dysplasias. Eur J Oral Sci. 2003;111(5):371–6.
38. Lexner MO, Bardow A, Hertz JM, et al. Whole saliva in X-linked hypohidrotic ectodermal dysplasia. Int J Paediatr Dent. 2007;17(3):155–62.
39. Villavisanis DF, Blum JD, Plana NM, Taub PJ, Taylor JA. Choosing a multidisciplinary cleft and craniofacial team: medical, surgical, and social considerations. Cleft Palate Craniofac J. 2024;61:518.
40. Stock NM, Marik P, Magee L, et al. Facilitating positive psychosocial outcomes in craniofacial team care: strategies for medical providers. Cleft Palate Craniofac J. 2020;57(3):333–43.
41. Ascha M, McDaniel J, Link I, et al. Social and support services offered by cleft and craniofacial teams: a national survey and institutional experience. J Craniofac Surg. 2016;27(2):356–60.

42. Lofgren CD, Wickstrom C, Sonesson M, Lagunas PT, Christersson C. A systematic review of methods to diagnose oral dryness and salivary gland function. BMC Oral Health. 2012;12:29.
43. Pillai S, Munguia-Lopez JG, Tran SD. Hydrogels for salivary gland tissue engineering. Gels. 2022;8(11):730.
44. Contessi Negrini N, Angelova Volponi A, Higgins CA, Sharpe PT, Celiz AD. Scaffold-based developmental tissue engineering strategies for ectodermal organ regeneration. Mater Today Bio. 2021;10:100107.
45. Clauss F, Maniere MC, Obry F, et al. Dento-craniofacial phenotypes and underlying molecular mechanisms in hypohidrotic ectodermal dysplasia (HED): a review. J Dent Res. 2008;87(12):1089–99.
46. Birgfeld CB, Glick P, Singh D, LaRossa D, Bartlett S. Midface growth in patients with ectrodactyly-ectodermal dysplasia-clefting syndrome. Plast Reconstr Surg. 2007;120(1):144–50.
47. Vink CP, Ockeloen CW, ten Kate S, et al. Variability in dentofacial phenotypes in four families with WNT10A mutations. Eur J Hum Genet. 2014;22(9):1063–70.
48. Lexner MO, Bardow A, Bjorn-Jorgensen J, et al. Anthropometric and cephalometric measurements in X-linked hypohidrotic ectodermal dysplasia. Orthod Craniofac Res. 2007;10(4):203–15.
49. Nguyen T, Phillips C, Frazier-Bower S, Wright T. Craniofacial variations in the tricho-dento-osseous syndrome. Clin Genet. 2013;83(4):375–9.
50. Bergendal B. Orodental manifestations in ectodermal dysplasia—a review. Am J Med Genet A. 2014;164A(10):2465–71.
51. Crawford PJM, Aldred JM, Clarke A. Clinical and radiographic dental findings in X linked hypohidrotic ectodermal dysplasia. J Med Genet. 1991;28:181–5.
52. Thesleff I, Vaahtokari A, Vainio S, Jowett A. Molecular mechanisms of cell and tissue interactions during early tooth development. Anat Rec. 1996;245:151–61.
53. Kangas AT, Evans AR, Thesleff I, Jernvall J. Nonindependence of mammalian dental characters. Nature. 2004;432(7014):211–4.
54. Kere J, Srivastava AK, Montonen O, et al. X-linked anhidrotic (hypohidrotic) ectodermal dysplasia is caused by mutation in a novel transmembrane protein. Nat Genet. 1996;13(4):409–16.
55. Casal ML, Lewis JR, Mauldin EA, et al. Significant correction of disease after postnatal administration of recombinant ectodysplasin A in canine X-linked ectodermal dysplasia. Am J Hum Genet. 2007;81(5):1050–6.
56. Lexner MO, Bardow A, Juncker I, et al. X-linked hypohidrotic ectodermal dysplasia. Genetic and dental findings in 67 Danish patients from 19 families. Clin Genet. 2008;74(3):252–9.
57. Gökdere S, Schneider H, Hehr U, et al. Functional and clinical analysis of five. Front Genet. 2022;13:934395.
58. Wright JT, Grange DK, Fete M. Hypohidrotic ectodermal dysplasia. In: Adam MP, Everman DB, Mirzaa GM, Pagon RA, Wallace SE, Bean LJH, et al., editors. GeneReviews; 1993.
59. Hudson CD, Witkop CJ. Autosomal dominant hypodontia with nail dysgenesis. Report of twenty-nine cases in six families. Oral Surg Oral Med Oral Pathol. 1975;39(3):409–23.
60. Wicomb GM, Stephen LX, Beighton P. Dental implications of tooth-nail dysplasia (Witkop syndrome): a report of an affected family and an approach to dental management. J Clin Pediatr Dent. 2004;28(2):107–12.
61. Mues G, Bonds J, Xiang L, et al. The WNT10A gene in ectodermal dysplasias and selective tooth agenesis. Am J Med Genet A. 2014;164A(10):2455–60.
62. Bergendal B, Norderyd J, Zhou X, Klar J, Dahl N. Abnormal primary and permanent dentitions with ectodermal symptoms predict WNT10A deficiency. BMC Med Genet. 2016;17(1):88.
63. Yu M, Liu Y, Liu H, et al. Distinct impacts of bi-allelic WNT10A mutations on the permanent and primary dentitions in odonto-onycho-dermal dysplasia. Am J Med Genet A. 2019;179(1):57–64.

64. Bohring A, Stamm T, Spaich C, et al. WNT10A mutations are a frequent cause of a broad spectrum of ectodermal dysplasias with sex-biased manifestation pattern in heterozygotes. Am J Hum Genet. 2009;85(1):97–105.
65. Yu T, Klein OD. Molecular and cellular mechanisms of tooth development, homeostasis and repair. Development. 2020;147(2):dev184754.
66. Guckes AD, Roberts MW, McCarthy GR. Pattern of permanent teeth present in individuals with ectodermal dysplasia and severe hypodontia suggests treatment with dental implants. Pediatr Dent. 1998;20(4):278–80.
67. Wright JT. Enamel phenotypes: genetic and environmental determinants. Genes (Basel). 2023;14(3):545.
68. Wright JT, Kula K, Hall K, Simmons JH, Hart TC. Analysis of the tricho-dento-osseous syndrome genotype and phenotype. Am J Med Genet. 1997;72(2):197–204.
69. Hart TC, Bowden DW, Bolyard J, et al. Genetic linkage of the tricho-dento-osseous syndrome to chromosome 17q21. Hum Mol Genet. 1997;6(13):2279–84.
70. Shapiro SD, Quattromani FL, Jorgenson RJ, Young RS. Tricho-dento-osseous syndrome: heterogeneity or clinical variability. Am J Med Genet. 1983;16(2):225–36.
71. Hassan MQ, Javed A, Morasso MI, et al. Dlx3 transcriptional regulation of osteoblast differentiation: temporal recruitment of Msx2, Dlx3, and Dlx5 homeodomain proteins to chromatin of the osteocalcin gene. Mol Cell Biol. 2004;24(20):9248–61.
72. Price JA, Bowden DW, Wright JT, Pettenati MJ, Hart TC. Identification of a mutation in DLX3 associated with tricho-dento-osseous (TDO) syndrome. Hum Mol Genet. 1998;7(3):563–9.
73. Price JA, Wright JT, Kula K, Bowden DW, Hart TC. A common DLX3 gene mutation is responsible for tricho-dento-osseous syndrome in Virginia and North Carolina families. J Med Genet. 1998;35:825–8.
74. Price JA, Wright JT, Crawford PC, Aldred MJ, Hart TC. Tricho-dento-osseous syndrome and amelogenesis imperfecta with taurodontism are genetically distinct conditions. Clin Genet. 1999;56:35–40.
75. Wright T. The molecular control of and clinical variations in root formation. Cells Tissues Organs. 2007;186(1):86–93.
76. Dissaux C, Ruffenach L, Bruant-Rodier C, et al. Cleft alveolar bone graft materials: literature review. Cleft Palate Craniofac J. 2022;59(3):336–46.
77. Bayat M, Khobyari MM, Dalband M, Momen-Heravi F. Full mouth implant rehabilitation of a patient with ectodermal dysplasia after orthognathic surgery, sinus and ridge augmentation: a clinical report. J Adv Prosthodont. 2011;3(2):96–100.
78. Omeish N, Nassif A, Feghali S, Vi-Fane B, Bosco J. Esthetic and functional rehabilitation of peg-shaped maxillary lateral incisors: practical recommendations. Clin Case Rep. 2022;10(3):e05507.
79. Waggoner WF. Anterior crowns for primary anterior teeth: an evidence based assessment of the literature. Eur Arch Paediatr Dent. 2006;7(2):53–7; discussion 57.
80. Kupietzky A, Waggoner WF, Galea J. The clinical and radiographic success of bonded resin composite strip crowns for primary incisors. Pediatr Dent. 2003;25(6):577–81.
81. Pena CE, Viotti RG, Dias WR, et al. Esthetic rehabilitation of anterior conoid teeth: comprehensive approach for improved and predictable results. Eur J Esthet Dent. 2009;4(3):210–24.
82. Vaghela LL, Patel MC, Bhatt RK, Patel CN, Joshi KR. Clinical performance and parental satisfaction with composite strip crown and prefabricated zirconia crown for primary anterior teeth: a randomized clinical trial. J Contemp Dent Pract. 2021;22(12):1462–70.
83. Elheeny AAH, Abdelmotelb MA. Oral health-related quality of life (OHRQOL) of preschool children's anterior teeth restored with zirconia crowns versus resin-bonded composite strip crowns: a 12-month prospective clinical trial. Clin Oral Investig. 2022;26(5):3923–38.
84. Alaki SM, Abdulhadi BS, AbdElBaki MA, Alamoudi NM. Comparing zirconia to anterior strip crowns in primary anterior teeth in children: a randomized clinical trial. BMC Oral Health. 2020;20(1):313.

85. Garcia PP, da Costa RG, Calgaro M, et al. Digital smile design and mock-up technique for esthetic treatment planning with porcelain laminate veneers. J Conserv Dent. 2018;21(4):455–8.
86. Whiteman YY. A communication guide for orthodontic-restorative collaborations: digital smile design outline tool. Dent Clin North Am. 2020;64(4):719–30.
87. Schmitz JH, Coffano R, Bruschi A. Restorative and orthodontic treatment of maxillary peg incisors: a clinical report. J Prosthet Dent. 2001;85(4):330–4.
88. Alberton SB, Alberton V, de Carvalho RV. Providing a harmonious smile with laminate veneers for a patient with peg-shaped lateral incisors. J Conserv Dent. 2017;20(3):210–3.
89. Kallala R, Nasri S, Adli A, et al. Peg-shaped lateral incisors treated with ceramic three-quarter crown. Case Rep Dent. 2021;2021:9412638.
90. Al-Ani AH, Antoun JS, Thomson WM, Merriman TR, Farella M. Hypodontia: an update on its etiology, classification, and clinical management. Biomed Res Int. 2017;2017:9378325.
91. Levy-Bercowski D, Abreu A, Parker C, Riggs B, Rockman R. Immediate vacuum formed overdenture for a pediatric patient with ectodermal dysplasia. J Dent Child (Chic). 2018;85(3):139–42.
92. Tong HJ, Tahmassebi JF. Management of a child with severe hypodontia in the mixed dentition stage of development. Eur Arch Paediatr Dent. 2014;15(6):449–54.
93. Maroulakos G, Artopoulou II, Angelopoulou MV, Emmanouil D. Removable partial dentures vs overdentures in children with ectodermal dysplasia: two case reports. Eur Arch Paediatr Dent. 2016;17(3):205–10.
94. Stephen A, Cengiz SB. The use of overdentures in the management of severe hypodontia associated with microdontia: a case report. J Clin Pediatr Dent. 2003;27(3):219–22.
95. Vergo TJ. Prosthodontics for pediatric patients with congenital/developmental orofacial anomalies: a long-term follow-up. J Prosthet Dent. 2001;86(4):342–7.
96. Török G, Saláta J, Ábrám E, et al. Prosthetic rehabilitation of a patient with ectrodactyly-ectodermal dysplasia-cleft lip/palate syndrome through a hybrid workflow: a case report with 2-year follow-up. Spec Care Dentist. 2023;44:96.
97. Peroz S, Peroz I, Beuer F, Sterzenbach G, von Stein-Lausnitz M. Digital versus conventional complete dentures: a randomized, controlled, blinded study. J Prosthet Dent. 2022;128(5):956–63.
98. Peroz S, Peroz I, Beuer F, von Stein-Lausnitz M, Sterzenbach G. Digital versus conventional complete dentures: a randomized, controlled, double-blinded crossover trial. J Prosthet Dent. 2022;128:956.
99. Zupancic Cepic L, Gruber R, Eder J, et al. Digital versus conventional dentures: a prospective, randomized cross-over study on clinical efficiency and patient satisfaction. J Clin Med. 2023;12(2):434.
100. Kang YJ, Oh KC, Kim GY, Moon HS. Comparative evaluation of digitally fabricated complete dentures versus conventional complete dentures: a randomized, single-blinded, cross-over clinical trial. J Prosthet Dent. 2024;132(2):408–18.
101. de Freitas RF, de Carvalho DK, da Fonte Porto Carreiro A, Barbosa GAS, Ferreira MAF. Mandibular implant-supported removable partial denture with distal extension: a systematic review. J Oral Rehabil. 2012;39(10):791–8.
102. Taylor M, Masood M, Mnatzaganian G. Longevity of complete dentures: a systematic review and meta-analysis. J Prosthet Dent. 2021;125(4):611–9.
103. Quintanilha LELP, Carneiro-Campos LE, Antunes LAA, et al. Prosthetic rehabilitation in a pediatric patient with hypohidrotic ectodermal dysplasia: a case report. Gen Dent. 2017;65(5):72–6.
104. Schnabl D, Grunert I, Schmuth M, Kapferer-Seebacher I. Prosthetic rehabilitation of patients with hypohidrotic ectodermal dysplasia: a systematic review. J Oral Rehabil. 2018;45(7):555–70.
105. Mello BZ, Silva TC, Rios D, et al. Mini-implants: alternative for oral rehabilitation of a child with ectodermal dysplasia. Braz Dent J. 2015;26(1):75–8.

106. Aydinbelge M, Gumus HO, Sekerci AE, Demetoğlu U, Etoz OA. Implants in children with hypohidrotic ectodermal dysplasia: an alternative approach to esthetic management: case report and review of the literature. Pediatr Dent. 2013;35(5):441–6.
107. Kramer FJ, Baethge C, Tschernitschek H. Implants in children with ectodermal dysplasia: a case report and literature review. Clin Oral Implants Res. 2007;18(1):140–6.
108. Knobloch LA, Larsen PE, Saponaro PC, L'Homme-Langlois E. Early implant placement for a patient with ectodermal dysplasia: thirteen years of clinical care. J Prosthet Dent. 2018;119(5):702–9.
109. Enlow DH. A morphogenetic analysis of facial growth. Am J Orthod. 1966;52(4):283–99.
110. Kurihara S, Enlow DH, Rangel RD. Remodeling reversals in anterior parts of the human mandible and maxilla. Angle Orthod. 1980;50(2):98–106.
111. Goker F, Grecchi E, Mancini EG, Del Fabbro M, Grecchi F. Zygomatic implant survival in 9 ectodermal dysplasia patients with 3.5- to 7-year follow-up. Oral Dis. 2020;26(8):1803–9.
112. Schneider H, Schweikl C, Faschingbauer F, Hadj-Rabia S, Schneider P. A causal treatment for X-linked hypohidrotic ectodermal dysplasia: long-term results of short-term perinatal ectodysplasin A1 replacement. Int J Mol Sci. 2023;24(8):7155.
113. Wright JT, Abbott BM, Salois MN, et al. Rare diseases of ectoderm: translating discovery to therapy. Am J Med Genet A. 2023;191(3):902–9.
114. Hashem A, Kelly A, O'Connell B, O'Sullivan M. Impact of moderate and severe hypodontia and amelogenesis imperfecta on quality of life and self-esteem of adult patients. J Dent. 2013;41(8):689–94.
115. Crossan E, O'Connell AC. Parental perception on oral health-related quality of life and dental features of ectodermal dysplasia and isolated hypodontia in children. BMC Oral Health. 2021;21(1):510.
116. Niekamp N, Kleinheinz J, Reissmann DR, Bohner L, Hanisch M. Subjective oral health-related quality of life and objective oral health in people with ectodermal dysplasia. Int J Environ Res Public Health. 2020;18(1):143.

Chapter 11
Oral and Dental Phenotype of Ectodermal Dysplasias

Johanna Norderyd and Hilde Nordgarden

Keywords Oligodontia · Bone defects · Prosthesis

11.1 Introduction

The oral cavity is lined with epithelium derived from the ectoderm. The development of structures derived from this cell layer is similar to the development of extraoral structures derived from epithelium. Tooth development is extensively studied in mammals and represents a common pattern for the development of ectodermal placodes deployed in diverse types of epithelium organogenesis, such as salivary glands, mammary glands, sweat glands, limb buds, and more [1].

Mutations in genes involved in the conserved molecular pathways regulating these developmental processes may affect oral tissues and cause a range of clinical phenotypes. When classifying and utilizing the phenotypes in diagnostics, it is essential that the clinical descriptions are accurate. In our experience, this is not always the case, as clinicians and researchers do not use the same descriptive terms for identical phenotypes, or even use the wrong nomenclature. One must also be aware that many of the anomalies described in this chapter are associated with each other and may represent a continuum of anomalies caused by the same genetic mutation [2]. This may explain the wide variation in phenotypes seen between individuals with the same genotype. Therefore, when an individual presents with dental or other oral anomalies that may be a manifestation of a genetic disorder, it is very important that a dentist with knowledge of and experience in genetic disorders makes the evaluation.

J. Norderyd
Centre for Oral Health, Jönköping University, Jönköping, Sweden

H. Nordgarden (✉)
National Competence Center for Oral Health in Rare Diagnoses, The TAKO Centre, Lovisenberg Diaconal Hospital, Oslo, Norway
e-mail: hilde.nordgarden@tako.no

G. Tadini et al. (eds.), *Multidisciplinary Approach to Ectodermal Dysplasia*,
https://doi.org/10.1007/978-3-031-75790-7_11

The term **hypodontia** (from Greek, *hypo*: less than normal) is often used to describe the congenital absence of one or more teeth, third molars (wisdom teeth) excluded. The term hypodontia is unspecific and includes all cases of congenitally missing teeth, regardless of number. While hypodontia is relatively uncommon in the primary dentition, agenesis of one or more permanent teeth is one of the most common developmental disturbances in humans [3], with a described prevalence of 2.5–6.9% [4].

The term **oligodontia** is more specific and describes the congenital absence of six or more teeth, third molars excluded. In Scandinavian studies, the prevalence of oligodontia is described to be 0.08–0.16% [5–7]. This phenotype is often associated with other dental developmental disturbances, such as microdontia (abnormally small teeth), abnormal tooth form, delayed tooth eruption, and disturbances in enamel formation and in aberrant jaw growth [8].

Anodontia describes the most serious form of hypodontia: total agenesis of teeth in the lower jaw, upper jaw, or both. This is a very rare phenotype.

In the part of the jaw where one or more teeth are missing, the alveolar bone will not develop normally. The more absent teeth, the less alveolar bone will develop. **Hypoplastic jawbone** is often described as a phenotype in ectodermal dysplasias (EDs), but is usually a secondary effect of hypodontia, oligodontia, or anodontia. **Widely spaced teeth are** also mentioned as a phenotype but are also a result of either small teeth (microdontia) and/or missing teeth (hypodontia). The same is the case for over-eruption of teeth when the occluding teeth are absent or when the occlusion in general is unstable because of many missing teeth (Fig. 11.1).

Different forms of ED may also have different **hypodontia patterns**. Heterozygous EDAR mutations and homozygous mutations in KREMEN1 are reported to cause congenital absence of maxillary lateral incisors and one or more of the mandibular incisors (often all four mandibular incisors) [9, 10]. Monoallelic mutations in WNT10A typically lead to agenesis of maxillary and mandibular premolars, whereas biallelic mutations in addition often also cause the absence of maxillary and mandibular molars [11].

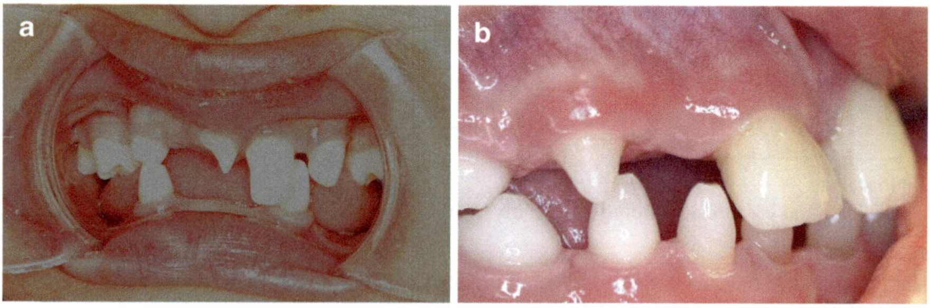

Fig. 11.1 (**a**) Over eruption of a central incisor in an individual with mutation in EDA1; (**b**) Over eruption of central incisors and an erupting peg-shaped canine in an individual with a WNT10A mutation

Microdontia describes teeth that are unusually small, although an established definition of microdontia does not exist. However, a Norwegian study concluded that the median tooth size of molars and central incisors in the upper jaw in individuals with oligodontia with or without ED was below or on the tenth percentile of size measures in healthy, Caucasian North Americans [12].

Abnormal tooth form: There are different morphological tooth deviations described in different EDs. The most commonly described deviation is peg-shaped incisors and canines, which is also described as a "microform" of hypodontia [13]. Other terms often used to describe variants of or different grades of peg-shaped teeth are conical, tapered, or screwdriver-shaped (Fig. 11.2).

However, there are other abnormal tooth forms found in some EDs, as, for example, seen in focal dermal hypoplasia/Goltz syndrome with accessory cusps, notched incisors, or generally malformed teeth (Fig. 11.3) or in incontinentia pigmenti (Fig. 11.4).

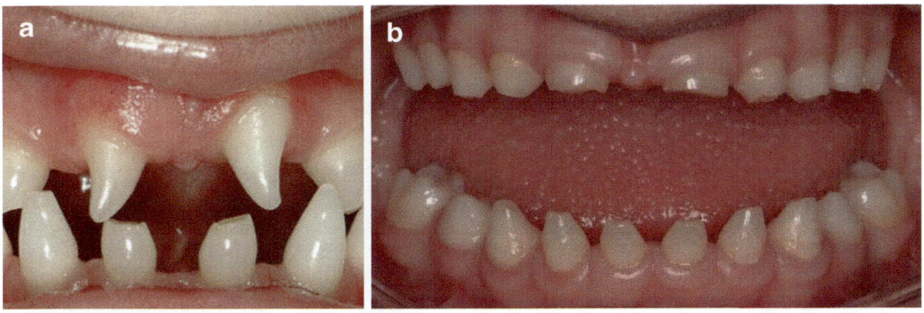

Fig. 11.2 (**a**) Peg shaped central incisors in an individual with mutation in WNT10a; (**b**) Peg shaped incisors in the lower jaw in an individual with mutation in WNT10A

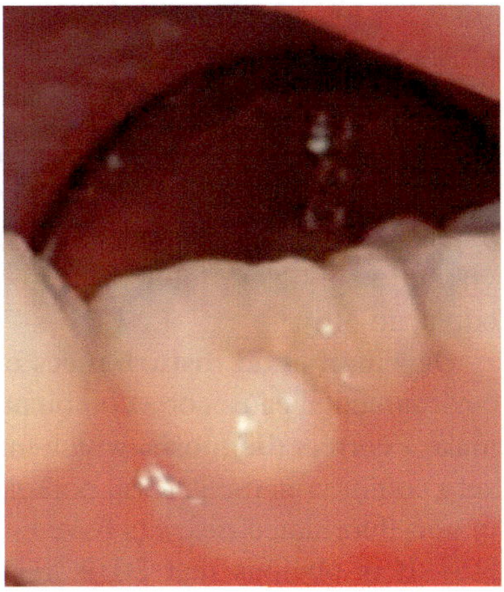

Fig. 11.3 A molar with an accessory buccal cusp in an individual with focal dermal hypoplasia (mutation in PORCN)

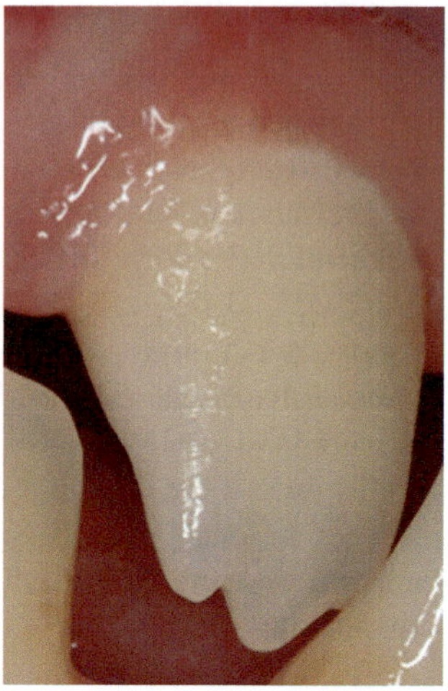

Fig. 11.4 Abnormal tooth form in an individual with incontinentia pigmenti (mutation in IKBKG)

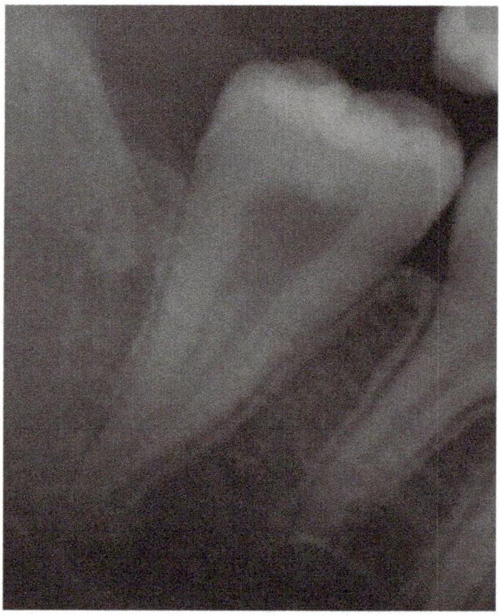

Fig. 11.5 A taurodont lower second molar in an individual with clinically diagnosed ectodermal dysplasia

Taurodontism is another variant of abnormal tooth form found in some EDs. It is the term for when the tooth crown-body length in relation to the root length in molars is altered. This is therefore only possible to discover through a dental radiograph (Fig. 11.5). A tooth crown-body root ratio of 0.9 or more is considered taurodontism [14].

Developmental disturbances of enamel (DDE) may have a genetic cause, an environmental cause, or a combination of these. Accurate description is essential to make a correct **diagnosis**, which may be difficult for untrained clinicians. DDE are very common in the general population. In fact, up to 50% of the population living in non-fluoridated districts have been shown to have one or more teeth with DDE [15]. It is obvious that DDE linked to EDs are caused by the relevant genetic mutation. However, it is necessary that the clinician involved in the diagnostic process also is familiar with DDE not linked to ED or other genetic conditions, such as molar-incisor hypomineralization (MIH), dental fluorosis, and sequela after dental trauma (these DDE are not described in this chapter). A correct diagnosis is important not only for the patients, but also for proper classification of oral phenotypes in EDs in the future.

Enamel hypoplasia means that a tooth has reduced thickness of enamel when erupting, as opposed to enamel lost in post-eruptive breakdown or dental caries. Enamel hypoplasia is caused by a disruption in the formation of enamel matrix during the odontogenesis. Enamel hypoplasia may manifest as pits, horizontal or vertical furrows, missing enamel on parts of the tooth crown, and generalized thin or total lack of enamel on the tooth crown (Fig. 11.6).

Enamel hypomineralization means that the enamel has normal thickness but reduced mineral content. Hence, it is a qualitative rather than a quantitative enamel disorder. It is caused by defects in the maturation phase of enamel development and may result in a less transparent or opaque enamel, often manifested as discolored enamel. The enamel has normal thickness upon eruption, but since it is less mineralized, it may, however, break down after exposure to tear and wear (Fig. 11.7).

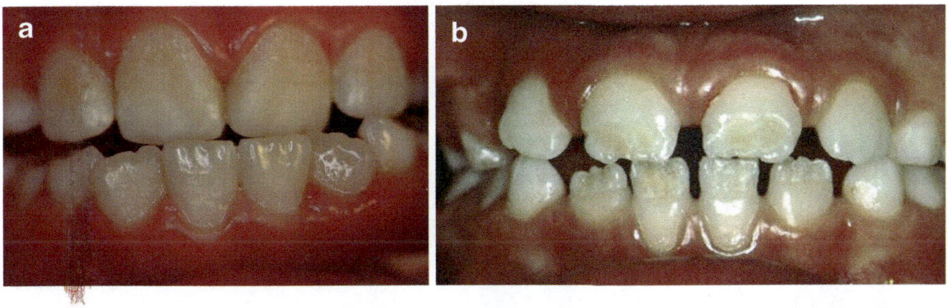

Fig. 11.6 (**a**) Example of enamel hypoplasia manifesting as pits, in particular in the cervical parts of the upper central incisors; (**b**) Example of enamel hypoplasia manifesting as missing enamel in parts of the dental crowns

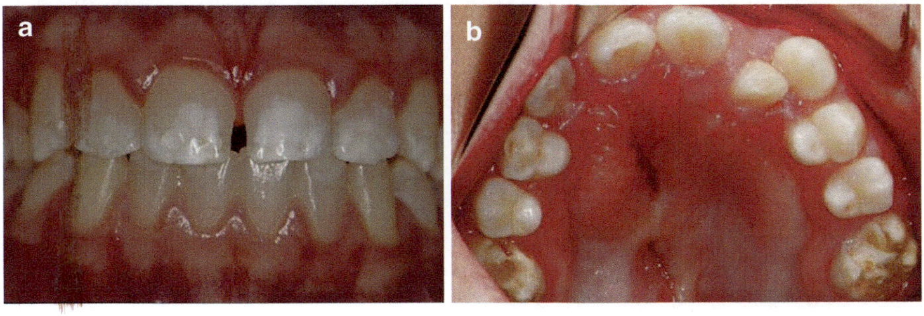

Fig. 11.7 Examples (**a**, **b**) of enamel hypomineralization manifesting as white spots as the enamel is less transparent

Sometimes, there is a combination of enamel hypoplasia and hypomineralization in the same tooth or dentition (Fig. 11.8).

When all teeth in an individual are affected by genetic DDE, the disorder is termed **amelogenesis imperfecta (AI)**. Amelogenesis imperfecta most often occurs as an isolated trait, but may also be associated with another genetic disease, such as some forms of ED. There are also different types of AI (hypoplasia, hypocalcification, hypomaturation, or combinations), although no specific type has been linked to ED (Fig. 11.9).

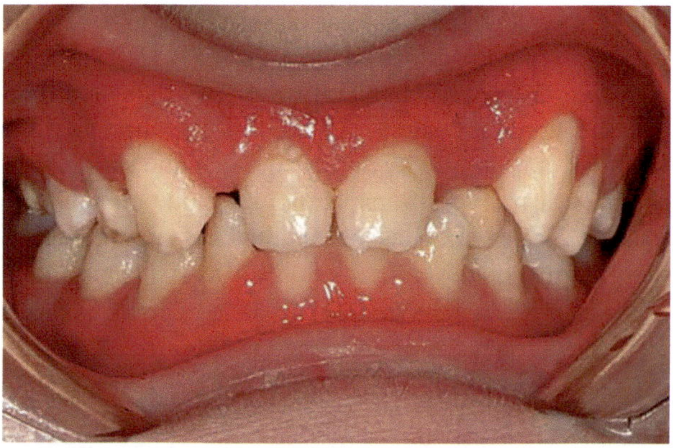

Fig. 11.8 Example of a combination of both enamel hypoplasias and enamel hypomineralization with post eruptive breakdown in an individual with a mutation in TP63

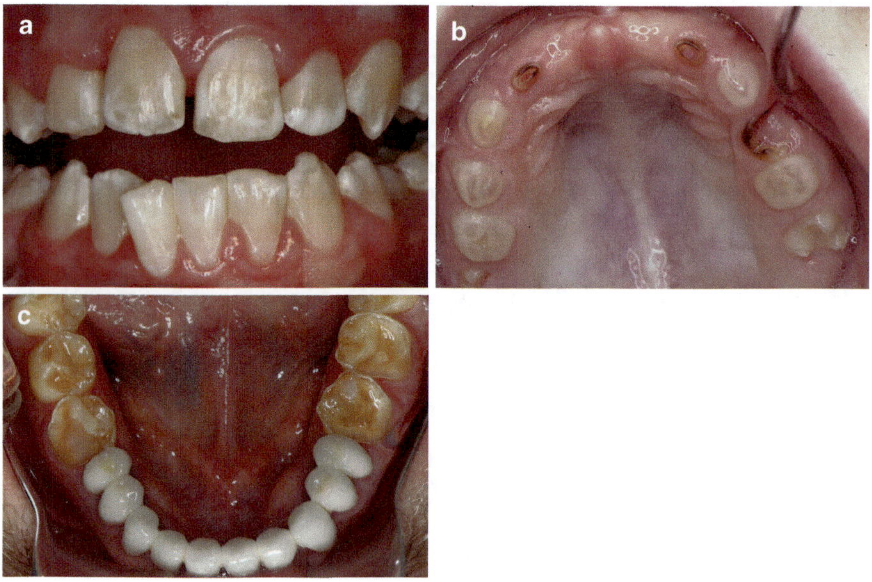

Fig. 11.9 (**a**) Example of amelogenesis imperfecta, hypomineralization type; (**b**) Amelogenesis imperfecta in a child affected by trichi-dento-osseus syndrome (mutation in DLX); (**c**) Amelogenesis imperfecta in an adult with tricho-dento-osseus sundrome. Note that anterior teeth have been rehabilitated with prosthetic crowns

Delayed Eruption: Reports of delayed tooth eruption are also found in some forms of ED, but an exact definition of delay does not exist. In the primary dentition, the variability in healthy children's age at the emergence of the individual teeth is relatively small (SD of 2–3 months). In the permanent dentition, the variability is considerably larger, with a standard deviation of 8–18 months. Consideration also has to be taken to the fact that tooth eruption in girls normally occurs significantly earlier than in boys, and in addition, that eruption times may vary with ethnicity. In order to determine whether the eruption is abnormally delayed or not, one therefore has to consider the standard deviation of the particular tooth in question, the child's gender, and ethnic background [16, 17].

Hypoplastic maxilla is a reported trait in a few EDs. This term indicates that the dimensions of the maxilla are abnormally small, usually creating a malocclusion or malalignment between the upper and lower teeth. It is unclear to the authors of this chapter, however, if the descriptions in the literature reflect a true maxillary hypoplasia or is a result of tooth agenesis and, thus, a reduced facial height.

Salivary secretions: As the salivary glands are ectodermal derivatives and their development is dependent on the same mechanisms as other ectodermal appendages, they are often affected in EDs. Subjective salivary problems have been reported by 37% of the members of the American National Foundation for Ectodermal Dysplasias (NFED), and mean salivary flow rates, when objectively measured, have been reported to be significantly reduced in individuals with EDs as a group [12] and in those with X-linked hypohidrotic ED (XLHED) [18]. Studies in mice with a murine EDA deficiency have shown that the submandibular glands exhibit less branching morphogenesis than in control mice [19]. In a male with XLHED and low salivary flow rates, examination with computed tomography suggested agenesis of both parotid and one submandibular gland [20]. Genetic mutations causing ED may also affect the quality of saliva, and one study demonstrated altered composition of salivary proteins and an elevated total concentration in a group of individuals affected by clinically diagnosed EDs [21]. An elevated level of NaCl in saliva from individuals with XLHED has also been shown [18], most likely caused by a reduced reabsorption of NaCl in the affected glands [22].

As the saliva has important functions, reduced salivary secretion may lead to secondary health problems. Saliva keeps the mouth moist and comfortable and facilitates talking, chewing, and swallowing. It aids in the defense against harmful oral microorganisms, protects dental enamel, and prevents tooth decay.

Lip malformations are reported in some EDs, such as a thin upper lip in tricho-rhinophalangeal syndrome. In addition, mutations in the genes TP63 and PVRL4 may cause cleft lip/palate.

Other oral manifestations are reported in EDs, such as oral papillomas, aberrant frenula, and jaw cysts in focal dermal hypoplasia [23]. Many other rare oral finds are seen in single case reports and are therefore not mentioned in this chapter, since it is difficult to assess whether they are true symptoms of the ED diagnosis or coincidental.

Tables 11.1 and 11.2 list hypodontia, abnormal tooth forms, and DDE in ED syndromes and syndromes partly associated with ED. The tables are based on the

Table 11.1 Hypodontia and other abnormal tooth forms in ectodermal dysplasia syndromes and syndromes partly associated with ectodermal dysplasia, as reported in OMIM and literature

Diagnosis (gene), OMIM no.	Hypodontia	Microdontia	Peg-shaped, conical, or tapered	Other tooth malformations	References
X-chromosome-linked hypohidrotic ectodermal/Christ-Siemens-Touraine syndrome/XLHED (*EDA*), 305100	X	X	X	Taurodontism	[24]
Ectodermal dysplasia, AD and AR/ECTD 10A and B (*EDAR*), 129490, 224900	X	X	X	Hypodontia pattern	[9, 24]
Ectodermal dysplasia, AD and AR/ ECTD 11A and B (*EDARADD*), 614940, 614941	X		X		[24, 25]
Incontinentia pigmenti (*IKBKG*), 308300	X	X	X	Accessory cusps, Notched incisors	[24, 26]
Ectodermal dysplasia and immunodeficiency 1/EDAID2 (*IKBKG*), 300291	X		X		[24]
Ectodermal dysplasia and immunodeficiency 2/EDAID2 (*NFKBIA*), 612132	X		X		[24]
Congenital heart defects and ectodermal dysplasia (*PKRD1*), 617364	X	X	X		[24, 27]
Focal dermal hypoplasia/Goltz-Gorlin syndrome (*PORCN*), 305600	X		X	Notched incisors, Cusp tips	[23, 24]
Odonto-onycho-dermal dysplasia/ Schöpf-Schulz-Passarge syndrome (*WNT10A*), 257980, 224750	X	X	X	Taurodontism, Hypodontia pattern	[24, 28]

(continued)

Table 11.1 (continued)

Diagnosis (gene), OMIM no.	Hypodontia	Microdontia	Peg-shaped, conical, or tapered	Other tooth malformations	References
Ectodermal dysplasia hair/tooth type/ ECTD13 (*KREMEN1*), 617392	X			Hypodontia pattern	[24]
Ulnar-mammary syndrome (*TBX3*), 181450	X				[24]
Ectodermal dysplasia with or without hypohidrosis (*LEF1*), 153245	X	X		Taurodontism	[29]
Ectodermal dysplasia with or without hypohidrosis (*LRP6*), 603507	X		X		[30]
Ectodermal dysplasia/ Witkop syndrome (*MSX1*), 189500	X	X	X		[24, 31]
Acro-dermato-ungual-lacrimal-tooth syndrome/ADULT (*TP63*), 103285	X	X	X		[24, 32]
Ectrodactyly-ectodermal dysplasia-cleft lip and palate syndrome/EEC (*TP63*), 604292	X	X	X	Barrel-shaped maxillary incisors	[24, 33]
Limb-mammary syndrome (*TP63*), 603543	X				[24]
Ankyloblepharon-ectodermal defects-cleft lip/palate/ Rapp-Hodgkin syndrome (*TP63*), 106260, 129400	X	X	X		[24]
Ectodermal dysplasia, ectrodactyly, macular dystrophy syndrome/ EEMS (*CDH3*), 225280	X	X			[24]

(continued)

Table 11.1 (continued)

Diagnosis (gene), OMIM no.	Hypodontia	Microdontia	Peg-shaped, conical, or tapered	Other tooth malformations	References
Hypohidrotic/hair/tooth/nail type ectodermal dysplasia/ECTD12 (*KDF1*), 617337	X				[24]
Tricho-dento-osseous syndrome (*DLX3*), 190320		X		Taurodontism	[24]
Ectodermal dysplasia-short stature syndrome (*GRHL2*), 616029	X				[24]
Cleft lip/palate-ectodermal dysplasia syndrome/CLPED1 (*PVRL1*), 225060	X	X			[24]
Ectodermal dysplasia-syndactyly syndrome (*PVRL4*), 613573		X	X		[24]
Oculo-dento-digital dysplasia (*GJA1*), 164200, 257850	X	X		Taurodontism	[24, 34]
Ectodermal dysplasia hair/tooth type with or without hypohidrosis/ECTD14 (*TSPEAR*), 618180	X		X		[24]
Trichorhinophalangeal syndrome, type I or type III (*TRPS1*), 190350	X	X		Supernumerary teeth	[24, 35]
Trichorhinophalangeal syndrome, type II/Langer-Giedion syndrome (*TRPS1, EXT1*), 150230	X				[24, 36]
Blepharocheilodontic syndrome 1 and 2 (*CDH1, CTNND1*), 119580, 617681	X		X	Notched incisors, Taurodontism, Hypodontia pattern	[24, 37]

(continued)

Table 11.1 (continued)

Diagnosis (gene), OMIM no.	Hypodontia	Microdontia	Peg-shaped, conical, or tapered	Other tooth malformations	References
Cranioectodermal dysplasia, types 1–4/Sensenbrenner syndrome (*IFT43, -52,-122, -140 WDR19, -35*), 218330	X	X	X	Dental fusion (in mice)	[24, 38]
Ellis-van Creveld syndrome (*EVC, EVC2*), 225500	X	X	X	Taurodontism, Natal teeth	[24, 39]
Weyers acrofacial dysostosis (*EVC. EVC2*), 193530	X	X	X	Single central incisor	[24]
Scalp-ear-nipple syndrome (*KCTD1*), 181270	X				[24]
Growth retardation, alopecia, pseudoanodontia, and optic atrophy syndrome/GAPO syndrome (*ANTXR1*), 230740	(X) Pseudoanodontia			Total failure of eruption	[24]
Carvajal syndrome (*DSP*), 605676	X				[40]
Gorlin-Chaudhry-Moss syndrome (*SLC25A24*), 612289	X	X			[24]
Johanson-–Blizzard syndrome (*UBR1*), 243800	X	X	X		[24, 41]
Lacrimo-auriculo-dento-digital syndrome/LADD (*FGFR3, -2, FGF10*), 149730	X	X	X		[24, 42]
Pycnodysostosis (*CTSK*), 265800	X				[24]
Schinzel-Giedion midface retraction syndrome (SETBP1), 269150				Macrodontia	[22, 43]

Table 11.2 Symptoms from enamel (DDE) in different ectodermal dysplasia syndromes and syndromes partly associated with ectodermal dysplasia, as reported in OMIM and literature

Diagnosis (gene), OMIM no.	Hypomineralization (qualitative defect)	Hypoplastic (quantitative defect)	Unclear/ incomplete description	Symptom based on single case report	References
Focal dermal hypoplasia or Goltz-Gorlin syndrome (PORCN), 305600	X	X			[23, 24]
Adult syndrome/ acro-dermato-ungual-lacrimal-tooth syndrome (*TP63*), 103285		X	Dysplastic teeth		[24, 44]
Tricho-dento-osseous syndrome (*DLX3*), 190320	X	X			[24, 45]
Ectodermal dysplasia-short stature syndrome (*GRHL2*), 616029		X		X	[24]
Ectodermal dysplasia-syndactyly syndrome (*PVRL4*), 613573		X			[24]
Oculo-dento-digital dysplasia (*GJA1*), 164200, 257850	X	X			[24, 46]
Keratitis-ichthyosis-deafness syndrome, AR (KIDAR), 242150	X				[24]
Cranioectodermal dysplasia, types 1–4/Sensenbrenner syndrome (*IFT43, -52,-122, -140 WDR19, -35*), 218330		X	Enamel dysplasia		[24, 47]

(continued)

Table 11.2 (continued)

Diagnosis (gene), OMIM no.	Hypomineralization (qualitative defect)	Hypoplastic (quantitative defect)	Unclear/ incomplete description	Symptom based on single case report	References
Dermatopathia pigmentosa reticularis/Naegeli syndrome (*KRT14*), 125595, 161000			Yellow discoloration, enamel defects		[24, 48]
Heimler syndrome 1 and 2 (*PEX1, PEX6*), 234580, 616617	X	X	Amelogenesis imperfecta, loss of enamel		[24]
LADD/Lacrimo-auriculo-dento-digital syndrome (*FGFR3, FGFR2 FGF10*), 149730		X			[24]
Kohlschütter-Tönz syndrome (RODGI), 226750	X	X			[24]

latest genetic classification of EDs [49], on clinical synopses in Online Mendelian Inheritance in Man (OMIM), and on literature search.

We have now described the most common oral phenotypes in EDs. For the affected individual, however, the secondary effect of congenital dental issues on **orofacial function** and **quality of life** is important to address. In one study, American and Swedish individuals with EDs reported difficulties with chewing and swallowing, dryness of the mouth, and speech. These difficulties directly relate to the abnormal development of teeth and salivary glands [50]. Another study of Norwegian patients with oligodontia, of which 75% also had clinical signs of ED, showed that the psychological burden of oligodontia is heavy, as they scored higher than healthy controls on measures on mental health-related quality of life [51]. When interviewing the same individuals, it was found that they often felt different from their peers, that the burden of dental treatment was significant, and that they missed a holistic approach from health personnel. They also reported a significant rise in self-esteem and that most of them had adopted useful coping strategies, which helped them tackle the many challenges their congenital disorder brought with it [52].

11.2 Summary

In order to get a correct dental/oral diagnosis in EDs, it is essential to include a dentist in the multiprofessional diagnostic team. In the following process of oral habilitation/rehabilitation, it is important to take the secondary effects on the individual patient's quality of life into account.

References

1. Chen J, Sun T, You Y, Lin B, Wu B, Wu J. Genome-wide identification of potential odontogenic genes involved in the dental epithelium-mesenchymal interaction during early odontogenesis. BMC Genomics. 2023;24(1):163.
2. Laugel-Haushalter V, Langer A, Marrie J, Fraulob V, Schuhbaur B, Koch-Phillips M, Dollé P, Bloch-Zupan A. From the transcription of genes involved in ectodermal dysplasias to the understanding of associated dental anomalies. Mol Syndromol. 2012;3(4):158–68.
3. Matalova E, Fleischmannova J, Sharpe PT, Tucker AS. Tooth agenesis: from molecular genetics to molecular dentistry. J Dent Res. 2008;87(7):617–23.
4. Polder BJ, Van't Hof MA, Van der Linden FP, Kuijpers-Jagtman AM. A meta-analysis of the prevalence of dental agenesis of permanent teeth. Community Dent Oral Epidemiol. 2004;32(3):217–26.
5. Rølling S, Poulsen S. Oligodontia in Danish schoolchildren. Acta Odontol Scand. 2001;59(2):111–2.
6. Nordgarden H, Jensen JL, Storhaug K. Reported prevalence of congenitally missing teeth in two Norwegian counties. Community Dent Health. 2002;19(4):258–61.
7. Bergendal B, Norderyd J, Bågesund M, Holst A. Signs and symptoms from ectodermal organs in young Swedish individuals with oligodontia. Int J Paediatr Dent. 2006;16(5):320–6.
8. Schalk-van der Weide Y, Steen WH, Bosman F. Distribution of missing teeth and tooth morphology in patients with oligodontia. ASDC J Dent Child. 1992;59(2):133–40.
9. Kieri CF, Bergendal B, Lind LK, Schmitt-Egenolf M, Stecksén-Blicks C. EDAR-induced hypohidrotic ectodermal dysplasia: a clinical study on signs and symptoms in individuals with a heterozygous c.1072C > T mutation. BMC Med Genet. 2014;16(15):57.
10. Issa YA, Kamal L, Abu Rayyan A, Dweik D, Pierce S, Lee MK, King M-C, Walsh T, Kanaan M. Mutation of KREMEN1, a modulator of Wnt signaling, is responsible for ectodermal dysplasia including oligodontia in Palestinian families. Eur J Hum Genet. 2016;24(10):1430–5.
11. Arzoo PS, Klar J, Bergendal B, Norderyd J, Dahl N. WNT10A mutations account for ¼ of population-based isolated oligodontia and show phenotypic correlations. Am J Med Genet A. 2014;164A(2):353–9.
12. Nordgarden H, Jensen JL, Storhaug K. Oligodontia is associated with extra-oral ectodermal symptoms and low whole salivary flow rates. Oral Dis. 2001;7(4):226–32.
13. Graber LW. Congenital absence of teeth: a review with emphasis on inheritance patterns. J Am Dent Assoc. 1978;96(2):226–75.
14. Kan WY, Seow WK, Holcombe T. Taurodontism in children with hypodontia and supernumerary teeth: a case control study. Pediatr Dent. 2010;32(2):134–40.
15. Dummer PM, Kingdon A, Kingdon R. Prevalence and distribution by tooth type and surface of developmental defects of dental enamel in a group of 15- to 16-year-old children in South Wales. Community Dent Health. 1990;7(4):369–77.
16. Lysell I, Magnusson B, Thilander B. Relations between the times of eruption of primary and permanent teeth. A longitudinal study. Acta Odontol Scand. 1969;27(3):271–81.

17. Helm S, Seidler B. Timing of permanent tooth emergence in Danish children. Community Dent Oral Epidemiol. 1974;2(3):122–9.
18. Lexner MO, Bardow A, Hertz JM, Almer L, Nauntofte B, Kreiborg S. Whole saliva in X-linked hypohidrotic ectodermal dysplasia. Int J Paediatr Dent. 2007;17(3):155–62.
19. Jaskoll T, Zhou Y-M, Trump G, Melnick M. Ectodysplasin receptor-mediated signaling is essential for embryonic submandibular salivary gland development. Anat Rec A Discov Mol Cell Evol Biol. 2003;271(2):322–31.
20. Nordgarden H, Johannessen S, Storhaug K, Jensen JL. Salivary gland involvement in hypohidrotic ectodermal dysplasia. Oral Dis. 1998;4(2):152–4.
21. Nordgarden H, Storhaug K, Lyngstadaas SP, Jensen JL. Salivary gland function in persons with ectodermal dysplasias. Eur J Oral Sci. 2003;111(5):371–6.
22. Mukaibo T, Munemasa T, Masaki C, Cui CY, Melvin JE. Defective NaCl reabsorption in salivary glands of Eda-Null X-LHED mice. J Dent Res. 2018;97(11):1244–51.
23. Wright JT, Puranik CP, Farrington F. Oral phenotype and variation in focal dermal hypoplasia. Am J Med Genet C Semin Med Genet. 2016;172C(1):52–8.
24. https://www.omim.org/. Accessed 4 May 2023.
25. Barbato E, Traversa A, Guarnieri R, Giovannetti A, Genovesi ML, Magliozzi MR, Paolacci S, Ciolfi A, Pizzi S, Di Giorgio R, Tartaglia M, Pizzuti A, Caputo V. Whole exome sequencing in an Italian family with isolated maxillary canine agenesis and canine eruption anomalies. Arch Oral Biol. 2018;91:96–102.
26. Bergendal B. Orodental manifestations in ectodermal dysplasia—a review. Am J Med Genet A. 2014;164A(10):2465–71.
27. Alghaith FA, Arts HH, Plourde FJ, Boswall A, Gulati P, McNeely PD, Acott PD, Wong KK, Dyack S. Increased intracranial pressure in a patient with congenital heart defect and ectodermal dysplasia (CHDED): extension of phenotype and review of literature. Am J Med Genet A. 2023;191(2):554–8.
28. Bergendal B, Norderyd J, Zhou X, Klar J, Dahl N. Abnormal primary and permanent dentitions with ectodermal symptoms predict WNT10A deficiency. BMC Med Genet. 2016;17(1):88.
29. Lévy J, Capri Y, Rachid M, Dupont C, Vermeesch JR, Devriendt K, Verloes A, Tabet AC, Bailleul-Forestier I. LEF1 haploinsufficiency causes ectodermal dysplasia. Clin Genet. 2020;97(4):595–600.
30. Chu KY, Wang YL, Chou YR, Chen JT, Wang YP, Simmer JP, Hu JC, Wang SK. Synergistic mutations of *LRP6* and *WNT10A* in familial tooth agenesis. J Pers Med. 2021;11(11):1217.
31. Wicomb GM, Stephen LX, Beighton P. Dental implications of tooth-nail dysplasia (Witkop syndrome): a report of an affected family and an approach to dental management. J Clin Pediatr Dent. 2004;28(2):107–12.
32. Whittington A, Stein S, Kenner-Bell B. Acro-dermato-ungual-lacrimal-tooth syndrome: an uncommon member of the ectodermal dysplasias. Pediatr Dermatol. 2016;33(5):e322–6.
33. Sripathomsawat W, Tanpaiboon P, Heering J, Dötsch V, Hennekam RC, Kantaputra P. Phenotypic analysis of Arg227 mutations of TP63 with emphasis on dental phenotype and micturition difficulties in EEC syndrome. Am J Med Genet A. 2011;155A(1):228–32.
34. Taşdelen E, Durmaz CD, Karabulut HG. Autosomal recessive oculodentodigital dysplasia: a case report and review of the literature. Cytogenet Genome Res. 2018;154(4):181–6.
35. Kantaputra PN, Coury SA, Tan WH. Impaired dentin mineralization, supernumerary teeth, hypoplastic mandibular condyles with long condylar necks, and a TRPS1 mutation. Arch Oral Biol. 2020;116:104735.
36. Katge FA, Rusawat BD, Shivasharan PR, Patil DP. Langer-Giedion syndrome: a rare case report. J Dent (Shiraz). 2016;17(3):238–41.
37. Awadh W, Kiukkonen A, Nieminen P, Arte S, Hurmerinta K, Rice DP. Blepharocheilodontic (BCD) syndrome: new insights on craniofacial and dental features. Am J Med Genet A. 2017;173(4):905–13.

38. Zannolli R, Mostardini R, Carpentieri ML, Gatti MG, Galluzzi P, Terrosi Vagnoli P, Giorgetti R, Calvieri S, Morgese G. Cranioectodermal dysplasia: a new patient with an inapparent, subtle phenotype. Pediatr Dermatol. 2001;18(4):332–5.
39. Tuna EB, Koruyucu M, Kürklü E, Çifter M, Gençay K, Seymen F, Tüysüz B. Oral and craniofacial manifestations of Ellis-van Creveld syndrome: case series. J Craniomaxillofac Surg. 2016;44(8):919–24.
40. Chalabreysse L, Senni F, Bruyère P, Aime B, Ollagnier C, Bozio A, Bouvagnet P. A new hypo/oligodontia syndrome: Carvajal/Naxos syndrome secondary to desmoplakin-dominant mutations. J Dent Res. 2011;90(1):58–64.
41. Daentl DL, Frías JL, Gilbert EF, Opitz JM. The Johanson-Blizzard syndrome: case report and autopsy findings. Am J Med Genet. 1979;3(2):129–35.
42. Guven Y, Rosti RO, Tuna EB, Kayserili H, Aktoren O. Orodental findings of a family with lacrimo-auriculo-dento digital (LADD) syndrome. Oral Surg Oral Med Oral Pathol Oral Radiol Endod. 2008;106(6):e33–44.
43. Cooke ME, Davidson LE, Livesey SL. Schinzel-Giedion syndrome: interesting facial and orodental features, and dental management. Int J Paediatr Dent. 2002;12(1):66–72.
44. Azzi L, Maurino V, Vinci R, Croveri F, Boggio A, Tagliabue A, Silvestre-Rangil J, Tettamanti L. ADULT syndrome: dental features of a very rare condition. J Biol Regul Homeost Agents. 2017;31(2 Suppl 1):61–5.
45. Al-Batayneh OB. Tricho-dento-osseous syndrome: diagnosis and dental management. Int J Dent. 2012;2012:514692.
46. Jensen ED. Generalised hypomineralisation of enamel in oculodentodigital dysplasia: comprehensive dental management of a case. BMJ Case Rep. 2021;14(1):e238079.
47. Hampl M, Cela P, Szabo-Rogers HL, Kunova Bosakova M, Dosedelova H, Krejci P, Buchtova M. Role of primary cilia in odontogenesis. J Dent Res. 2017;96(9):965–74.
48. Sprecher E, Itin P, Whittock NV, McGrath JA, Meyer R, DiGiovanna JJ, Bale SJ, Uitto J, Richard G. Refined mapping of Naegeli-Franceschetti-Jadassohn syndrome to a 6 cM interval on chromosome 17q11.2-q21 and investigation of candidate genes. J Invest Dermatol. 2002;119(3):692–8.
49. Peschel N, Wright JT, Koster MI, Clarke AJ, Tadini G, Fete M, Hadj-Rabia S, Sybert VP, Norderyd J, Maier-Wohlfart S, Fete TJ, Pagnan N, Visinoni AF, Schneider H. Molecular pathway-based classification of ectodermal dysplasias: first five-yearly update. Genes (Basel). 2022;13(12):2327.
50. Bergendal B, McAllister A, Stecksén-Blicks C. Orofacial dysfunctions in ectodermal dysplasias measured using the nordic orofacial test-screening protocol. Acta Odontol Scand. 2009;67(6):377–81.
51. Saltnes SS, Jensen JL, Sæves R, Nordgarden H, Geirdal AØ. Associations between ectodermal dysplasia, psychological distress and quality of life in a group of adults with oligodontia. Acta Odontol Scand. 2017;75(8):564–72.
52. Saltnes SS, Geirdal AØ, Saeves R, Jensen JL, Nordgarden H. Experiences of daily life and oral rehabilitation in oligodontia—a qualitative study. Acta Odontol Scand. 2019;77(3):197–204.

Chapter 12
Ocular Manifestation in Hypohidrotic Ectodermal Dysplasia

Michele Callea, Vito Romano, Stefano Bignotti, Stefano Pensiero, and Colin Eric Willoughby

Keywords Dry eye · Meibomian glands · Glaucoma

12.1 Introduction

The term ectodermal dysplasia (ED) is defined as a heterogeneous group of heritable, congenital, and rare disorders affecting several tissues of ectodermal origin, which are characterized by alterations in two or more ectodermal structures that involve the hair, teeth, nails, and sweat gland function, in association with malformations in other organs and systems [1, 2]. Pure ED is manifested by defects in ectodermal structures alone, while ED syndromes are defined by the combination of ectodermal defects in association with other anomalies. The overall prevalence of ED syndromes is unknown, but appears rare, with a presumed cumulative frequency of approximately 7/10,000 [1]. More than 170 clinically and/or genetically distinct EDs have been catalogued, and the mode of inheritance varies among the different disorders. The current classification of ED is based on clinical features (e.g.,

M. Callea (✉)
Pediatric Dentistry and Special Dental Care Unit, Meyer Children's Hospital IRCCS, Florence, Italy
e-mail: michele.callea@meyer.it

V. Romano · S. Bignotti
Eye Unit, ASST Spedali Civili di Brescia, Piazzale Spedali Civili, Brescia, Italy

Eye Unit, Department of Medical and Surgical Specialties, Radiological Sciences, and Public Health, University of Brescia, Brescia, Italy

S. Pensiero
Ophthalmology Unit, IRCCS Burlo Garofolo, Trieste, Italy

C. E. Willoughby
Genomic Medicine, Biomedical Sciences Research Institute, Ulster University, Coleraine, UK

G. Tadini et al. (eds.), *Multidisciplinary Approach to Ectodermal Dysplasia*,
https://doi.org/10.1007/978-3-031-75790-7_12

hypohidrotic or anhidrotic forms), although a genetic classification, which led to the identification of genes encoding the EDs, has been reviewed and widely used in clinical practice [1–4]. All reviewed genes were known to be responsible for ED considering their molecular and biological functions and supported a new approach to ED classification, integrating both molecular-genetic data and corresponding clinical findings. A clinical-genetic classification of ED was proposed, expanding it to other entities in which no causative genes have been identified based on the phenotype, and speculating on possible candidate genes suggested by associated "non-ectodermal" features [3]. Basically, two different nosological groups were proposed, each likely to result from mutations in genes with similar function, and possibly involved in the same mechanisms of regulation of development and/or pathogenesis. This classification allows a different approach to the patient affected by any form of ED using major clinical features to guide the physician to a grouping by underlying mechanisms [3].

12.2 Hypohidrotic Ectodermal Dysplasia

The most common form of ED is hypohidrotic ectodermal dysplasia (HED or Christ-Siemens-Touraine syndrome), which is characterized by hypodontia, hypotrichosis, and partial or total eccrine sweat gland deficiency. HED is a heterogeneous group of disorders and is estimated to affect at least 1 in 17,000 people worldwide [4]. The most prevalent form of HED is inherited as an X-linked recessive pattern; however, autosomal dominant and autosomal recessive forms of the disorder have been described, albeit at a much lower frequency [5].

HED is caused by mutations that affect components of a tumor necrosis factor (TNF)-like signaling pathway. Activation of this pathway is initiated by binding of the TNF-like ligand ectodysplasin (EDA) to its transmembrane receptor (EDAR). This connects to a canonical TNF signaling cascade through a dedicated adaptor protein, ultimately leading to the stimulation of NF-κB [6]. The gene responsible for X-linked HED (ED1, hypohidrotic, X-linked, OMIM 305100) is named *EDA* (ED1, OMIM 300451) and produces ectodysplasin-A, a protein that is involved in the normal development of ectodermal appendages including hair, teeth, and sweat glands. Defects in the molecular structure of ectodysplasin-A may inhibit the action of enzymes necessary for normal development of the ectoderm and/or its interaction with the underlying mesoderm. Mutations in *EDAR* (ectodysplasin-A receptor, OMIM 604095, that forms a ligand-receptor pair with ectodysplasin) and *EDARADD* (EDAR-associated death domain, OMIM 606603, that interacts with the death domain of EDAR and links the receptor to signaling pathways downstream) are known to be associated with both autosomal dominant and autosomal recessive forms of HED (ED, hypohidrotic/hair/nail type, autosomal dominant, OMIM 129490, and ED, hypohidrotic/hair/tooth type, autosomal recessive, OMIM 224900, for *EDAR*; and ED, hypohidrotic/hair/tooth type, OMIM 614940, and ED, hypohidrotic/hair/tooth type, autosomal recessive, OMIM 614941, for *EDARADD*).

Among HED, there are some ED syndromes that may manifest in association with midfacial defects, mainly cleft lip, cleft palate, or both. The most commonly recognized entities are EEC syndrome (ED, ectrodactyly, and clefting), Hay-Wells syndrome (ankyloblepharon, ED, and cleft lip/palate syndrome), and Rapp-Hodgkin syndrome, all of which are caused by mutations in the same the *TP63* gene [4].

12.3 Clinical Features

Neonates with HED can present with peeling skin, like "post-mature" babies; sweating, although present, is greatly deficient, leading to episodes of hyperthermia. More often, diagnosis is delayed until the teeth fail to erupt at the expected age (6–9 months) or the teeth that erupt are conical in shape. Patients have a peculiar facies, characterized by periorbital hyperpigmentation, depressed nasal bridge (saddle nose deformity), and appearance of the midface retrusion. They tend to have sparse scalp and body hair (hypotrichosis) that is often light-colored, brittle, and slow-growing, and absent or sparse eyebrows and eyelashes. The epidermis is xerotic, with patches of hyperkeratosis and/or eczematous. Because of eccrine gland function deficiency, they suffer from frequent respiratory tract infections and changes in nasal secretions from concretions (solidified secretions in the nasal and aural passages) in early infancy to large mucous clots [7]. Common manifestations include chronic infections such as rhinitis, pharyngitis, and otitis media, epistaxis, hearing loss, and dysphonia. As a consequence of gastroenteric gland hypoplasia, these patients suffer from dysphagia and constipation. Physical growth and psychomotor development are otherwise within normal limits. There is a typical ocular phenotype associated with HED which is discussed below.

In X-linked HED, the affected are males, but female carriers may present with mild features such as a few missing or abnormal teeth, sparse hair, and some problems with sweat gland function. Female carriers may display a Blaschkoid distribution of hypohidrosis (the lesions arranged in whorls and streaks corresponding to the lines of Blaschko, which represent pathways of epidermal cell migration and proliferation during the development of the fetus) as a result of lyonization and somatic mosaicism for the abnormal X chromosome [4].

12.4 Ocular Features

In anhidrotic/HED, ocular involvement clearly affects ectodermal structures of origin, that is, eyebrows and eyelashes, corneal epithelium, lens, and lacrimal apparatus, especially the meibomian glands that may be absent or have missing orifices and secretions (Fig. 12.1) [8]. The ocular features may range from mild to vision-threatening pathology. The typical clinical picture [9] is characterized by the reduction of eyebrows and eyelashes, recurrent inflammation of the eyelids, trichiasis,

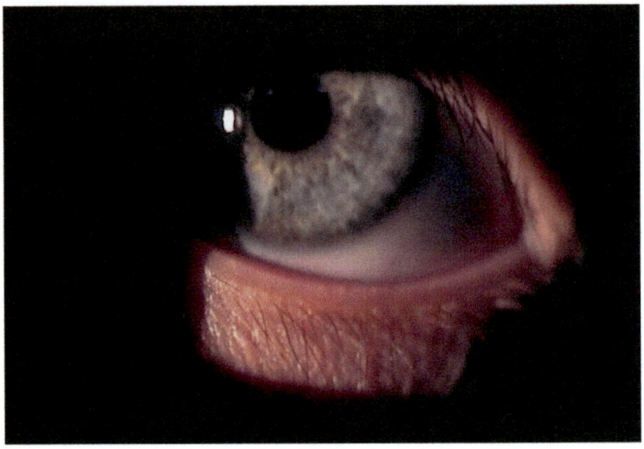

Fig. 12.1 Lid margin with the absence of meibomian gland orifices

features of dry eyes with burning, photophobia, and redness. Complications may include corneal scarring, ulcers, and perforation resulting from the combined effect of dysplasia, tear deficiency, and eye infection [4]. Chronic conjunctivitis and blepharitis and other signs of dry eye syndrome are caused by quantitative and/or qualitative alterations of the tear physiology [10].

Rarer ocular manifestations in HED are bilateral or unilateral [11] congenital cataract, chorioretinal atrophy, absence of lacrimal puncta, and atresia (or narrowing) of the nasolacrimal duct [9]. HED, characterized by a large susceptibility to infections, especially airway infections, can sometimes present serious intraocular infections, like bilateral panuveitis [12]. A case of a child with HED, confirmed by molecular diagnosis, who presented with infantile bilateral glaucoma has been reported [13, 14]. Finally, a single clinical report described a male with clinical manifestation of HED and keratoconus, a progressive eye disease that gradually causes thinning of the cornea [15].

Dry eye disease (DED) is the most common ocular problem in HED patients, present in about 30% of cases [16–18]. According to the most recent consensus, dry eye is a "multifactorial disease of the ocular surface, characterized by loss of homeostasis of the tear film and accompanied by ocular symptoms, in which an etiological role is played by instability and hyperosmolarity of the tear film, inflammation and damage to the ocular surface and neurosensory abnormalities" [19]. Since 2007, DED has been recognized as a multifactorial complex disease in which the disorder of the homeostasis of the tear film represents the basic process in its development [19]. According to the pathophysiological classification scheme of DEWS II [19], there are two predominant categories of DED: aqueous-deficient dry eye (ADDE) and evaporative dry eye (EDE) with the last one being the more common one. A fundamental mechanism in the development of DED is hyperosmolarity of tears. Hyperosmolarity leads to inflammation and damage of the ocular surface because it causes apoptosis of epithelial cells and goblet cells leading to tear film instability and increase in hyperosmolarity creating a vicious cycle [19]. Damaged epithelial cells activate the inflammatory cascade through cytokines (interleukin (IL)-1α,

IL-1β, TNF-α, and MMP-9) and MAPK and NF-κB of activated B-cell singling pathways [20]. This results in goblet cell death and disruption of the glycocalyx with loss of corneal barrier function, promoting more inflammation and creating a vicious cycle.

In HED, alteration of the meibomian glands is present in 95% of cases, with total or partial absence of the glands [16, 17] (normally allocated to the stratum fibrous, or tarsus, of the eyelid) and the orifices of the excretory channels, located in the posterior lip of the lid margin. The tear film alteration present in HED must be therefore mainly classified as meibomian gland dysfunction (MGD) [21]. MGD is often complicated by posterior blepharitis, an inflammation of the posterior lid margin, since this is primarily a disease related to the evaporation of the water content of the tears due to the lack of the lipid layer of the tear film. A reduction in aqueous secretion of lacrimal glands, evaluated using the Schirmer test and tear lysozyme measurements, has been reported in HED patients [15]. Wetting of less than 5 mm of the strip is normally considered to suggest aqueous tear deficiency. Lysozyme is a protein secreted by lacrimal glands; it is thought that its production decreases parallel the secretion of aqueous tears by the lacrimal glands [21–24]. Patients with combined lipid and aqueous tear abnormalities in HED are more likely to have severe dry eye state disease [25].

We clinically assessed 6 HED families for evidence of aqueous tear deficiency (tear meniscus <0.2 mm) and lipid abnormalities (tear break-up time (TBUT) <10 s) (Table 12.1). All affected males and carrier females (11/11 subjects) had meibomian gland anomalies with a reduction in number or complete absence. This resulted in an EDE in all cases of variable severity resulting in conjunctiva and occasionally corneal staining indicating epithelial damage. Aqueous tear deficiency was detected in 7 of 11 subjects. In the presence of meibomian gland dropout (reduced secretion of meibomian lipid) but normal aqueous production, there is an approximately threefold increase in tear evaporation rates [26], while in the presence of meibomian gland dropout and aqueous tear deficiency, the evaporation rate was increased by almost fourfold [26]. MGD increases tear electrolytes uniformly, consistent with a purely evaporative effect, while in lacrimal gland dysfunction, sodium concentration rises disproportionately [27, 28]. HED patients with combined lipid and aqueous tear abnormalities were more likely to have severe DED.

Kaercher et al. [29] evaluated eight infants, 12 boys, and 14 male adults with X-linked HED and 12 healthy control subjects to a panel of ocular tests. Meibography had 100% sensitivity and specificity for identifying X-linked HED. Infrared thermography, a completely noninvasive procedure, revealed a typical pattern for male subjects with X-linked HED, however less sensitive (86% for adults and 67% for children) than meibography or a combination of established routine tests. In adults, ocular surface disease index and noninvasive measurement of tear film break-up time were the best single routine tests (sensitivity of 86% and 71%, respectively), whereas increased tear osmolarity appeared as a rather unspecific ophthalmic symptom. In children, noninvasive measurement of tear film break-up time was the most

Table 12.1 Ocular surface of patients with HED

	Age	Disease status	Meibomian glands	TBUT (s)	TM (mm)	Tear film anomaly[a]	Conjunctival staining	Corneal PEEs	Corneal ulceration	Corneal NVs	Corneal scarring	Cataract
EDA001_1	33	CF	Reduced	4 R + L	<0.2 R + L	L, A	Nasal	–	–	–	–	+
EDA002_1	20	Affected	Reduced (2 present RUL only)	2 R + L	>0.4 R + L	L	Temporal	Central	–	Micropannus	–	+
EDA002_2	46	CF	Reduced	4 (R); 3 (L)	0.2–0.4	L	Nasal/temporal	Central	–	–	–	–
EDA002_3	51	CF	Reduced	1 R + L	<0.2	L, A	–	Inferior	–	–	–	–
EDA003	7	CF	Reduced	6 R + L	<0.2 R + L	L, A	Nasal/inferior	Inferior	–	–	–	–
EDA004	73	Affected	Reduced	7 (R);4(L)	<0.2 R + L	L, A	Interpalpebral/ inferior	Central	–	–	–	Age-related
EDA005_1	41	CF	Reduced	5 R + L	<0.2 mm	L, A	–	Inferior	–	–	–	–
EDA005_2	11	Affected	Absent	2 R + L	0.2 mm	L, A	Nasal/inferior	Inferior	–	–	–	–
EDA006_1	33	CF	Reduced	7 R + L	0.4 mm	L	–	–	–	–	–	–
EDA006_2	9	Affected	Absent	8 R + L	>0.4	Mild L	–	–	–	–	–	–
EDA006_3	44	Affected	Reduced	6 (R);8 (L)	0.2	L, A	–	–	–	–	–	–

CF carrier female
[a] Tear film anomaly: lipid defect (L), aqueous deficiency (A)

convincing routine test (sensitivity of 91%). Therefore, meibography is the most reliable ophthalmic examination to establish a clinical diagnosis in individuals with suspected HED, even before genetic test results are available. Tear film tests and ocular surface staining are very helpful for estimating the severity of ocular surface disease in individuals with known X-linked HED.

The clinical picture of HED is therefore mainly characterized by EDE, with keratitis and corneal ulcers associated with a (primitive) inability to corneal re-epithelialization [22]. Consequent corneal opacities (leukomas, pannus), which clearly increase in size and density with age, are present in approximately 19% of cases [23].

The management of corneal ulceration and subsequent scarring is challenging in HED.

Studies have shown that EDE significantly increases the production of MMP-9, MAPKs, IL-1a, IL-1b, and TNF-a, with damage to corneal epithelial barrier functions [20]. MMP-9, leading to lysis of tight junction in apical epithelium, seems to play an important role in corneal barrier disruption in dry eye [30]. Control of infection risk and inflammation caused by EDE is therefore essential in the management of HED. Supporting the ocular surface prophylactically from the time of diagnosis of HED is paramount and includes regular eyelid hygiene and installation of preservative-free tear substitutes containing lipids [31].

Here, we describe the role of drugs with immunomodulatory functions and a possible role in the management of the disease. Corticosteroids have a wide anti-inflammatory action. Dexamethasone can inhibit the synthesis of MMP-9 and the activation of MAPKs induced by IL-1b in corneal fibroblasts [32]. Similarly, methylprednisolone seems to preserve corneal epithelial barrier function because it lowers production and action of MMP-9 both in vivo and in vitro [20, 33], but it also lowers IL-1a, IL-1b, and TNF-a expression. The short-term use of topical corticosteroids is effective in modulating the inflammatory response in patients with dry eye-related sequelae with improvement in the TBUT and Schirmer test [34]. However, dosing, frequency, and duration of the treatment need further investigation.

Doxycycline is a broad-spectrum antibiotic of the tetracycline class. In ophthalmology, it is used in different pathologies like persistent epithelial defects and erosions and ocular rosacea [33, 35]. Oral doxycycline may have a role in management of HED-related ocular manifestation. In fact, results from various studies show a lowering effect on MAPK activation and on MMP-9, IL-1a, IL-1b, and TNF-a production [20, 36, 37]. Low-dose doxycycline 20 mg p.o. twice daily seems to have similar efficacy with fewer side effects compared to high-dose doxycycline (200 mg p.o. twice daily) in DED [38].

Cyclosporin-A (CsA) inhibits the calcineurin-phosphatase pathway and reduces the transcription of T-cell-activating cytokines, such as IL-4 and IL-2 (IL-2), and it also reduces the expression of proinflammatory cytokines, such as IL-1β, IL-6, TNF-α) [39]. CsA is associated with an increase in the density of conjunctival goblet cells and has immunomodulatory action [19]. CsA emulsion has been approved by FDA for the treatment of dry eye. Moreover, topical CsA is well tolerated and has a low systemic absorption rate with no critical side effects, which is essential, because long-term treatment is necessary in patients with HED syndrome [40]. No studies have reported the efficacy of topical CsA in HED.

12.5 Conclusion

HED results in ophthalmic manifestations, and the ocular features are characterized by EDE, with keratitis and corneal ulcers associated with a (primitive) inability to corneal re-epithelialization. Patients with HED require a multi-disciplinary approach, and the ophthalmologist has a role to play in preventing and treating the ocular impact of HED. Careful prophylactic treatment to protect and maintain the ocular surface is paramount to prevent sight-threatening complications. Improvements in our understanding and management options in DED can transfer into the ophthalmic care of HED, but further clinical trials are required to direct evidence-based eye care.

References

1. Mark BJ, Becker BA, Halloran DR, Bree AF, Sindwani R, Fete MD, Motil KJ, Srun SW, Fete TJ. Prevalence of atopic disorders and immunodeficiency in patients with ectodermal dysplasia syndromes. Ann Allergy Asthma Immunol. 2012;108:435–8.
2. Visinoni AF, Lisboa-Costa T, Pagnan NA, Chautard-Freire-Maia EA. Ectodermal dysplasias: clinical and molecular review. Am J Med Genet A. 2009;149A:1980–2002.
3. Priolo M, Laganà C. Ectodermal dysplasias: a new clinical-genetic classification. J Med Genet. 2001;38:579–85.
4. Tyagi P, Tyagi V, Hashim AA. Ocular and non-ocular manifestations of hypohidrotic ectodermal dysplasia. BMJ Case Rep. 2011;2011:bcr0120113731.
5. Lind LK, Stecksén-Blicks C, Lejon K, Schmitt-Egenolf M. EDAR mutation in autosomal dominant hypohidrotic ectodermal dysplasia in two Swedish families. BMC Med Genet. 2006;7:80.
6. Headon DJ. Ectodysplasin signaling in cutaneous appendage development: dose, duration, and diversity. J Invest Dermatol. 2009;129:817–9.
7. Wright JT, Grange DK, Richter MK. Hypohidrotic ectodermal dysplasia. GeneReviews.
8. Clarke A. Hypohidrotic ectodermal dysplasia. J Med Genet. 1987;24:659–63.
9. Kaercher T. Ocular symptoms and signs in patients with ectodermal dysplasia syndromes. Graefes Arch Clin Exp Ophthalmol. 2004;242:495–500.
10. Dietz J, Kaercher T, Schneider AT, Zimmermann T, Huttner K, Johnson R, Schneider H. Early respiratory and ocular involvement in X-linked hypohidrotic ectodermal dysplasia. Eur J Pediatr. 2013;172:1023–31.
11. Viljoen DL, Winship WS. A new form of hypohidrotic ectodermal dysplasia. Am J Med Genet. 1988;31:25–32.
12. Rodriguez N, Eliott D, Garcia-Valenzuela E, Baker J. Bilateral panuveitis in a child with hypohidrotic ectodermal dysplasia. Am J Ophthalmol. 2002;34:443–5.
13. Callea M, Vinciguerra A, Willoughby CE, Deroma L, Clarich G. Infantile bilateral glaucoma in a child with ectodermal dysplasia. Ophthalmic Genet. 2013;34:58–60.

14. Keklikci U, Yavuz I, Tunik S, Ulku ZB, Akdeniz S. Ophthalmic manifestations in patients with ectodermal dysplasia syndromes. Adv Clin Exp Med. 2014;23:605–10.
15. Piccione M, Serra G, Sanfilippo C, Andreucci E, Sani I, Corsello G. A new mutation in EDA gene in X-linked hypohidrotic ectodermal dysplasia associated with keratoconus. Minerva Pediatr. 2012;64:59–64.
16. Ekins MB, Waring GO 3rd. Absent meibomian glands and reduced corneal sensation in hypohidrotic ectodermal dysplasia. J Pediatr Ophthalmol Strabismus. 1981;18:44–7.
17. Ezzine Sebai N, Khaled A, Kharfi M, Bouzgarrou A, M'halla H, Jones M, Fazaa B, Kamoun MR. Anhidrotic/hypohidrotic ectodermal dysplasia: ten cases. Tunis Med. 2009;87:805–9.
18. Allali J, Roche O, Monnet D, Brezin A, Renard G, Dufier JL. Anhidrotic ectodermal dysplasia: "congenital ameibomia". J Fr Ophtalmol. 2007;30:525–8.
19. Craig JP, Nelson JD, Azar DT, Belmonte C, Bron AJ, Chauhan SK, de Paiva CS, Gomes JAP, Hammitt KM, Jones L, Nichols JJ, Nichols KK, Novack GD, Stapleton FJ, Willcox MDP, Wolffsohn JS, Sullivan DA. TFOS DEWS II report executive summary. Ocul Surf. 2017;15(4):802–12. https://doi.org/10.1016/j.jtos.2017.08.003.
20. De Paiva CS, Corrales RM, Villarreal AL, Farley WJ, Li DQ, Stern ME, Pflugfelder SC. Corticosteroid and doxycycline suppress MMP-9 and inflammatory cytokine expression, MAPK activation in the corneal epithelium in experimental dry eye. Exp Eye Res. 2006;83(3):526–35. https://doi.org/10.1016/j.exer.2006.02.004.
21. Nelson JD, Shimazaki J, Benitez-del-Castillo JM, Craig JP, McCulley JP, Den S, Foulks GN. The international workshop on meibomian gland dysfunction: report of the definition and classification subcommittee. Invest Ophthalmol Vis Sci. 2011;52:1930–7.
22. Beckerman BL. Lacrimal anomalies in anhidrotic ectodermal dysplasia. Am J Ophthalmol. 1973;75:728–30.
23. Wilson FM 2nd, Grayson M, Pieroni D. Corneal changes in ectodermal dysplasia. Case report, histopathology, and differential diagnosis. Am J Ophthalmol. 1973;75:17–27.
24. Kaercher T, Bron AJ. Classification and diagnosis of dry eye. Dev Ophthalmol. 2008;41:36–53.
25. Di Iorio E, Kaye SB, Ponzin D, Barbaro V, Ferrari S, Böhm E, Nardiello P, Castaldo G, McGrath JA, Willoughby CE. Limbal stem cell deficiency and ocular phenotype in ectrodactyly-ectodermal dysplasia-clefting syndrome caused by p63 mutations. Ophthalmology. 2012;119:74–83.
26. Mathers WD. Ocular evaporation in meibomian gland dysfunction and dry eye. Ophthalmology. 1993;100(3):347–51. https://doi.org/10.1016/s0161-6420(93)31643-x.
27. Gilbard JP, Rossi SR, Heyda KG. Tear film and ocular surface changes after closure of the meibomian gland orifices in the rabbit. Ophthalmology. 1989;96(8):1180–6. https://doi.org/10.1016/s0161-6420(89)32753-9.
28. Gilbard JP. Human tear film electrolyte concentrations in health and dry-eye disease. Int Ophthalmol Clin. 1994;34(1):27–36. https://doi.org/10.1097/00004397-199403410-00005. PMID: 8169071.
29. Kaercher T, Dietz J, Jacobi C, Berz R, Schneider H. Diagnosis of X-linked hypohidrotic ectodermal dysplasia by meibography and infrared thermography of the eye. Curr Eye Res. 2015;40:884–90.
30. Pflugfelder SC, Farley W, Luo L, Chen LZ, de Paiva CS, Olmos LC, Li DQ, Fini ME. Matrix metalloproteinase-9 knockout confers resistance to corneal epithelial barrier disruption in experimental dry eye. Am J Pathol. 2005;166(1):61–71. https://doi.org/10.1016/S0002-9440(10)62232-8.
31. Geerling G, Tauber J, Baudouin C, Goto E, Matsumoto Y, O'Brien T, Rolando M, Tsubota K, Nichols KK. The international workshop on meibomian gland dysfunction: report of the subcommittee on management and treatment of meibomian gland dysfunction. Invest Ophthalmol Vis Sci. 2011;52:2050–64.
32. Li DQ, Chen Z, Song XJ, Luo L, Pflugfelder SC. Stimulation of matrix metalloproteinases by hyperosmolarity via a JNK pathway in human corneal epithelial cells. Invest Ophthalmol Vis Sci. 2004;45:4302–11.

33. Dursun D, Kim MC, Solomon A, Pflugfelder SC. Treatment of recalcitrant recurrent corneal erosions with inhibitors of matrix metalloproteinase-9, doxycycline and corticosteroids. Am J Ophthalmol. 2001;132:8–13.
34. Prinz J, Maffulli N, Fuest M, Walter P, Bell A, Migliorini F. Efficacy of topical administration of corticosteroids for the management of dry eye disease: systematic review and meta-analysis. Life (Basel). 2022;12(11):1932.
35. Akpek EK, Merchant A, Pinar V, Foster CS. Ocular rosacea: patient characteristics and follow-up. Ophthalmology. 1997;104:1863–7.
36. Li DQ, Lokeshwar BL, Solomon A, Monroy D, Ji Z, Pflugfelder SC. Regulation of MMP-9 production by human corneal epithelial cells. Exp Eye Res. 2001;73:449–59.
37. Sobrin L, Liu Z, Monroy DC, Solomon A, Selzer MG, Lokeshwar BL, Pflugfelder SC. Regulation of MMP-9 activity in human tear fluid and corneal epithelial culture supernatant. Invest Ophthalmol Vis Sci. 2000;41:1703–9.
38. Yoo S-E, Lee D-C, Chang M-H. The effect of low-dose doxycycline therapy in chronic meibomian gland dysfunction. Korean J Ophthalmol. 2005;19(4):258–63.
39. Periman LM, Mah FS, Karpecki PM. A review of the mechanism of action of cyclosporine A: the role of cyclosporine A in dry eye disease and recent formulation developments. Clin Ophthalmol. 2020;14:4187–200.
40. Kymionis GD, Bouzoukis DI, Diakonis VF, Siganos C. Treatment of chronic dry eye: focus on cyclosporine. Clin Ophthalmol. 2008;2(4):829–36.
41. Yagi Y, Andoh A, Inatomi O, Tsujikawa T, Fujiyama Y. Inflammatory responses induced by interleukin-17 family members in human colonic subepithelial myofibroblasts. J Gastroenterol. 2007;42(9):746–53.
42. Corrales RM, de Paiva CS, Li DQ, Farley WJ, Henriksson JT, Bergmanson JPG, Pflugfelder SC. Entrapment of conjunctival goblet cells by desiccation-induced cornification. Invest Ophthalmol Vis Sci. 2011;52(6):3492–9.
43. Pflugfelder SC, Maskin SL, Anderson B, Chodosh J, Holland EJ, De Paiva CS, Bartels SP, Micuda T, Proskin HM, Vogel R. A randomized, double-masked, placebo-controlled, multicenter comparison of loteprednol etabonate ophthalmic suspension, 0.5%, and placebo for treatment of keratoconjunctivitis sicca in patients with delayed tear clearance. Am J Ophthalmol. 2004;138(3):444–57. https://doi.org/10.1016/j.ajo.2004.04.052.

Chapter 13
Otorhinolaryngologic Manifestations in Hypohidrotic Ectodermal Dysplasia

Michele Callea, Piercesare Grimaldi, and Roberto Teggi

Keywords Keratin debris · Nasal crusting · Fibroscopy

Hypohidrotic ectodermal dysplasia (HED) [1, 2] is a rare genetic disorder that affects the development of ectodermal structures such as hair, teeth, and sweat glands. The condition is caused by mutations in the EDA gene, which provides instructions for making a protein called ectodysplasin-A [3]. The absence or reduced levels of this protein can lead to various physical manifestations, including ear, nose, and throat (ENT) abnormalities [4].

The manifestations of HED [3] vary in severity and can range from mild to severe. In severe cases, individuals may experience significant ENT abnormalities that can impact their quality of life. In this chapter, we will discuss the different ENT manifestations of HED and their impact on affected individuals.

13.1 Ear Manifestations

HED can cause various ear abnormalities, including abnormal ear shape, small ear size, and a lack of ear canals. These abnormalities can result in conductive hearing loss, which occurs when sound waves cannot reach the inner ear properly [5]. Individuals with HED may also experience recurrent ear infections due to the lack of proper ear canal ventilation.

M. Callea (✉)
Pediatric Dentistry and Special Dental Care Unit, Meyer Children Hospital IRCCS, Florence, Italy
e-mail: michele.callea@meyer.it

P. Grimaldi
University of Turin, Turin, Italy

R. Teggi
San Raffaele Scientific Institute—"Vita e Salute" University, Milan, Italy

G. Tadini et al. (eds.), *Multidisciplinary Approach to Ectodermal Dysplasia*,
https://doi.org/10.1007/978-3-031-75790-7_13

Moreover, individuals with HED may have malformed or absent middle ear bones, which can further contribute to hearing loss. In severe cases, hearing loss can lead to speech and language delays, educational difficulties, and social isolation. In some cases, hearing aids or cochlear implants may be necessary to improve hearing.

13.2 Nose Manifestations

HED can also cause various nose abnormalities, including a small or underdeveloped nasal bone, a flattened nasal bridge, and narrow nasal passages. These abnormalities can cause breathing difficulties, particularly during exercise or sleep. Individuals with HED may also be more prone to recurrent sinus infections due to the narrowed nasal passages and impaired mucociliary clearance (Fig. 13.1).

In severe cases, individuals with HED may require nasal surgery to improve breathing and reduce the risk of infections. This may include nasal septoplasty to straighten the nasal septum or turbinectomy to remove the enlarged nasal turbinates.

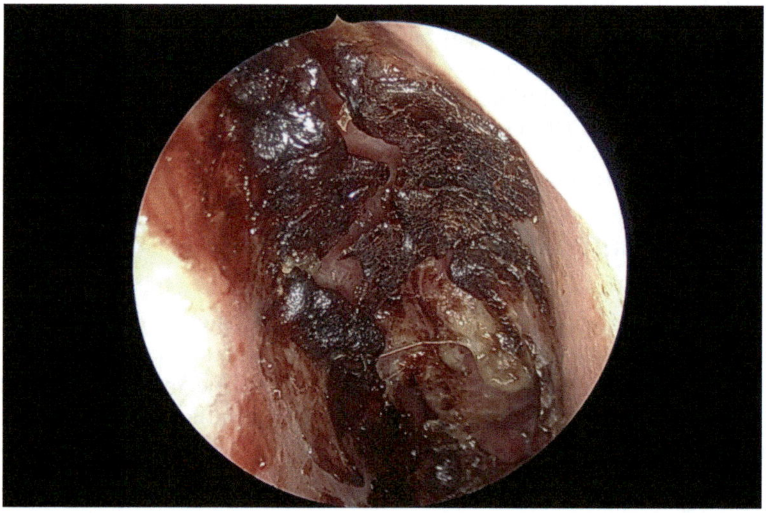

Fig. 13.1 Nasal crusting, narrowed nasal passages, and impaired mucociliary clearance

13.3 Throat Manifestations

HED can also cause various throat abnormalities, including a small jaw and a high-arched palate. These abnormalities can cause difficulty with swallowing and speaking. Individuals with HED may also be more prone to dental problems due to the lack of teeth and abnormal tooth development, which can further contribute to speech difficulties.

Moreover, individuals with HED may have reduced saliva production, which can lead to dry mouth and an increased risk of dental decay and gum disease. In severe cases, individuals may require dental implants or dentures to improve chewing, speech, and overall oral health.

In addition to the physical manifestations of HED, individuals with the condition may also experience psychosocial challenges. For instance, individuals with hearing loss may struggle with communication and social interactions, which can lead to social isolation and depression [6]. Similarly, individuals with speech difficulties may feel self-conscious and struggle to express themselves effectively, which can impact their self-esteem and overall quality of life.

Early diagnosis and appropriate management can help improve the outcomes and quality of life for individuals with HED. A multidisciplinary approach involving ENT specialists, audiologists, speech therapists, and dental professionals is necessary to provide comprehensive care for individuals with HED. For instance, hearing aids or cochlear implants may be necessary to improve hearing, while speech therapy may help improve communication skills. Similarly, dental professionals can provide preventive and restorative care to improve oral health and speech.

In conclusion, HED is a rare genetic disorder that can cause various ENT abnormalities, including ENT manifestations. These abnormalities can have a significant impact on affected individuals' quality of life, particularly their hearing, breathing, and speech. However, with appropriate care and management, individuals with HED can lead fulfilling and productive lives [7]. More research is necessary to better understand the pathophysiology of HED and develop more effective treatments to improve outcomes for affected individuals [8]. Additionally, greater awareness and education about HED can help reduce stigma and improve social support for individuals with the condition and their families.

Future research may also explore the potential for gene therapy and other innovative treatments to address the underlying genetic defects that cause HED. Gene therapy involves replacing or repairing the defective gene responsible for the condition, potentially leading to a cure. While gene therapy is still in the early stages of development, it holds promise for treating genetic disorders like HED.

In conclusion, HED is a rare genetic disorder that can cause a range of physical and psychosocial challenges, particularly in the ENT system. However, with early diagnosis and appropriate management, individuals with HED can lead fulfilling and productive lives. A multidisciplinary approach involving ENT specialists, audiologists, speech therapists, and dental professionals is necessary to provide comprehensive care for affected individuals. Further research and innovation in treatments, including gene therapy, may offer hope for a cure and improved outcomes for those with HED.

References

1. Bildik T, Ozbaran B, Kose S, Koturoglu G, Gokce B, Gunaydin A, Altintas I. Hypohidrotic ectodermal dysplasia: a multidisciplinary approach. Int J Psychiatry Med. 2012;44:225–40. https://doi.org/10.2190/PM.44.3.d.
2. Wright JT, Grange DK, Fete M. Hypohidrotic ectodermal dysplasia. In: Adam MP, Mirzaa GM, Pagon RA, Wallace SE, Bean LJ, Gripp KW, Amemiya A, editors. GeneReviews®. Seattle: University of Washington; 1993.
3. Meshram G, Kaur N, Hura K. A case report of hypohidrotic ectodermal dysplasia: a mini-review with latest updates. J Family Med Prim Care. 2018;7:264. https://doi.org/10.4103/jfmpc.jfmpc_20_17.
4. García-Martín P, Hernández-Martín A, Torrelo A. Displasias ectodérmicas: revisión clínica y molecular. Actas Dermosifiliogr. 2013;104:451–70. https://doi.org/10.1016/j.ad.2012.07.012.
5. Bagdey SP, Moharil RB, Dive A, Bodhade A. Hypohidrotic ectodermal dysplasia: a case report with review and latest updates. J Oral Maxillofac Pathol. 2022;26:S12–6. https://doi.org/10.4103/jomfp.jomfp_287_21.
6. D'Souza RN, Klein OD. Unraveling the molecular mechanisms that lead to supernumerary teeth in mice and men: current concepts and novel approaches. Cells Tissues Organs. 2007;186:60–9. https://doi.org/10.1159/000102681.
7. Bayram Y, Karaca E, Coban Akdemir Z, Yilmaz EO, Tayfun GA, Aydin H, Torun D, Bozdogan ST, Gezdirici A, Isikay S, et al. Molecular etiology of arthrogryposis in multiple families of mostly Turkish origin. J Clin Invest. 2016;126:762–78. https://doi.org/10.1172/JCI84457.
8. Clarke A. Hypohidrotic ectodermal dysplasia. J Med Genet. 1987;24:659–63. https://doi.org/10.1136/jmg.24.11.659.

Chapter 14
Broad Phenotypic Spectrum of Ectodermal Dysplasias in Childhood and Adolescence

Laura Guazzarotti

Keywords EDA1 pathway · WNT pathway · Phenotypes

Ectodermal dysplasias (EDs) represent a clinically and genetically heterogeneous group of diseases characterized by abnormal development of two or more ectodermal-derived structures such as hair, teeth, nails, and sweat and mucous glands [1–3]. The ectodermal-derived structure defects can be associated with more complex malformations of other organs and systems such as skeletal, heart, and external and internal genitalia that outline more complex syndromes [4–6]. The prevalence of the different forms of ED altogether is highly variable in literature due to the continuous expansion of description of different phenotypes.

The more common clinical-genetic form is the hypohidrotic ectodermal dysplasia (HED) due to mutations in the EDA gene, located on chromosome Xq12-13.1 (XLHED, OMIM 300451). The EDA gene encodes the tumor necrosis factor's protein ectodysplasin-A, working together with its receptor (EDAR, OMIM 604095) located on chromosome 2q11-q13 and with the EDAR-associated death domain gene (EDARADD, OMIM 606603) located on chromosome 1q42-q43, in the same signaling pathway.

The mutations of these three genes, resulting in the alteration of the same signal transduction pathway, often lead to overlapping phenotypes but with different inheritance and gender transmission [7–13].

The more severe clinical expression of ED tissues is present in XLHED where, besides the triad of major signs comprising abnormal or missing teeth (hypodontia or oligodontia), inability to sweat (anhidrosis or hypohidrosis), and sparse hair (hypotrichosis), minor ectodermal-derived tissue alterations are present in a large percentage of patients including severe skin abnormalities, nail dystrophy, allergic manifestations, recurrent respiratory infections for dryness of airways and mucous membranes, tear film, and ocular surface disturbances [14, 15]. Almost half of the XLHED young patients present with moderate-to-marked conjunctival and corneal

L. Guazzarotti (✉)
Pediatric Endocrinology Unit, University of Padova, Padova, Italy

G. Tadini et al. (eds.), *Multidisciplinary Approach to Ectodermal Dysplasia*,
https://doi.org/10.1007/978-3-031-75790-7_14

staining, severe corneal punctate epithelial erosions, filamentary keratitis, eyelid abnormalities, and a rapid tear film break-up time (TFBUT). The absence or dysfunction of meibomian glands leads to the absence in the lipid layer of the tear film resulting in a rapid tear break-up time (TBUT) and an evaporative dry eye [16]. These alterations, alone or in association with other underlying abnormalities, result in impairment of the ocular surface that generally develops during the second decade of life and require a rigorous ophthalmological follow-up to avoid more severe complications such as corneal ulceration or pannus [16]. Several clinical reports have described also rare severe eye alterations associated with EDs (subretinal fibrosis and uveitis, retinal detachment, macular dystrophy, glaucoma, and coloboma of the optic nerve) [17–20].

A decrease in or the absence of mucous glands in the pharynx, larynx, trachea, and bronchi is a common finding in XLHED patients [21], leading to the susceptibility to develop respiratory infections, and nasal and hearing problems during childhood.

Hypoplasia of mucous glands causes otologic problems ranging from impacted cerumen to complications of recurrent otitis media to hearing loss. In patients with HED, respiratory infections are present with a higher prevalence than the general pediatric population, affecting both the upper and lower respiratory tracts, due to the impairment of mucous gland secretion in the aerodigestive tract [22, 23].

Conductive hearing loss is present with higher frequency than the general pediatric population [22] probably due to the detection of endotympanic transudate or to the presence of abundant wax in the external auditory canal and the history of recurrent otitis media. Therefore, the ear, nose, and throat (ENT) follow-up is mandatory.

A high percentage of HED patients show allergic manifestations; atopic dermatitis is the most frequent with a positive skin prick test followed by rhinoconjunctivitis and asthma. Rarely may be present also food allergy. About a quarter of young patients with allergic disorders showed a plasma level of total serum IgE higher than the normal range for age. A high incidence of atopic disease in certain subsets of ED has been reported as a result of altered lipid profile in the stratum corneum [24]. It has been proposed that epidermal barrier dysfunction is a primary event in the development of allergy [25].

Several years ago, some studies have suggested substantial risk (10–50%) for delayed mental development, due to hyperthermic brain damage [26] or to a condition of chronic illness in XLHED subjects. In these studies, the neuropsychological disorders were reported by parents and not evaluated by a medical examination; moreover, both children with XLHED and autosomal HED/HED of unknown origin were considered. In one study performed by our group a decade ago in a large population of XLHED subjects ranging from 2 to 20 years, a 15% of them showed a neurodevelopmental delay such as cognitive and psychomotor delay. Psychiatric disorders like anxiety, hyperactivity, and deflection of humor were also found in 13% of patients [23].

These data, overall related to neurodevelopmental disorders, are decreasing, due to the reduction in disease diagnosis times and improvement in the quality of care, but psychiatric disorders are still described as the social anxiety disorder (SAD) and body dysmorphic disorder (BDD), highly distressing adolescent-onset disorder that may lead to social isolation, development of comorbid mental health disorders, and suicidality.

Therefore, psychological support is necessary in these young patients, especially during adolescence [27]. The WNT10A gene located on chromosome 2q35 (OMIM 606268) has been shown to be the second most common gene implicated in ED phenotypes, after EDA gene, with both autosomal dominant and recessive inheritance [28–32]. The WNT10A gene, implicated in the Wnt/beta-catenin pathway, works together with the ectodysplasin signaling pathway having a crucial role in tooth morphogenesis and in the development of other ectodermal structures, showing often milder but overlapping phenotypes of the EDA-EDAR-EDARADD gene pathway [33–35].

Two more complex phenotypes have been identified associated with recessive inheritance of WNT10A mutations, the odonto-onycho-dermal dysplasia (OODD) syndrome [28, 36, 37], and the Schopf-Schulz-Passarge syndrome (SSPS) [28, 38].

The TP63 gene, located on chromosome 3 (q28), encodes the p63 transcription factor. The p63 mRNA has been described in a variety of tissues including skin, placenta, skeletal muscle, heart, thymus, trachea, gonads, and uterus.

Different mutations of TP63 have been demonstrated to underlie very different phenotypes associated with abnormal development of ectodermal-derived structures. The previously described different syndromes are now referred to as p63-linked conditions [39] such as ectrodactyly, ED and cleft lip/palate (EEC) syndrome; ankyloblepharon-ectodermal defects-cleft lip/palate (AEC) syndrome; acro-dermato-ungual-lacrimal-tooth (ADULT) syndrome; and isolated malformations such as split hand/foot malformation (SHFM4) and isolated cleft lip or cleft palate. Morphogenetic studies performed in p63+/+ and p63−/− mice indicate a requirement for TP63 gene function in genital tract development, specifically in urorectal septation and modeling of external genitalia, as well as epithelial cell differentiation in the vagina, cervix, and urinary tract. These data explain the wide phenotypic expression of this gene deficiency.

One of the phenotypes linked to TP63 is the limb-mammary syndrome (LMS), an autosomal dominant disorder characterized by ectodermal derivative disorders, mammary and nipple anomalies, hand/foot or cleft lip/palate malformations, and urogenital abnormalities, presenting in different associations. Extremely variable and complex clinical phenotypes reflect the combination of different pathogenic mechanisms that may be associated with the different variants of the TP63 gene in the expression of the various p63 isoforms. The urogenital abnormalities present in the p63-linked condition include micropenis, hypospadias, external female genital hypoplasia, and vaginal septum that have to be evaluated in p63-deficient young subjects. Otherwise, in the presence of anomalies of the urogenital tract, the presence of ectodermal derivative anomalies has to be evaluated to reach an underlying genetic diagnosis. A few descriptions of uterus and ovary dysgenesia have been also reported [40, 41]. In the last years, TP63 mutations have been associated also with less severe nonsyndromic phenotypes with no clefting or hand/foot anomalies [42–44].

Recently, a novel variant of the TP63 gene has been segregated in a family with recurrence of a nonsyndromic limb-mammary phenotype characterized by ectodermal derivative anomalies, supernumerary nipple, and a symptomatic dysplasia of the uterine cervix [45–49].

References

1. Freire-Maia N, Cat I, Raponegaidzinski R. An ectodermal dysplasia syndrome of alopecia, onychodysplasia, hypohidrosis, hyperkeratosis, deafness and other manifestations. Hum Hered. 1977;27(2):127–33. https://doi.org/10.1159/000152861.
2. Joly-Tonetti N, Viñuelas J, Gandrillon O, Lamartine J. Differential miRNA expression profiles in proliferating or differentiated keratinocytes in response to gamma irradiation. BMC Genomics. 2013;14:184. https://doi.org/10.1186/1471-2164-14-184.
3. Visinoni AF, Lisboa-Costa T, Pagnan NA, Chautard-Freire-Maia EA. Ectodermal dysplasias: clinical and molecular review. Am J Med Genet A. 2009;149A(9):1980–2002. https://doi.org/10.1002/ajmg.a.32864.
4. Dhanrajani PJ, Jiffry AO. Management of ectodermal dysplasia: a literature review. Dent Update. 1998;25(2):73–5.
5. Pinheiro M, Freire-Maia N. Ectodermal dysplasias: a clinical classification and a causal review. Am J Med Genet. 1994;53(2):153–62. https://doi.org/10.1002/ajmg.1320530207.
6. Priolo M, Silengo M, Lerone M, Ravazzolo R. Ectodermal dysplasias: not only 'skin' deep. Clin Genet. 2000;58(6):415–30.
7. Monreal AW, Ferguson BM, Headon DJ, Street SL, Overbeek PA, Zonana J. Mutations in the human homologue of mouse dl cause autosomal recessive and dominant hypohidrotic ectodermal dysplasia. Nat Genet. 1999;22(4):366–9. https://doi.org/10.1038/11937.
8. Yan M, Wang LC, Hymowitz SG, et al. Two-amino acid molecular switch in an epithelial morphogen that regulates binding to two distinct receptors. Science. 2000;290(5491):523–7. https://doi.org/10.1126/science.290.5491.523.
9. Headon DJ, Emmal SA, Ferguson BM, et al. Gene defect in ectodermal dysplasia implicates a death domain adapter in development. Nature. 2001;414(6866):913–6. https://doi.org/10.1038/414913a.
10. Koppinen P, Pispa J, Laurikkala J, Thesleff I, Mikkola ML. Signaling and subcellular localization of the TNF receptor EDAR. Exp Cell Res. 2001;269(2):180–92. https://doi.org/10.1006/excr.2001.5331.
11. Kumar A, Eby MT, Sinha S, Jasmin A, Chaudhary PM. The ectodermal dysplasia receptor activates the nuclear factor-kappaB, JNK, and cell death pathways and binds to ectodysplasin A. J Biol Chem. 2001;276(4):2668–77. https://doi.org/10.1074/jbc.M008356200.
12. Bal E, Baala L, Cluzeau C, et al. Autosomal dominant anhidrotic ectodermal dysplasias at the EDARADD locus. Hum Mutat. 2007;28(7):703–9. https://doi.org/10.1002/humu.20500.
13. van der Hout AH, Oudesluijs GG, Venema A, et al. Mutation screening of the ectodysplasin—A receptor gene EDAR in hypohidrotic ectodermal dysplasia. Eur J Hum Genet. 2008;16(6):673–9. https://doi.org/10.1038/sj.ejhg.5202012.
14. Fan H, Ye X, Shi L, et al. Mutations in the EDA gene are responsible for X-linked hypohidrotic ectodermal dysplasia and hypodontia in Chinese kindreds. Eur J Oral Sci. 2008;116(5):412–7. https://doi.org/10.1111/j.1600-0722.2008.00555.x.
15. Keller MD, Petersen M, Ong P, et al. Hypohidrotic ectodermal dysplasia and immunodeficiency with coincident NEMO and EDA mutations. Front Immunol. 2011;2:61. https://doi.org/10.3389/fimmu.2011.00061.
16. Kaercher T. Ocular symptoms and signs in patients with ectodermal dysplasia syndromes. Graefes Arch Clin Exp Ophthalmol. 2004;242:495–500.

17. Huffman RI, Huang JJ. Subretinal fibrosis and uveitis syndrome in a patient with ectodermal dysplasia. Ocul Immunol Inflamm. 2009;17:348–50.
18. Wald KJ, Hirose T. Ectodermal dysplasia, ectrodactyly, and clefting syndrome and bilateral retinal detachment. Arch Ophthalmol. 1993;111:734.
19. Hayakawa M, Yanashima K, Kato K, Nakajima A, Yamauchi H. Association of ectodermal dysplasia, ectrodactyly and macular dystrophy: EEM syndrome (case report). Ophthalmic Paediatr Genet. 1989;10:287–92.
20. Callea M, Vinciguerra A, Willoughby CE, Deroma L, Clarich G. Infantile bilateral glaucoma in a child with ectodermal dysplasia. Ophthalmic Genet. 2013;34:58–60.
21. Clarke A, Phillips DI, Brown R, Harper PS. Clinical aspects of X linked hypohidrotic ectodermal dysplasia. Arch Dis Child. 1987;62:989–96.
22. Yildirim M, Yorgancilar E, Gun R, Topcu I. Ectodermal dysplasia: otolaryngologic evaluation of 23 cases. Ear Nose Throat J. 2012;91:28–33.
23. Guazzarotti L, Tadini G, Mancini GE, et al. Phenotypic heterogeneity and mutational spectrum in a cohort of 45 Italian males subjects with X-linked ectodermal dysplasia. Clin Genet. 2015;87:338. https://doi.org/10.1111/cge.12404.
24. Jungersted JM, Høgh JK, Hellgren LI. Ceramide profile in hypohidrotic ectodermal dysplasia. Clin Exp Dermatol. 2012;37:153–5.
25. Cork MJ, Danby SG, Vasilopoulos Y, et al. Epidermal barrier dysfunction in atopic dermatitis. J Invest Dermatol. 2009;129:1892–908.
26. Blüschke G, Nüsken KD, Schneider H. Prevalence and prevention of severe complications of hypohidrotic ectodermal dysplasia in infancy. Early Hum Dev. 2010;86(7):397–9. https://doi.org/10.1016/j.earlhumdev.2010.04.008.
27. Hammond BA, Reeve EA. A case of body dysmorphic disorder in an adolescent with hypohidrotic ectodermal dysplasia. Pediatr Dermatol. 2020;37(5):896–9. https://doi.org/10.1111/pde.14255.
28. Bohring A, Stamm T, Spaich C, et al. WNT10A mutations are a frequent cause of a broad spectrum of ectodermal dysplasias with sex-biased manifestation pattern in heterozygotes. Am J Hum Genet. 2009;85(1):97–105. https://doi.org/10.1016/j.ajhg.2009.06.001.
29. Van Geel M, Gattas M, Kesler Y, et al. Phenotypic variability associated with WNT10A nonsense mutations. Br J Dermatol. 2010;162(6):1403–6. https://doi.org/10.1111/j.1365-2133.2010.09703.x.
30. Cluzeau C, Hadj-Rabia S, Jambou M, et al. Only four genes (EDA1, EDAR, EDARADD, and WNT10A) account for 90% of hypohidrotic/anhidrotic ectodermal dysplasia cases. Hum Mutat. 2011;32(1):70–2. https://doi.org/10.1002/humu.21384.
31. Plaisancié J, Bailleul-Forestier I, Gaston V, et al. Mutations in WNT10A are frequently involved in oligodontia associated with minor signs of ectodermal dysplasia. Am J Med Genet A. 2013;161A(4):671–8. https://doi.org/10.1002/ajmg.a.35747.
32. Nagy N, Wedgeworth E, Hamada T, White JM, Hashimoto T, McGrath JA. Schöpf-Schulz-Passarge syndrome resulting from a homozygous nonsense mutation in WNT10A. J Dermatol Sci. 2010;58(3):220–2. https://doi.org/10.1016/j.jdermsci.2010.03.012.
33. Guazzarotti L, Tadini G, Mancini GE, et al. WNT10A gene is the second molecular candidate in a cohort of young Italian subjects with ectodermal derivative impairment (EDI). Clin Genet. 2018;93(3):693–8. https://doi.org/10.1111/cge.13147.
34. Cluzeau C, Marrakchi S, Picard C, Munnich A, Smahi A, Turki H. First homozygous large deletion in EDARADD gene associated with a severe form of anhidrotic ectodermal dysplasia. J Eur Acad Dermatol Venereol. 2019;33(2):e55–7. https://doi.org/10.1111/jdv.15182.
35. Plaisancié J, Ragge NK, Dollfus H, et al. FOXE3 mutations: genotype-phenotype correlations. Clin Genet. 2018;93(4):837–45. https://doi.org/10.1111/cge.13177.
36. Adaimy L, Chouery E, Megarbane H, et al. Mutation in WNT10A is associated with an autosomal recessive ectodermal dysplasia: the odonto-onycho-dermal dysplasia. Am J Hum Genet. 2007;81(4):821–8. https://doi.org/10.1086/520064.

37. Nawaz S, Klar J, Wajid M, et al. WNT10A missense mutation associated with a complete odonto-onycho-dermal dysplasia syndrome. Eur J Hum Genet. 2009;17(12):1600–5. https://doi.org/10.1038/ejhg.2009.81.
38. Tziotzios C, Petrof G, Liu L, et al. Clinical features and WNT10A mutations in seven unrelated cases of Schöpf-Schulz-Passarge syndrome. Br J Dermatol. 2014;171(5):1211–4. https://doi.org/10.1111/bjd.13158.
39. Rinne T, Brunner HG, van Bokhoven H. p63-associated disorders. Cell Cycle. 2007;6(3):262–8. https://doi.org/10.4161/cc.6.3.3796.
40. Guazzarotti L, Caprio C, Rinne TK, et al. Limb-mammary syndrome (LMS) associated with internal female genitalia dysgenesia: a new genotype/phenotype correlation? Am J Med Genet A. 2008;146A(15):2001–4. https://doi.org/10.1002/ajmg.a.32371.
41. Ergin H, Semerci CN, Karakuş YT, et al. The EEC syndrome and SHFM: report of two cases and mutation analysis of p63 gene. Turk J Pediatr. 2010;52(5):529–33.
42. Alves LU, Pardono E, Otto PA, Mingroni Netto RC. A novel c.1037C>G (p.Ala346Gly) mutation in TP63 as cause of the ectrodactyly-ectodermal dysplasia and cleft lip/palate (EEC) syndrome. Genet Mol Biol. 2015;38(1):37–41. https://doi.org/10.1590/S1415-4757381201401.
43. Tajir M, Lyahyai J, Guaoua S, El Alloussi M, Sefiani A. Ankyloblepharon-ectodermal defects-cleft lip-palate syndrome due to a novel missense mutation in the SAM domain of the TP63 gene. Balkan J Med Genet. 2020;23(1):95–8. https://doi.org/10.2478/bjmg-2020-0013.
44. Gonzalez F, Loidi L, Abalo-Lojo JM. Novel variant in the TP63 gene associated to ankyloblepharon-ectodermal dysplasia-cleft lip/palate (AEC) syndrome. Ophthalmic Genet. 2017;38(3):277–80. https://doi.org/10.1080/13816810.2016.1210649.
45. Soares E, Zhou H. Master regulatory role of p63 in epidermal development and disease. Cell Mol Life Sci. 2018;75(7):1179–90. https://doi.org/10.1007/s00018-017-2701-z.
46. Maillard A, Alby C, Gabison E, et al. P63-related disorders: dermatological characteristics in 22 patients. Exp Dermatol. 2019;28(10):1190–5. https://doi.org/10.1111/exd.14045.
47. Rinne T, Clements SE, Lamme E, et al. A novel translation re-initiation mechanism for the p63 gene revealed by amino-terminal truncating mutations in Rapp-Hodgkin/Hay-Wells-like syndromes. Hum Mol Genet. 2008;17(13):1968–77. https://doi.org/10.1093/hmg/ddn094.
48. Cunha GR, Robboy SJ, Kurita T, et al. Development of the human female reproductive tract. Differentiation. 2018;103:46–65. https://doi.org/10.1016/j.diff.2018.09.001.
49. Kurita T, Mills AA, Cunha GR. Roles of p63 in the diethylstilbestrol-induced cervicovaginal adenosis. Development. 2004;131(7):1639–49. https://doi.org/10.1242/dev.01038.

Chapter 15
ED Practical Management

Gianluca Tadini and Michela Brena

Keywords Heat intolerance · Devices · Prosthesis

15.1 Socio-political Issues

Relevance of the recognition for ectodermal dysplasia's (ED) patients, families, and Associations from the health services and the assignment to ED for the status of "rare disease" are mandatory. This socio-political recognition is noteworthy for specific "therapeutic plans," devoted to assure to ED patients medical therapies and devices (i.e., health service gratuity for dental therapies and prosthesis, air conditioning…) and surgery when needed.

15.2 Registries

With the same intent, the creation of epidemiological registries is mandatory. Health services require the number of patients for each subgroup of ED in order to plan strategies and expenses. To our knowledge, few countries have a specific registry of patients. It shall be very important in the future that centers for care, patients, and their families, and associations could cooperate in order to know the effective number of affected ED patients for each country.

G. Tadini · M. Brena (✉)
Pediatric Dermatology Unit, Department of Clinical Sciences and Community Health, Fondazione IRCCS Ca' Granda Ospedale Maggiore Policlinico, Milan, Italy

Center for Inherited Cutaneous Diseases, University of Milan, Milan, Italy
e-mail: gtadinicmce@unimi.it; michela.brena@policlinico.mi.it

G. Tadini et al. (eds.), *Multidisciplinary Approach to Ectodermal Dysplasia*,
https://doi.org/10.1007/978-3-031-75790-7_15

15.3 Medical Centers

A list of selected centers for care for ED should be available. Due to the fact that ED requires a multidisciplinary approach, the selected centers must offer a complete multidisciplinary staff.

Specialists for ED are the following:

Neonatal Care Unit and Pediatricians

Dermatologist

Odontostomatologist

Medical Geneticist

Ophthalmologist

Orthopedics

General Surgeon

Neurologist, Psychologist

Radiologist, Echotomographist

Selected centers may be centralized in major hospitals to assure complete staff for the diagnosis, neonatal care, and follow-up.

15.4 Prenatal Diagnosis

During the last decade, the molecular pathogenesis is available for almost all the different subtypes of ED and prenatal diagnosis in family at risk for severe forms is performed in respect of the current laws present in each country, with substantial differences [1]. Geneticists may offer the evaluation and coordinate the procedures (usually with chorionic villus examination at the 10–11th week of gestation).

15.5 Diagnosis and Skin Management

For EDA1 families with molecular established diagnosis, specific molecular therapies are available during pregnancy.

Echotomographists are able to establish diagnosis of EDA1- and WNT-related ED by looking, that is, for alveolar bones and the formations of dental buds or of p63-related ED by looking for malformation of hands and feet in the first trimester of gestation.

A multidisciplinary approach of specific age-related or organ-related disorders.

Many ED patients, especially when affected from EDA1 pathway ED, present at birth with a collodion-baby-like presentation with a pattern similar to late gestation skin that may be hyperkeratotic, configuring a differential diagnosis with patients suffering from ichthyosis.

Usually, the peculiar "facies" and absence of appendages facilitate the recognition. This phenotype requires attention to avoid the risk of infection and sepsis.

During late spring and summer, ED patients may present at birth with high temperatures and a higher risk of heat intolerance that may be recognized and urgently treated. Similar febrile episodes, even less severe, are visible also during fall and winter. Assessment for febrile episodes starts from the exclusion of infections and sepsis. Untreatable and non-infectious-related episodes of fever in a neonate with skin disorders and characteristic facies lead to the diagnosis of heat intolerance related to EDs. These heat intolerance episodes may be present in all subtypes of ED, even though they are the hallmark of EDA1 pathway-related subtypes, and less frequently in other pathway-related phenotypes (WNT- and p63- and TSPEAR-related ED). During infancy and adulthood, heat intolerance episodes rarely cause febrile convulsions. Cold bath or shower is the first aid treatment. If needed, these episodes may be managed with hospitalization.

Once the diagnosis is established, the neonatologist modulates temperature and humidity of the neonatological devices in order to avoid overheating. Multidisciplinary approach is required since birth.

Specifically for p63-related ED, an ophthalmologist is required to correct ankyloblepharon when needed and orthopedics may be involved to assure correct the diagnosis of split hand and foot malformations. Maxillofacial surgeons and odontostomatologists establish precocious diagnosis and treatment for lips and palate malformations.

Some patients with p63 molecular defects present at birth with large and dramatic loss of substance in the midline skin all over the body. They must be treated early to avoid infections with advanced polyurethane medications or withcord blood-derived platelet gel or with PRIMA-1/APR246 DNA correction approach.

In early infancy and childhood especially for EDA1-related phenotypes, a clinical picture with generalized xerosis and atopic dermatitis is frequently visible. In many cases, orbital involvement may lead to a severe atopic-like pigmentation of the orbital areas that is highly characteristic of the EDA1 pathway-related ED. For that, atopic-like dermatitis is frequently needed to alternate therapies (low potency topical steroids and calcineurin inhibitors) and emollients that must be carefully chosen: creams and emulsions are preferable. Ointments may contribute to accelerate heat intolerance for their occlusive properties when large body sites are treated. Topical therapies must be tailored, and often, different body sites may require different emollients. Urea preparations are needed when hyperkeratosis is present, especially in friction areas of arms and legs. Atopic signs may persist throughout life: severe cases are rare, but on the contrary, they require upgrade of therapies with antihistaminic and steroids per os. Refractory patients may be treated with dupilumab and JAK-inhibitors like tofacitinib [2].

Onychodystrophy is usually not severe and limited to koilonychia in the majority of EDA1-related ED patients, and treatments are not requested. For the p63 subset, some patients need urea preparations to modulate thickness. Surgical treatment and

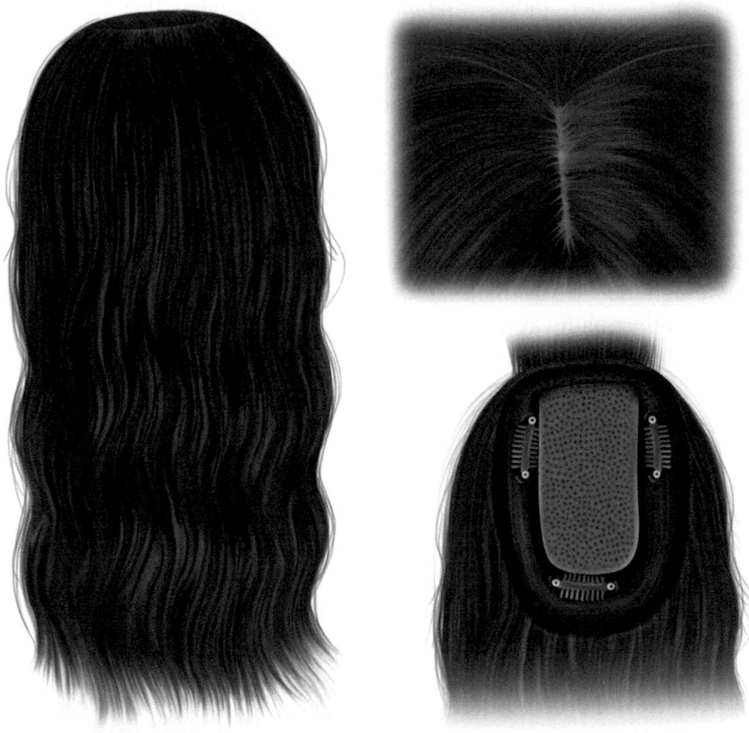

Fig. 15.1 Wigs preferred by female patients

nail substitutions are anecdotal. Sulfur-rich amino acids are useful in case of nail fragility.

EDA1 female carriers at birth may present with severe heat intolerance, dry skin, and dull sparse hair. Recognition of female carriers requires careful skin inspection in order to detect mosaicism. This pattern is not obvious to recognize and is characterized by alternate streaks of presence and absence of skin appendages distributed along Blaschko's lines, especially visible on the back and buttocks. The same pattern of mosaicism is visible also in true mosaic males with postzygotic mutations in the genes of the EDA1 pathway.

Hair distribution is highly perturbed in most cases of ED and is not confined to EDA1 pathway patients. Hypotrichosis and hypotrophy and the absence of eyelashes and eyebrows may lead to major discomfort since scholar age and in youngsters and adults, and require, especially in females, psychological support. Many young female patients and adults claim prosthesis that may diminish aesthetic disturbances. Wigs is the choice in about a third of female patients (Fig. 15.1). At this level, we recommend to pay attention to the materials and especially to the

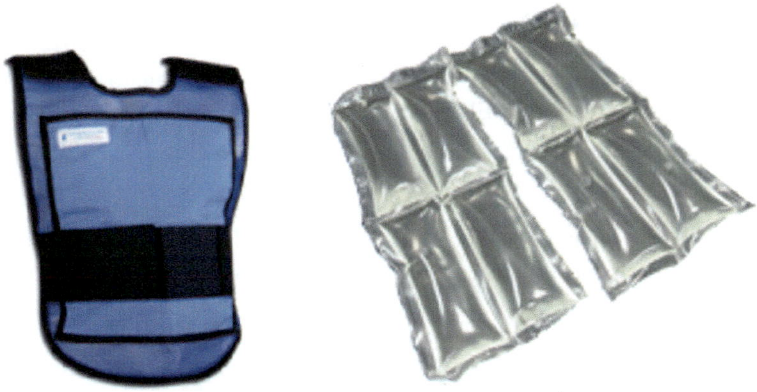

Fig. 15.2 Example of medical cooling vest (Courtesy of Elite Medical Distributors LTD, 2024, All Rights Reserved)

"interface" skin prosthesis to avoid irritation. Glues and other similar substances must be avoided. Young and adult males may suffer discomfort in beard distribution patterns.

For young and adults, heat intolerance for all ED subtypes is a major item: since childhood, facilities to avoid overheating are mandatory for hot climates and seasons. Air conditioning must be assured at home, school, and transportation, and in adult age, the same facilities must be present during job. Sometimes, guidance for employment and specific choice of duties and/or of special schedules are adopted to decrease the risk of heat intolerance episodes at work. Special clothing is available also to decrease discomfort during job hours (Fig. 15.2). Same devices are useful for recreation and sport. These clothes are conceived to have normal-appearing external pattern, but they hide internally a cavity that could be refrigerated and inserted into the fabric cloth, assuring modulations of temperature along sport or job efforts.

For all ED patients, sun protection is mandatory in order to avoid the risk of development of precancerous lesions.

15.6 Management of Internal Organs Disorders

There is an increased risk for atopy and allergies, due to the different permeability of skin and other epithelia, in particular for aerial allergens and dust, but severe involvement is very rare, and standard therapies are usually enough to cope with these hypersensibility problems. Seasonal worsening may be treated with antihistaminic drugs. Steroids and bronchodilatation drugs are rarely necessary. Minor concerns are for xerostomia and poor nasal mucus secretion that may lead to acute and chronic rhinitis. Test for diagnosis of specific allergies may help to find specific hypersensitivity and to target vaccination approach.

There is a controversial report in the literature with regard to a suspected increased risk for infection in ED patients. In our cohort of 300 patients followed during a period of 40 years, we did not find any report for high sensibility to bacterial infections. ED patients may undergo vaccination plans without any risk since early infancy.

Stipsis is due to a paucity of secretory intestinal cells that are ectodermal derivatives and may be managed easily with standard therapy including an appropriate diet regimen.

Some pubertal disorders are reported, usually dealing with delayed puberty in females. In a small subset of p63-related ED, major developmental defects of internal genitalia are reported. In these ED subsets, pelvic echotomography is suggested for early diagnosis.

In our experience, pregnancy and delivery are uneventful in ED patients. Nevertheless, mammary glands and nipples may be hypotrophic or even absent, leading to obvious problems for breast-feeding. Mammary and nipple defects are source of self-esteem and social disturbances. Rarely, plastic surgery approach may be helpful to solve these impasses with nipple reconstruction and mammary prosthesis.

Concerning the p63 subset of ED, orthopedic and plastic surgery corrections of major defects of development of hand and foot osseous rays may be requested in order to avoid practical problems of touch and prension and of standing, walking, and performances for foot defects.

Nectin-related ED during early infancy is suggested to remove skin membranes that create pseudosyndactyly allowing normal prension that is very important in the first years of life.

In p63 and Nectin ED, defects of lips and palate must be corrected early to assure normal feeding. This approach is prepared by radiological studies, and the cooperation of odontostomatologists, plastic surgeons, and maxillofacial surgeons is required.

References

1. Peschel N, Wright JT, Koster MI, et al. Molecular pathway-based classification of ectodermal dysplasias: first five-yearly update. Genes (Basel). 2022;13(12):2327. https://doi.org/10.3390/genes13122327.
2. Li X, Wu X, Elston DM, Zhang J, Zhou C. Hypohidrotic ectodermal dysplasia with c.28delG mutation in ectodysplasin A gene and severe atopic dermatitis treated successfully with tofacitinib. Acta Derm Venereol. 2021;101(1):adv00352. https://doi.org/10.2340/00015555-3693.

Chapter 16
Molecular Therapies

Holm Schneider and Pascal Schneider

Keywords Molecular therapy · Ectodysplasin A · Neonatal Fc receptor · p63 PRIMA-1^{MET}

16.1 Introduction

Recent advances in translational research linked to molecular genetic findings have increased the therapeutic opportunities for a number of ectodermal dysplasias. Most genes known to regulate the position, shape, or number of structures derived from the embryonic ectoderm play crucial roles in the mediation of cell communication, which is generally considered the most important mechanism driving embryonic development [1]. Integration of genomics has been instrumental in explaining complex sequential interactions between epithelium and mesenchyme that direct ectodermal differentiation. This is reflected by the new classification system for ectodermal dysplasias based on the molecular pathways rather than just the anatomical structures affected (see Chap. 2). It also stimulated extensive studies on the prenatal development of vertebrates that have led to a more comprehensive understanding of the interplay between the many genes involved and the developmental windows during which their expression is required. Timely replacement of a missing signaling molecule thus appeared to be a promising therapeutic strategy.

In X-linked hypohidrotic ectodermal dysplasia (XLHED), the genetic deficiency of ectodysplasin A1 (EDA1) may even be overcome before birth by administration

H. Schneider (✉)
Department of Pediatrics & Center for Ectodermal Dysplasias,
University of Erlangen-Nürnberg, Erlangen, Germany
e-mail: Holm.Schneider@uk-erlangen.de

P. Schneider
Department of Immunobiology, University of Lausanne, Lausanne, Switzerland
e-mail: pascal.schneider@unil.ch

G. Tadini et al. (eds.), *Multidisciplinary Approach to Ectodermal Dysplasia*,
https://doi.org/10.1007/978-3-031-75790-7_16

of a recombinant protein. This has been shown at least for the key problem of male subjects with XLHED, the nearly complete absence of sweat glands and perspiration that can lead to life-threatening hyperthermia. Prenatal treatment of six affected boys by injection of an EDA1 replacement protein into the amniotic fluid consistently induced the development of functional sweat glands [2, 3]. Normal ability to perspire has already persisted for 8 years in the two oldest subjects, and the absence of circulating EDA1 proved that these children would have been unable to perspire if they had been left untreated [3]. The novel approach is currently being evaluated in a worldwide clinical study, which constitutes the first attempt to investigate a pharmacotherapy of genetic disease in patients in utero. If successful, knowledge transfer to the treatment of other congenital disorders will be facilitated.

For ectodermal dysplasias caused by pathogenic variants of the gene *TP63* (encoding the transcription factor p63), the typical skin and corneal lesions may be amenable to cell therapy using genetically corrected autologous stem cells. Last but not least, small molecule drugs are being increasingly used to improve wound healing, the outcome of prosthodontic treatment, the longevity of dental implants, the results of cleft lip and cleft palate surgery, or ocular surface regeneration. Similar small molecule therapies might also be developed for the treatment of other manifestations of ectodermal dysplasias.

16.2 EDA1 Replacement Therapy

Most male patients hemizygous for pathogenic variants of the ectodysplasin A (*EDA*) gene carry null mutations of the signaling protein EDA1. The congenital absence of sweat glands [4] causes their main clinical problem. Sweating is essential for human thermoregulation, especially during outdoor activities on sunny days, during febrile infections, or in hot environments. Although infants with XLHED are at the highest risk of hyperthermia [5], the inability to sweat remains dangerous throughout life (Hammersen et al. 2011*). Notably, another cardinal symptom, oligodontia, allows noninvasive prenatal diagnosis as early as 5 months before birth by tooth bud counting during a routine fetal ultrasound scan [6, 7].

In mice affected by XLHED, treatment with a recombinant protein resembling the defective EDA1 molecule was investigated already in 2002; it was effective, but administration proved to be time-critical [8]. This recombinant protein, Fc-EDA, combined the receptor-binding domain of EDA1 and the Fc domain of human immunoglobulin G1 (IgG1). After further animal studies, Fc-EDA was evaluated first in a Phase I clinical trial in adults with XLHED who received 5 doses of the drug intravenously (ClinicalTrials.gov identifier: NCT01564225). No relevant side effects, except for the formation of antidrug antibodies, were observed [9]. In 2013, a clinical trial in newborn males with XLHED was initiated, which showed Fc-EDA to be safe but ineffective. No sweat ducts could be detected after postnatal dosing, and the subjects were unable to perspire. We reasoned that if there was any chance of success in human patients, we would need to administer the drug within the natural time window of sweat gland formation.

In humans, the development of eccrine sweat glands normally occurs in utero. Glandular structures begin to form in palmoplantar skin and a bit later (around gestational week 20) across the rest of the body with the formation of a placode in the epidermis. This placode soon undergoes solid cylindrical downgrowth into the mesenchyme. Once long enough a lumen develops, the duct end begins to coil and becomes surrounded by myoepithelial cells. At 30 weeks of gestation, most sweat glands have already completed the critical portion of development but still lack sympathetic innervation [10]. Thus, in order to rescue sweat gland formation, minimally invasive delivery of Fc-EDA at the end of the second trimester of pregnancy (Fig. 16.1a and b) appeared to be the most reasonable and, considering the procedural risks to the fetus, also the safest approach.

Important is that the Fc component of our replacement protein enables a new drug delivery method using the neonatal Fc receptor (FcRn). In mammals, including human babies, FcRn is situated in small bowel epithelia and mediates the uptake of maternal antibodies from breast milk. It binds the Fc portion of such antibodies and transports them across the intestinal epithelium into the baby's blood [11]. FcRn-mediated transcytosis (Fig. 16.1c) is already operational in the fetus in the third trimester of pregnancy when a fetus regularly swallows amniotic fluid. In Tabby mice, a naturally occurring animal model of XLHED, prenatal administration of

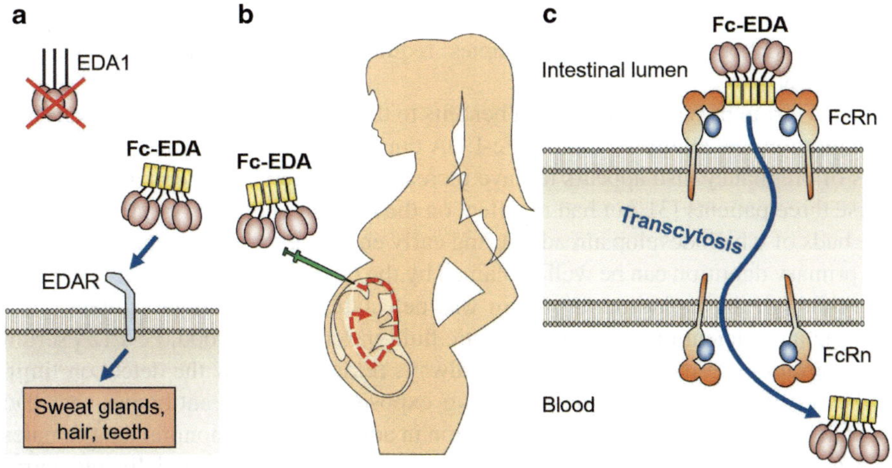

Fig. 16.1 Protein replacement therapy for X-linked hypohidrotic ectodermal dysplasia. (**a**) Genetic deficiency of ectodysplasin A1 (EDA1) can be at least partially corrected by administration of Fc-EDA, a recombinant protein containing the receptor-binding domain of EDA1 fused to the Fc portion of IgG1, which is used for timely stimulation of the intact EDA receptor (EDAR) in patients with XLHED to initiate the development of skin appendages and teeth. (**b**) Fc-EDA is delivered to an affected fetus by injection into the amniotic fluid and is taken up by fetal swallowing. (**c**) It hijacks the neonatal Fc receptor (FcRn) in the intestine to enter the fetal circulation

Fc-EDA into the amniotic cavity of affected embryos was shown to prevent the disease completely [12]. This treatment only corrected the development of hair, teeth, and sweat glands in the presence of intact FcRn, proving that the therapeutic route of the drug is systemic rather than through a direct effect on the skin and oral epithelia [2]. In dogs with XLHED, minimally invasive delivery of Fc-EDA into the amniotic fluid also rescued the formation of skin appendages and teeth [13].

The first prenatal treatments of affected humans (on a named-patient basis) took place in 2016. Monochorionic, diamniotic twins carrying an *EDA* mutation that results in an insoluble EDA1 protein with complete loss of function were treated by repeated injection of Fc-EDA into the amniotic cavities at gestational weeks 26 and 31 [2]. Postnatally, the most impressive finding was the normal sweat duct density on the soles of the feet, while we did not observe any sweat ducts in the untreated older brother. The twins' ability to perspire, quantified by measuring pilocarpine-induced sweat production, also proved to be normal. To date, pilocarpine-induced sweating has remained at roughly the same level and no hyperthermic episodes or XLHED-related hospitalizations have occurred. There are good reasons to assume that once sweat glands are normally formed they will work permanently.

Half a year later, we treated another affected boy who received, however, only one dose of Fc-EDA in utero at gestational week 26. This boy developed slightly fewer sweat glands and produced less sweat than the treated twins, suggesting an advantage of repeated dosing [2]. The drug product administered intra-amniotically represents a first-in-class protein replacement molecule that acts as a substitute for the missing EDA1 in unborn patients. This is the first use of drug therapy to trigger a developmental step that then corrects—at least partially—a developmental genetic disorder. Other protein-based therapies require prolonged, and often lifelong, application.

Apart from providing significant benefits to the development of sweat glands and perspiration, the administration of Fc-EDA during the late second and third trimesters of pregnancy also appears to have increased the number of permanent teeth in these three patients [3], but had no effect on the number and shape of primary teeth, the buds of which develop already during early embryogenesis. The missing impact on primary dentition can be well explained by the timing of treatment with Fc-EDA.

Although the replacement protein was detectable in cord blood samples, confirming an efficient uptake from amniotic fluid into the fetal blood, Fc-EDA serum concentrations in the pregnant women always remained below the detection limit, indicating minimal if any maternal drug exposure. Antidrug antibodies that had been found after intravenous administration in adult males and nonpregnant females did not appear to be elicited in the mother when Fc-EDA was delivered intra-amniotically [9].

Transillumination of the treated infants' eyelids revealed a larger number of meibomian glands than usually present in subjects with XLHED [2]. In all three treated boys, we observed increased, basically normal saliva production. Thus, the prenatal therapy does not only rescue sweat gland development but also seem to have an impact on the function of other eccrine glands. This became even more evident when patients who had been treated as neonates or prenatally at our center were compared at the age of 5 years: The first group showed the classical symptoms of XLHED, including oligodontia, anhidrosis, hyperthermic episodes, dry eyes, frequent nosebleeds, airway infections, lack of saliva, a hoarse voice, and dry skin. Patients treated prenatally, in contrast, have so far experienced neither hyperthermic episodes during the summer nor any significant eye, nose, airway, or throat issues. The twins are now 7 years old and very active also during the summer, and efficient thermal sweating could be documented by infrared thermography when having a sauna with their parents [3].

Three more affected fetuses received Fc-EDA on a named-patient basis repeatedly between gestational weeks 25 and 31 and are now able to sweat as efficiently as the infants treated before. A pivotal, genotype-controlled, multicenter clinical trial of fetal therapy that could lead to an approval of the new drug (ClinicalTrials.gov identifier: NCT04980638) is now recruiting patients: The efficacy and safety of Fc-EDA as a prenatal pharmacotherapy for male subjects with XLHED is being investigated, benefitting from the PRIME scheme of the European Medicines Agency and breakthrough therapy designation by the FDA. In this study, fetuses are treated with up to three injections of Fc-EDA, trying to confirm the clinical improvements observed in the first 6 boys treated in utero. The efficacy endpoints at the age of 6 months will be compared to data from untreated affected relatives [14].

Thus, drug targeting via FcRn appears to be a promising way to cure a so far immedicable genetic deficiency: the life-threatening inability to sweat associated with XLHED. The same drug delivery route might also be usable for the treatment of other disorders of early development.

16.3 Treatment of Cutaneous and Ocular Lesions Resulting from p63 Deficiency

Translational research has also been paving the way to more effective regenerative therapies for the typical tissue defects observed in patients with ankyloblepharon-ectodermal dysplasia-cleft lip/palate (AEC) syndrome and ectrodactyly-ectodermal dysplasia-cleft lip/palate (EEC) syndrome. In children affected by AEC syndrome, treatment of chronic skin erosions based on the expansion and grafting of genetically corrected autologous keratinocytes might be feasible and has been discussed [15]. This may involve the generation of patient-specific induced pluripotent stem cells, correction of the disease-causing *TP63* mutation with genome editing techniques, subsequent differentiation of corrected stem cells into keratinocytes, and production of keratinocyte sheets to be transplanted onto the chronic wound, a technically very challenging and time-consuming approach. Alternatively, such keratinocyte sheets could also be produced from patient-derived epidermal stem cells defined by their expression of p63 (reviewed in [16]), as shown recently by the successful regeneration of almost an entire, fully functional epidermis on a child with severe junctional epidermolysis bullosa [17, 18] (Fig. 16.2a). In this respect, the CRISPR/Cas genome editing system may hold a lot of promise. Novel engineered CRISPR-associated endonucleases allow for much higher specificity and fewer off-target effects than previous systems, which have improved gene editing for autosomal dominant diseases that cannot be tackled by alternative allele-specific gene therapy [20].

Furthermore, the small molecule drug PRIMA-1^{MET}, a p53 reactivator that has been tested in clinical trials for the treatment of malignant neoplastic disease, was shown to rescue epidermal differentiation and to improve wound healing in two patients with AEC syndrome when applied topically to affected regions of the skin

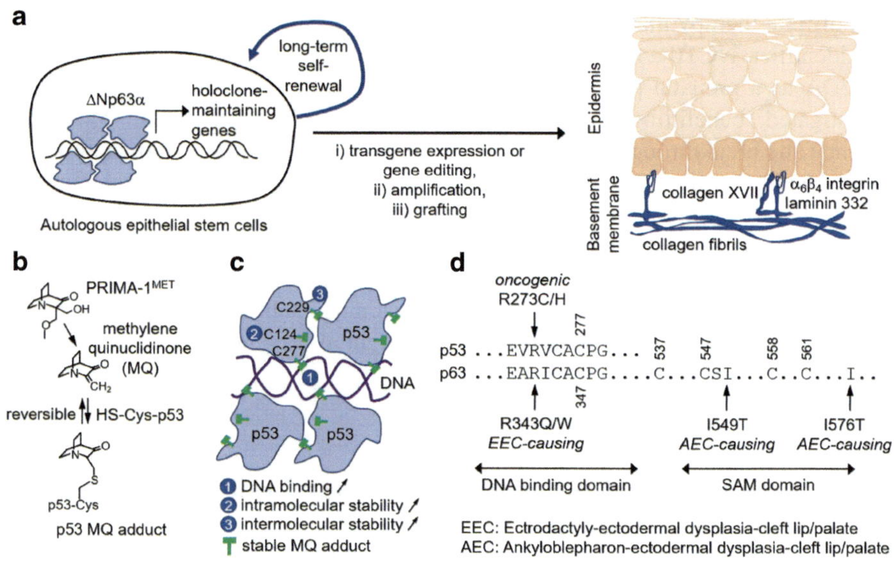

Fig. 16.2 Epithelial stem cell therapy of skin disorders and putative mechanism of action of p53 reactivator PRIMA-1^{MET}. (**a**) Epithelial stem cells capable of long-term self-renewal form holoclones in culture that are characterized by high-level expression of the transcription factor ΔNp63α. The introduction of a corrective transgene in such stem cells, followed by amplification and grafting of epithelial sheets onto skin wounds, corrected the epidermis-anchoring defect in a patient with junctional epidermolysis bullosa (who was lacking the beta-chain of the anchoring protein laminin 332). (**b**) The molecule PRIMA-1^{MET} is the precursor of methylene quinuclidinone (MQ) that can reactivate oncogenic mutants of the transcription factor p53 by forming reversible adducts on free cysteine residues. (**c**) Crystal structures of p53 tetramers bound to DNA revealed stable MQ adducts on C124, C229, and C277 that were selected in the structure because they stabilize intra- and intermolecular interactions, including p53-DNA interactions in oncogenic p53 R273H or R273C mutants (scheme drawn from data of [19]). (**d**) Amino acid C277 of p53 (UniProt accession number P04937-1), which is key for the reactivation of oncogenic p53 mutants R273H or R273C, is conserved also in the sequence of p63 (C347, UniProt accession number Q9H3D4-1) and adjacent to EEC-causing *TP63* mutations R343Q and R343W. The mutations I549T and I576T in the SAM domain of p63, both causing AEC syndrome, are located close to free cysteine residues that might similarly be involved in the mechanism of action of PRIMA-1^{MET} which restored epithelialization of nonhealing skin erosions in two patients with *TP63* mutations I549T and I576T, respectively

[21]. Although the mechanism of action has remained unclear, experimental evidence for transcriptional reactivation of several (but not all) p63-dependent genes in patient-derived induced pluripotent stem cells treated with PRIMA-1^{MET} in vitro [21] suggests that the drug could have restored transcriptionally active p63 through addition of methylene quinuclidinone (MQ) on free cysteine residues in the vicinity of the mutated amino acids, as shown previously for p53 [19] (Fig. 16.2b–d).

Similar strategies might be used to treat nonhealing corneal abrasions in the eyes of patients with EEC or AEC syndrome. Such lesions that may finally result in loss of vision [22] have been a great therapeutic challenge. The primary cause of the slow corneal healing process appears to be a malfunction and later disappearance of limbal stem cells [23]. These cells are crucial for corneal epithelial regeneration and for the maintenance of a physical barrier between the clear, avascular cornea and the vascularized conjunctiva. Human limbal stem cells can be harvested and cultured for transplantation [24]. Autologous, ex vivo expanded epithelial cells containing limbal stem cells were approved some years ago as an advanced therapy medicinal product to treat severe limbal stem cell deficiency [25]. Regeneration of the cornea with this method has led to the recovery of vision in numerous patients and is one of the first examples of a successful stem cell therapy [16, 25]. Considering the healthy marriage of gene and stem cell therapy in other fields [26], merging the two also for the treatment of corneal lesions in EEC or AEC syndrome with patient-derived, genetically corrected limbal stem cells seems to be auspicious.

References

1. Thesleff I. Developmental biology and building a tooth. Quintessence Int. 2003;34:613–20.
2. Schneider H, Faschingbauer F, Schuepbach-Mallepell S, Korber I, Wohlfart S, Dick A, et al. Prenatal correction of X-linked hypohidrotic ectodermal dysplasia. N Engl J Med. 2018;378:1604–10. https://doi.org/10.1056/NEJMoa1714322.
3. Schneider H, Hadj-Rabia S, Faschingbauer F, Bodemer C, Grange DK, Norton M, et al. Protocol for the phase 2 EDELIFE trial investigating the efficacy and safety of intra-amniotic ER004 administration to male subjects with X-linked hypohidrotic ectodermal dysplasia. Genes (Basel). 2023a;14:153. https://doi.org/10.3390/genes14010153.
4. Schneider H, Hammersen J, Preisler-Adams S, Huttner K, Rascher W, Bohring A. Sweating ability and genotype in individuals with X-linked hypohidrotic ectodermal dysplasia. J Med Genet. 2011;48:426–32. https://doi.org/10.1136/jmg.2010.084012.
5. Blüschke G, Nüsken KD, Schneider H. Prevalence and prevention of severe complications of hypohidrotic ectodermal dysplasia in infancy. Early Hum Dev. 2010;86:397–9. https://doi.org/10.1016/j.earlhumdev.2010.04.008.
6. Hammersen J, Wohlfart S, Goecke T, Köninger A, Stepan H, Gallinat R, et al. Reliability of prenatal detection of X-linked hypohidrotic ectodermal dysplasia by tooth germ sonography. Prenat Diagn. 2019;39:796–805. https://doi.org/10.1002/pd.5384.
7. Wünsche S, Jüngert J, Faschingbauer F, Mommsen H, Goecke T, Schwanitz K, et al. Noninvasive prenatal diagnosis of hypohidrotic ectodermal dysplasia by tooth germ sonography. Ultraschall Med. 2015;36:381–5. https://doi.org/10.1055/s-0034-1384933.
8. Gaide O, Schneider P. Permanent correction of an inherited ectodermal dysplasia with recombinant EDA. Nat Med. 2003;9:614–8. https://doi.org/10.1038/nm861.

9. Körber I, Klein O, Morhart P, Faschingbauer F, Grange D, Clarke A, et al. Safety and immunogenicity of Fc-EDA, a recombinant ectodysplasin A1 replacement protein, in human subjects. Br J Clin Pharmacol. 2020;86:2063–9. https://doi.org/10.1111/bcp.14301.
10. Ersch J, Stallmach T. Assessing gestational age from histology of fetal skin: an autopsy study of 379 fetuses. Obstet Gynecol. 1999;94:753–7. https://doi.org/10.1016/s0029-7844(99)00379-8.
11. Martins JP, Kennedy PJ, Santos HA, Barrias C, Sarmento B. A comprehensive review of the neonatal Fc receptor and its application in drug delivery. Pharmacol Ther. 2016;161:22–39. https://doi.org/10.1016/j.pharmthera.2016.03.007.
12. Hermes K, Schneider P, Krieg P, Dang A, Huttner K, Schneider H. Prenatal therapy in developmental disorders: drug targeting via intra-amniotic injection to treat X-linked hypohidrotic ectodermal dysplasia. J Invest Dermatol. 2014;134:2985–7. https://doi.org/10.1038/jid.2014.264.
13. Margolis CA, Schneider P, Huttner K, Kirby N, Houser TP, Wildman L, et al. Prenatal treatment of X-linked hypohidrotic ectodermal dysplasia using recombinant ectodysplasin in a canine model. J Pharmacol Exp Ther. 2019;370:806–13. https://doi.org/10.1124/jpet.118.256040.
14. Schneider H, Schweikl C, Faschingbauer F, Hadj-Rabia S, Schneider P. A causal treatment for X-linked hypohidrotic ectodermal dysplasia: long-term results of short-term perinatal ectodysplasin A1 replacement. Int J Mol Sci. 2023b;24:7155. https://doi.org/10.3390/ijms24087155.
15. Koch PJ, Koster M. Rare genetic disorders: novel treatment strategies and insights into the human body. Front Genet. 2021;12:714764. https://doi.org/10.3389/fgene.2021.714764.
16. De Luca M, Aiuti A, Cossu G, Parmar M, Pellegrini G, Robey PG. Advances in stem cell research and therapeutic development. Nat Cell Biol. 2019;21:801–11. https://doi.org/10.1038/s41556-019-0344-z.
17. Hirsch T, Rothoeft T, Teig N, Bauer JW, Pellegrini G, De Rosa L, et al. Regeneration of the entire human epidermis using transgenic stem cells. Nature. 2017;551:327–32. https://doi.org/10.1038/nature24487.
18. Kueckelhaus M, Rothoeft T, De Rosa L, Yeni B, Ohmann T, Maier C, et al. Transgenic epidermal cultures for junctional epidermolysis bullosa—5-year outcomes. N Engl J Med. 2021;385:2264–70. https://doi.org/10.1056/NEJMoa2108544.
19. Degtjarik O, Golovenko D, Diskin-Posner Y, Abrahmsen L, Rozenberg H, Shakked Z. Structural basis of reactivation of oncogenic p53 mutants by a small molecule: methylene quinuclidinone (MQ). Nat Commun. 2021;12:7057. https://doi.org/10.1038/s41467-021-27142-6.
20. Caruso SM, Quinn PMJ, Lopes da Costa B, Tsang SH. CRISPR/Cas therapeutic strategies for autosomal dominant disorders. J Clin Invest. 2022;132:e158287. https://doi.org/10.1172/JCI158287.
21. Aberdam E, Roux LN, Secretan PH, Boralevi F, Schlatter J, Morice-Picard F, et al. Improvement of epidermal covering on AEC patients with severe skin erosions by PRIMA-1(MET)/APR-246. Cell Death Dis. 2020;11:30. https://doi.org/10.1038/s41419-020-2223-8.
22. Felipe AF, Abazari A, Hammersmith KM, Rapuano CJ, Nagra PK, Peiro BM. Corneal changes in ectrodactyly-ectodermal dysplasia-cleft lip and palate syndrome: case series and literature review. Int Ophthalmol. 2012;32:475–80. https://doi.org/10.1007/s10792-012-9585-6.
23. Di Iorio E, Kaye SB, Ponzin D, Barbaro V, Ferrari S, Bohm E, et al. Limbal stem cell deficiency and ocular phenotype in ectrodactyly-ectodermal dysplasia-clefting syndrome caused by p63 mutations. Ophthalmology. 2012;119:74–83. https://doi.org/10.1016/j.ophtha.2011.06.044.
24. Rama P, Matuska S, Paganoni G, Spinelli A, De Luca M, Pellegrini G. Limbal stem-cell therapy and long-term corneal regeneration. N Engl J Med. 2010;363:147–55. https://doi.org/10.1056/NEJMoa09059.
25. Pellegrini G, Ardigo D, Milazzo G, Iotti G, Guatelli P, Pelosi D, et al. Navigating market authorization: the path Holoclar took to become the first stem cell product approved in the European Union. Stem Cells Transl Med. 2018;7:146–54. https://doi.org/10.1002/sctm.17-0003.
26. Nogrady B. Stem-cell and genetic therapies make a healthy marriage. Nature. 2019;569:S23–5. https://doi.org/10.1038/d41586-019-01442-w.

Chapter 17
Patient Advocacy Organizations: One Story of Success

Mary Fete

Keywords Families · Patient organizations · Global assistance

Patient advocacy organizations play a vital role for individuals and families living with rare disorders. They have the unique ability to connect patients to support services, other affected families, providers, treatment options, and research opportunities, while also serving as a hub for accurate and dependable information related to the disorders. Above all, these organizations and their leaders must always have the highest level of ethical integrity to provide the best services for the communities they serve.

Patient advocacy organizations are catalysts that bring attention to the disorder and advance understanding of the condition. Who else is going to lead those initiatives? Governments and health care systems do not have the capacity to play this role for all medical conditions. Without patient advocacy groups, affected individuals and their families are left to navigate the rocky waters of specialized health care and treatments alone. Together, families and patient advocacy organizations must lead the effort to advocate for change and a better quality of life.

17.1 NFED History

The National Foundation for Ectodermal Dysplasias (NFED) stands as one example of how important patient advocacy organizations are to everyone connected to a rare disorder—providers, researchers, patients, and patient families.

Nothing was really known for hundreds of years about ectodermal dysplasias. The first known descriptions of clinical cases that might correspond to what we would now classify as ectodermal dysplasias date back to 1792. Charles Darwin

M. Fete (✉)
National Foundation for Ectodermal Dysplasias, Fairview Heights, IL, USA
e-mail: mary@nfed.org

G. Tadini et al. (eds.), *Multidisciplinary Approach to Ectodermal Dysplasia*,
https://doi.org/10.1007/978-3-031-75790-7_17

cited cases of ectodermal dysplasia in his book published in 1875, *The Variations of Animals and Plants Under Domestication* [1]. In 1929, Dr. A. A. Weech was the first to coin the term "ectodermal dysplasia" in the medical literature [2]. However, it wasn't until the NFED was formed in 1981, as the first patient support group for ectodermal dysplasias, that there has been significant improvement in the understanding, management, and treatment of the conditions.

Mary Kaye Richter founded the NFED and was a pioneer in the ectodermal dysplasia community. Her mission began on April 28, 1978, when her third child, Charley Richter, was born. Charley was born with dry scaly skin and a flat nose—he just looked "different" than her other two children. He also overheated easily. When Charley did not develop teeth normally, the astute mom knew that something was not right and took him to the dentist in search of answers. The dentist diagnosed him with hypohidrotic ectodermal dysplasia, which is characterized by hypohidrosis, hypodontia, and hypotrichosis, among other symptoms.

17.2 Knowledge Is Power

Like many parents of children newly diagnosed with a rare disorder, Mary Kaye quickly learned that there was very little information in the medical literature and no organization she could turn to for help. Understanding that knowledge is power, she knew she had a lot to learn to best take care of Charley. Due to the lack of medical literature on the disorder, doctors recommended she find another family with a child with ectodermal dysplasia to learn more.

Mary Kaye began her quest for information by writing dental schools across the country in search of other affected individuals. Soon, she had connected with a dozen families who all shared a desire to create a community. They founded the NFED in Mascoutah, Illinois, on December 24, 1981, with Mary Kaye serving as an executive director. She envisioned a better life for her son and all individuals with ectodermal dysplasias. This sentiment lies at the heart of the Foundation's mission to the present day.

The reality is that discovering new knowledge about rare disorders typically falls to the patient advocacy organizations, which are generally founded and driven by affected individuals and their families. These families share a vision for a better future for themselves and others who are affected.

By working together, affected individuals and the associated patient advocacy groups can drive forward research and develop necessary resources for their community. Their efforts ensure that we continue to learn more about their disorders so they know how to manage their condition.

17.3 Education

An important role of patient advocacy groups is to be a source of accurate and comprehensive information in order to educate, raise awareness about the medical condition, and improve diagnosis and treatment. Given the scarcity of information available when the organization was founded, education has always been the NFED's paramount goal. Understanding the complexity of this large group of disorders with a wide range of manifestations proved to be a challenge for the Foundation in its early years.

The NFED has always focused its quest to find answers on its families' needs. To find these answers, the organization collaborates with credible medical and scientific advisors to explore the issues, provide guidelines, and develop educational resources based on published science.

Mary Kaye often said the best advice she got when founding the NFED was to form a Scientific Advisory Council (SAC). She recruited the best researchers and medical and dental professionals, who specialized in treating the wide range of symptoms found in the ectodermal dysplasias, to volunteer. The SAC has been instrumental throughout NFED's history in listening to families, identifying educational needs, directing the focus of the research program, and developing appropriate educational resources. They developed processes to ensure the quality and accuracy of NFED's content.

The importance of professional advisors to patient advocacy organizations cannot be overstated. It is ethically imperative for these organizations to be cautious and publish health information that is backed by research and not based on anecdotal stories. This professionally vetted information can then be disseminated through printed guides, a website, and webinars, and at family gatherings. Patient advocacy organizations can also educate medical and dental professionals through webinars, professional conferences, and printed and electronic information.

17.4 Vision/Passion

Patient advocacy organizations require an extraordinary amount of time, work, and resources to survive and be successful. They need leaders who are savvy strategists and gifted communicators who can articulate their vision and recruit others to work for the cause. Leaders must understand how the medical and research communities operate. They should attend conferences to learn from and network with providers who share an interest in the disorder to help advance their mission.

The NFED was fortunate that Mary Kaye did this successfully from the very beginning. Her passion inspired people to help, and this network of supporters sustained and grew the Foundation. That culture has continued throughout the Foundation's history.

17.5 Representing Patients

Patient advocacy organizations operate on the philosophy that the patient is the most important voice. Often times with ectodermal dysplasias, families know more than doctors about the condition and hold the key to better understanding of their condition. The patient advocacy organizations' role is to listen to the families to understand their stories, needs, and concerns and to serve as a representative of those voices to other entities to achieve the mission.

17.6 National Programs/Policies

The needs of individuals with rare conditions are often overlooked in conversations addressing national programs, policy-making, or education curriculum. Patient advocate leaders have opportunities to add their voice to discussions by serving on national committees both in the United States and in Europe.

Organizations must research and learn what committees or organizations in their country address solutions to the issues their families face and find a way to collaborate. For example, NFED executive directors have served on the National Advisory Dental Research Council at the National Institute of Dental and Craniofacial Research to help address the needs of special care patient populations.

Participating and networking at this level raises the profile of the ectodermal dysplasias and the patient advocacy group. It can also connect leaders with resources such as interested researchers, awareness opportunities, and funding sources that will further help the organization. Sometimes, the best way to advocate for the needs of a specific patient population is to broaden the scope and include the needs of all patients with rare conditions, rather than a single condition, in the discussions, solutions, and program. In this way, many patient populations can be positively impacted, including the organization's specific patient population.

17.7 NFED Impact

The NFED has enjoyed many accomplishments. Today, the Foundation is the largest patient organization for ectodermal dysplasias in the world, with over 10,000 affected individuals in over 90 countries in its database.

For over four decades, the NFED has been the worldwide expert on ectodermal dysplasias and the only advocacy organization in the United States dedicated to those living with these disorders. Rather than having a singular focus such as research or support, the NFED offers numerous, comprehensive services to meet families' varied needs. The number of services offered by the Foundation has grown over time as it has developed greater financial resources and increased staffing. There is always more that the NFED could do if it had the capacity.

Mary Kaye saw the value of patient advocacy organizations long before they became as prevalent as they are today. Because of the NFED's success, many people came to her for help or advice on how to start their own advocacy organization. She also helped many other patient groups for ectodermal dysplasias get started outside of the United States. Patient advocacy groups and leaders have a responsibility to share information and mentor other new groups who share the common goal of helping the families they represent.

Patient advocacy groups who are just beginning must consider the type and level of support they can provide with the resources they have. It takes an extraordinary amount of time and money to do it well. This cannot be underestimated. Mary Kaye often told people who came to her for advice about starting a patient advocacy group: "Don't do it. It will take over your life." She knew from experience! But, the ectodermal dysplasia community is prospering to this day because she had the tenacity to do it.

17.8 International Collaboration

As of 2023, there are ectodermal dysplasia organizations or support groups in 38 different countries across the world. Leaders from many of these organizations formed a coalition called the Ectodermal Dysplasia International Network (EDIN) to foster information sharing and collaboration. EDIN was formally organized as a nonprofit coalition, registered in France, in 2022.

The goal of EDIN is to increase awareness of ectodermal dysplasias worldwide and support other ectodermal dysplasia groups. They collaborate on various research and advocacy projects, bringing together scientists and health care providers from around the world to share their knowledge. United, these organizations advocate for the global ectodermal dysplasia community, and their collaborative efforts generate an even greater impact for this community.

17.9 Support Services

Providing support services is an important role for patient advocacy organizations. Each program should address the unique needs of its families. Living with ectodermal dysplasias can be challenging for families for many different reasons. The organization's caring staff can provide empathy and emotional support that a family may not get anywhere else.

At the NFED, a staff member answers the phone instead of an automated phone service. This practice connects a patient or family to immediate help and one-on-one support from someone who cares about them. This is incredibly important to families when they receive the initial diagnosis. Helping families who are newly diagnosed and welcoming them into the community can make an enormous difference in how individuals cope, seek information, and manage their initial needs. By connecting with a patient advocacy organization, they are immediately connected to resources.

Patient advocacy organizations have the power to what few other types of organizations can connect families to others who share their condition. This provides them with a network of support and the opportunity to learn from each other as they share tips and ideas.

Holding family conferences or gatherings is a critical component of supporting families and is often the most important thing that a patient advocacy group can do. Bringing families together is very powerful. Individuals can support each other and develop lifelong friendships. These relationships are empowering and can teach individuals to advocate for themselves or their child. The community can help families learn what's possible for their child and themselves. An informal conversation can be life-changing for someone and help them realize they are not alone.

Patient advocacy organizations have a role in empowering individuals to advocate for themselves and their children in workplaces, schools, and everyday life situations. They often have tool kits that they can provide their community to make advocating easier and more successful. Staff can provide hope and encourage optimism by helping parents understand what's possible for their child. The NFED has always maintained a philosophy that parents can expect great things for their child. Their positive attitude can greatly influence how a child copes with the condition and how it can increase their self-esteem.

17.10 Treatment

Another way a patient advocacy organization can serve families is to help them access treatment. The NFED strongly advocates that children affected by ectodermal dysplasias start school with a full set of teeth and receive ongoing dental care. It's well documented that teeth improve digestion, health, speech, and self-esteem.

Finding doctors and dentists who are knowledgeable and willing to treat the unique symptoms associated with the disorder can be difficult. Patient advocacy groups can help identify medical, dental, and social services. They can also help families access and navigate insurance coverage for treatment, if applicable in their country. The NFED takes this a step further and has developed a network of treatment centers and referral sources for families.

Many patient advocacy organizations provide funding to help families access the care they need. Depending on the health care system of the country, the patient advocacy group can work to improve a patient's access to see care providers at affordable costs. For example, the NFED is working to get a federal law passed in the United States that would provide insurance benefits for the medically necessary care caused not only by ectodermal dysplasias but also by any congenital anomaly. If passed, this legislation would decrease the financial barriers patients face to get the care they need.

17.11 Research

Patient advocacy organizations are typically the catalyst for research in their rare disease space and have the opportunity to substantially advance research that benefits their patient population. They must lead, support, and finance research for that medical condition to identify better treatments, expand knowledge, and, where possible, find treatments and cures. Patient needs can help inform the organization's research agenda.

From its founding, NFED leadership understood that research would be critical to the rest of its mission. It was clear to Mary Kaye and the SAC that if the NFED was not the catalyst for ectodermal dysplasia research, no one else would be. Early NFED efforts of patient surveys later developed into a robust research program that provided investigators with seed grants to fund their projects.

The NFED could also provide researchers with one very important resource—access to patients. Because the conditions are rare and individuals are scattered geographically, the NFED was a central place where an investigator could more easily find people to volunteer for their research project. To protect the patients, the SAC rigorously reviews all research proposals before granting such access.

The NFED continues to lead ectodermal dysplasia research efforts and has invested more than $three million in research, supported more than 180 studies, and sponsored 15 research conferences. The results have been significant and helped make enormous strides in our quest to better understand and treat ectodermal dysplasias. The 50+ syndromes have been categorized, genes have been identified, and treatment protocols have been developed.

The NFED's greatest success in its research program has been the development of a potential treatment, ER004, for the most common type of ectodermal dysplasia, X-linked hypohidrotic ectodermal dysplasia (XLHED). The potential treatment is being tested in the EDELIFE clinical trial to determine its safety and possible health benefits in boys affected by XLHED. ER004 is a synthetic protein that was developed (with support from the NFED) to replace the protein that is missing in individuals affected by XLHED. Early findings show that the in utero therapy has restored sweat gland function and improved other symptoms in affected boys, which is extraordinary!

If approved, this cutting-edge therapy would be the first of its kind to correct a genetic condition before birth, and ER004 would be the first commercially available treatment for XLHED. This is truly remarkable! Hopefully, before this book edition is published, this will be a reality. The key message is that patient advocacy organizations can drive research in a very powerful way.

Research takes years, even decades. Patient advocacy organizations can expect for there to be many stops and starts along the journey toward success. It's important to never give up and be strongly committed to the end goal. Mary Kaye's determination to find answers will impact not only future generations of her own family but also those of all XLHED families. This can happen for other patient advocacy groups, too.

17.12 Conclusion

The NFED is but one example of how a small patient advocacy organization can have a profound impact on a rare disease community. As the organization's founder, Mary Kaye was the ultimate patient advocate who demonstrated the importance of the affected individual's role in advancing research, genetics, and medical and dental literature. She gave voice to an entire community of people with rare conditions whose needs had largely been ignored. She inspired her staff and successors to do the same.

Mary Kaye is certainly not the only person to create a successful patient advocacy group. But, she stands as a shining example of someone who built a legacy that serves as a beacon of light and hope for other founders who aspire to make a difference. She laid the groundwork and built the organization in a way that enabled the NFED to thrive and network to prosper even after her retirement.

Mary Kaye taught all of us who are patient advocates to be relentless in our efforts to find answers, to provide support and love to affected families, and to find treatments and cures for ectodermal dysplasias. All patient advocacy organizations has the enormous opportunity and privilege to change the lives of patients affected by ectodermal dysplasias in a very positive way.

References

1. Felsher Z. Hereditary ectodermal dysplasia: report of a case, with experimental study. Arch Dermatol Syphilol. 1944;49(6):410–4. https://doi.org/10.1001/archderm.1944.01510120024005.
2. Weech AA. Hereditary ectodermal dysplasia (congenital ectodermal defect): a report of two cases. Am J Dis Child. 1929;37(4):766–90. https://doi.org/10.1001/archpedi.1929.01930040075005.

GPSR Compliance

The European Union's (EU) General Product Safety Regulation (GPSR) is a set of rules that requires consumer products to be safe and our obligations to ensure this.

If you have any concerns about our products, you can contact us on ProductSafety@springernature.com

In case Publisher is established outside the EU, the EU authorized representative is:

Springer Nature Customer Service Center GmbH
Europaplatz 3
69115 Heidelberg, Germany

Batch number: 10732044

Printed by Printforce, the Netherlands